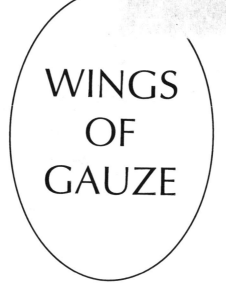

WINGS
OF
GAUZE

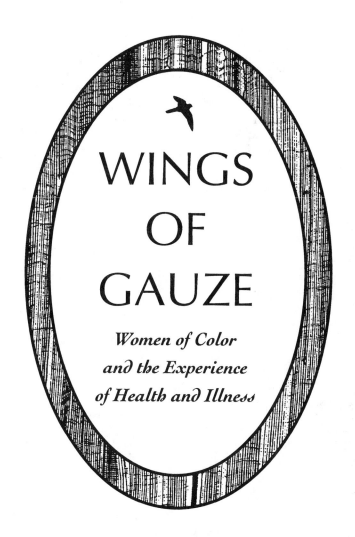

WINGS
OF
GAUZE

Women of Color
and the Experience
of Health and Illness

Edited by
Barbara Bair
and Susan E. Cayleff

WAYNE STATE UNIVERSITY PRESS

DETROIT

Library of Congress Cataloging-in-Publication Data

Wings of gauze: women of color and the experience of health and illness /
  edited by Barbara Bair and Susan E. Cayleff.
     p. cm.
  Includes bibliographical references and index.
  ISBN 0-8143-2301-4 (alk. paper). — ISBN 0-8143-2302-2 (pbk. :
alk. paper)
    1. Minority women—Medical care—Social aspects—United States.
2. Minority women—Health and hygiene—Social aspects—United
States.   I. Bair, Barbara, 1955– . II. Cayleff, Susan E., 1954– .
RA564.86.W55   1993
362.1′08′693—dc20   92-46308

Designer: Mary Krzewinski

CONTENTS

3 HISTORICAL PERSPECTIVES AND THE PROVISION OF CARE: QUESTIONS OF EMPOWERMENT AND SOCIAL CONTROL

4 BREAST CANCER: IMAGES OF SELF

5 COMMUNITY ACTION AND PUBLIC HEALTH POLICY

FOREWORD

Poetic and factual, much like the lives of women, these voices speak to us about the health and illness experiences of women of color. Not a bland collection varying on just one theme, these essays are as diverse and provocative as the life experiences and academic views of the authors. These writers understand and convey that women of color are defined by the complex experiences of culture, oppression, and exploitation. African American, Latina, Native American, and Asian American women share commonalties as they celebrate their strength and resistance. In defense of themselves and their loved ones, they display courage and wisdom and a steadfast will to survive, not merely alone, but as central to their communities. They are women who have always understood that they are the collective memory and keepers of culture. The writers bring personal experiences and research, sharing their survival strategies, taking us to deeper levels of feeling and understanding.

Several authors describe the role of traditional healing in their communities. At one time, many groups had respected and effective traditional healers, men and women. Women were midwives and healers, helpers and sisters. But the dominant white European society has waged an intense cultural assault, depriving the people of their knowledge, and also denying access to the best conventional medicine. Lacking access, women of color receive medical care later than their white sisters for preventable diseases such as cervical cancer. For far too many, the diagnosis of diabetes, breast cancer, and other conditions that are only successfully controlled in earlier stages comes too late. All too often professionals blame women for their ill health, invoking "life style" issues. Physicians discuss how to manage the "non compliant" patient, rarely addressing the insurmountable barriers placed on her road to care.

With piercing insight, the authors of this rich collection fully understand and communicate to us the indivisibility of women's harsh social and economic life conditions and their health. Health care is but one component. Of greater weight in determining health are economic status, education, rewarding work, decent housing, safe neighborhoods, and freedom from discrimination for women and children. The greatest enemies are poverty, violence, joblessness, homelessness, and lack of control.

Racism affects our vision as does a faulty lens, constantly distorting the "others" and their reality. Here, in scholarly and graceful texts, the authors provide us with correction. If we read with care we may grasp what women of color are distilling from their personal and collective realities. We will grow stronger as we identify more deeply with one another.

Helen Rodriguez-Trias, M.D.
President, American Public Health Association

PREFACE

Nikky Finney's "On Wings Made of Gauze" lends its power to the title of this anthology and captures the complexity of the themes presented in its pages. The poem—as, we hope, the book itself—is open to discussion and several kinds of interpretations. It can be read as a presentation of a woman who has experienced the demands of providing and the pangs of physical illness and substance abuse/use. The theme of black people who can fly, thus escaping bondage or pain, pervades the African-American oral tradition. Finney builds on that folk knowledge in her poem. It can be read as a poem about a woman who transforms her pain into psychic transcendence, in turn suggesting to others the magical power to remake and redefine. Her wings made of gauze, the stuff of bandages, signaling the presence of wounds, are images of victimization and suffering. They are also images of self-reinvention, at once delicate and transformative. The unnamed woman of the poem, who has hands that ache and a soul that soars in the moonlight, symbolizes the interplay of mind and body in conceptualizing and defining "health" and "illness" that is fundamental to this collection.

We hope this book will be of interest to students in the humanities and social sciences, to health professionals and policy makers, and to all readers concerned about the issues of health, the status of women of color, and the cultural diversity of American society.

Nikky Finney, "On Wings Made of Gauze"

she lived not in a shoe
but on wings made of gauze
and when she left on midnight rides
she wrapped herself in moonbeams
to help light the way

her life before
had been tied to clotheslines
to shoestrings
of all sizes
of different hues

11

and after her life
no one cried
cause no one knew
how deeply her hands ached
and now when she's remembered
it's for the warm beer she guzzled
from tattered war canteens
and talk is still
how carelessly but gracefully
she flings them from the sky

in the evenings
if the light is right
quickly may you lift your eyes
and see her riding by
silhouetted by the moon
she rides boldly with no hands
as if life had no more boundaries
as if living held no more cautions

and in the mornings
if you walk quickly
before the others arrive
you may find one of her tattered canteens
scattered about the underbrush
and if you lift it gently to your lips
you'll find she didn't drink it all
she never does
she's left some for you
who've always been afraid of heights
and never had the courage
to fly

INTRODUCTION

Time is a crucial element in the treatment of cancer, and I had to decide
which chances I would take, and why. I think of what this means to
other Black women living with cancer, to all women in general. Most
of all I think of how important it is for us to share with each other the
powers buried within the breaking silence about our bodies and our
health, even though we have been schooled to be secret and stoical
about pain and disease. But that stoicism and silence does not serve us
nor our communities, only the forces of things as they are.

—Audre Lorde, "A Burst of Light: Living with Cancer"[1]

What we call "illness" and "health" are both private bodily matters
and public social constructs based on notions of relative value. For women
of color, conditions of "health" or "illness" are inextricably tied to a multiple
consciousness of their history, their status within a dominant society that affords them a secondary role, and their place within communities of color that
offer both alternative sources of strength and internal problems induced by a
history of repression. Women of color make up a disproportionate number of
the nation's poor. They habitually live with illness and pain for which middle-
class women, suffering the same ailments, receive care. They are chronically
put in positions—scrubbing floors, walking long distances between buses,
bending in fields, performing repetitive tasks on assembly lines, working
exposed to hazardous materials, making dinners for families from too-empty
pots, facing violence both arbitrary and personal, using emergency rooms
as clinics, speaking with practitioners who do not know their language or
grasp the full meaning of their concerns—that endanger their health and
offer improper recourse for their illnesses. Many carry in the present time the
legacy of the past: slavery, genocide, relocation, ghettoization, and unequal
protection under the law. As a result, women of color face out of proportion to
their numbers the pressing problems and consequences of infant mortality and
poor pediatric care, drug and alcohol abuse, hypertension and cardiovascular
disease, high blood pressure, psychological stress, stroke, diabetes, breast

13

cancer, lupus, physical endangerment and homicide, and the likelihood that they will die at a younger age than whites. They are far less likely than whites to breast feed, in part because of hospital policies and pressure from infant formula manufacturers, and thus they are more likely to be caring for babies with a higher incidence of diarrhea, respiratory infection, and malnutrition. They have fewer options in the availability of birth control, prenatal care, and abortion services. They are far less likely than privileged whites to have access to expensive fertility services and such other forms of high-technology testing and treatment as heart bypass surgery or kidney transplants, and they are more likely to be labeled as "proper" candidates for sterilization. When suffering from pneumonia, often a consequence of other ailments, they are less likely than whites to receive intensive treatment. Federal cutbacks in public programs have coincided with the rising incidence of infectious diseases in inner city communities, including syphilis, tuberculosis, and measles. Over half of the women in the United States who are HIV-positive or suffer from the AIDS virus are women of color. Minority women are less likely to have personal physicians, to have quality health insurance coverage, or to be treated with respect and understanding in negotiating with health care institutions. However, many also have as resources belief systems and traditions of caretaking, expertise, and mutual understanding that broaden dominant ways of perceiving well- or ill-being in the world. Thus their stories are about both oppression and empowerment, victimization as well as the strength to reshape and redefine.

Byllye Avery, describing the path she took to founding the National Black Women's Health Project in Atlanta, has spoken of the conspiracy of silence that has enveloped black women and the intimate realities that shape their health and their lives.[2] Through work like hers; through self-help groups, crisis and community health centers staffed by people of color; through the publication of more writings by women of color; and through the growing voices of dissent in the institutional levels of public health, public policy, medicine and the academy, the silence is being broken. This book is one contribution to that process.

The essays featured in this book represent the experiences of African-American, Native-American, Latina, and Southeast-Asian-American women. Written by scholars in the social sciences and the humanities, community activists, and health professionals, these essays illustrate a variety of approaches from a range of academic disciplines, theoretical models, and individual perspectives. They testify to the many layers of women's experience and are written in the spirit of broadening our understanding of the connections that exist between those many experiences and the seemingly different health issues and cultural standpoints that frame them. All contributions in this book were written expressly for this publication, as a response to a call for papers. The response has defined the specific topics presented here.

Overarching themes emerge from the essays, linking individual topics together. The essays in Part One—and, indeed, throughout the collection—contribute to our awareness that women's definitions of health and illness are not linear, clinical, or individuated. They emerge out of socioeconomic conditions and from an ever-present consciousness of race and of the consequences of racism. Women of color's concepts of personal illness or health are twinned with their own awareness of themselves as caretakers: caretakers for themselves; for their own bodies and world views; and caretakers for the wholeness, safety, confidence, and security of those close to them. Their ideas of well-being have personal meanings that transcend internal boundaries between mind and body and external limits between the self and others. Health is related to self-help and self-worth, to the ability to create alternatives, and to access to resources and power.

The majority of contributors to this book are people of color; there are also essays written by Anglo-Americans. The majority of authors are women; there are also contributions written or co-authored by men. In addition to these different types of voices and standpoints, there are also important variations of style or mode of expression. Some essays are non-linear, subjective and expressive. Personal narratives literally conflate subject and object. Other essays, especially those prepared from a social science perspective, adhere to more conventional models and strive to be linear and "objective," to speak with authority from without instead of (or as well as) from within. In all cases the goals in creating this book were to let the subjective voices of women of color speak through the texts as much as possible and allow their perspectives to shape the interpretations offered by the authors.

The essays also seek to decenter the Anglo-American experiences and ways of seeing that have dominated discussions of health. To date, with some very notable exceptions, the outpouring of feminist scholarship about women's health and the history of health care has focused primarily on the experiences of white, middle-class women. Literature by health professionals about people of color has generally focused upon illness and perceived deviance from white-defined norms rather than upon the political economy of health and alternative concepts of well-being. It has also focused on men rather than women, and on African Americans to the exclusion of other people of color. The essays here contribute to a shift away from the standard paradigm of scholarship and subject matter that puts women of color at the margins and perceives them as a deviant "other" or as a "problem." Instead, most of these essays seek to make women of color and their own perceptions the central reality.

This book also addresses issues of culture and identity. The collected essays challenge monolithic concepts of culture that define "people of color" as singularly African-American, or that speak of single "black" or "Hispanic," "Asian" or "Indian" points of view. As the authors of some of the following essays point out, for example, "Latina" experience varies by regional heritage (South American, Central American, Caribbean) and national origin, rural or urban living, occupation, and relation to neo-colonial history. There are both similarities and differences in the health needs and concerns of Latinas employed in field labor or living in migrant labor camps or Latinas employed as household workers in cities or in middle-class pursuits. Similarly, African-Americans, Asians, and Native Americans all enjoy multiple identities based on such elements as origin, migration, orientation, sexual preference, gender, and class.

While displaying some of the richness and variety of the experience of people of color, the essays in this book also point toward ways in which experiences converge and coalitions can be formed. For example, Mexican-American and Southeast-Asian-American women share much in common in terms of the traditional cosmologies of health that inform their modern caretaking. Native-American women and African-American women share much in common in their respective histories as healers and midwives and in the spiritual sense brought to lay medical practice.

Essays in this book look at the politics of cultural interpretations from several sides. Some advocate the introduction of cultural diversity and specificity into medical practice and into concepts of health previously dominated by ideas and practices that excluded people of nonwhite heritage. Others question whether a focus on culture puts a benign, reformist face on the more important underlying issues of power, racism, and socioeconomic privilege, subverting opportunities for greater change. Still others argue from the standpoint of cultural nationalism. Closely related is the issue of consciousness. Some contributors argue that good psychological and physical health for people of color is dependent on a healthy sense of racial consciousness, one that looks away from dominant Anglo-American standards of beauty and worth and replaces them with standards of value from one's own history and heritage. Black feminist theorist Bell Hooks has referred to this process as the decolonization of the mind; in this volume, Frenzella Elaine De Lancey details what poet and teacher Sonia Sanchez has called "cracking the skull." Part of the process of "cracking the skull" is to look at old assumptions with new eyes and to become open to alternative explanations, visions, and goals that may challenge those old ways of seeing. It creates the groundwork for self-initiative and group empowerment. Discussing the essays in this book can help bring about just such a process.

Talk of cultural difference can lead to affirmation of the multiplicity and richness of our specific experiences, and to both new appreciation and a better critique of our American culture as a whole. It can help us think about gender and how men and women in the same culture may experience different realities. It can also help us think about positive ways in which the affirmation of culture long denied encourages health and indicates ways that suffering can be alleviated.

The emphasis in this collection is on changing perception, giving voice, and addressing the issues of racial discrimation. There is also discussion of solutions: ways to personal empowerment and better health; ways of changing outreach to more equitably instill the benefits of preventive education; ways of altering the structures of care offered through health institutions; and ways to think about self-help.

The title of this book emerged from Ama R. Saran's personal narrative about gathering her own healing means about her during hospitalization for surgery. Those resources included friends and written texts, health food, and familiar, beautiful things. Among the texts that Saran found sustaining was Nikky Finney's book of poetry, *On Wings Made of Gauze*. Finney's poem "On Wings Made of Gauze" is reprinted as the preface of this collection. Wings of gauze represent the two-sidedness of women of color's experience of health and illness: the side of victimization and pain, and the side of healing and self-empowerment. Wings of gauze connote woundedness and fraility. They also connote self-help and metamorphosis: the power to heal, recover, and transcend. They symbolize the dual message of this collection of essays.

Notes

1. Audre Lorde, "A Burst of Light: Living with Cancer," in *A Burst of Light: Essays by Audre Lorde* (Ithaca, N.Y.: Firebrand Books, 1988), pp. 118–119. See also Lorde, *The Cancer Journals* (San Francisco: Spinsters/Aunt Lute, 1980). Lorde writes of her experiences, feelings, political analysis, and personal decisions regarding treatment for breast and liver cancer.

2. Byllye Y. Avery, "Breathing Life into Ourselves: The Evolution of the National Black Women's Health Project," *Sojourner* 14, no. 5 (January 1989); reprinted in Evelyn C. White, *The Black Woman's Health Book: Speaking for Ourselves* (Seattle: Seal Press, 1990), pp. 4–10. The National Black Women's Health Project is located at 1237 Gordon Street, SW, Atlanta, Georgia, 30310.

PART 1

COPING AND CARETAKING: RETHINKING THE BOUNDARIES OF PHYSICAL/PSYCHOLOGICAL HEALTH

Introduction

The six essays in Part One introduce us to two themes present throughout this volume: the interconnectedness of psychological and somatic health, and the socioeconomic underpinnings of disease. Part One also begins discussion of ways in which women cope with illness and serve as caretakers of others who are ill.

The first essay is a personal narrative by Ama R. Saran that testifies to the importance of psychosocial aspects of care. In preparation for a stay in the hospital, Saran summons "guardian spirits" to help her during her impending surgery and recovery. She hints of the physical facts of her situation—symptoms of pain, planned abdominal surgery—and of her scheduled admission to the hospital, but the center of her appeal is to largely intangible aesthetic, spiritual, and emotional elements that will aid her in healing. The things she names as important to her are those considered marginal by most medical practitioners. She refers to the restorative effects of beauty, smell, sound, touch, and the spoken and written word; to the importance of familiar, evocative and beloved things; and to the curative factors supplied by visitors—humor, massage, nourishing food, gentleness, and attitudes of acceptance. In presenting her holistic litany, Saran counters the alienating aspects of institutional health care. An empowered patient, she introduces optimal conditions for her own recovery and, in doing so, exercises an agency that revises the hospital's standard routine of care.

Saran stresses that individual perspective, self-help, and looking to the support of others are large parts in the maintenance of health. She also emphasizes the positive psychosomatic role that reading Afrocentric creative writing—literature that reaches back to the experiences of African ancestors and biographical narratives of exemplary black women's lives—can play in overcoming illness. Reading affirming materials offers sustenance and reinforces the reader's power to deconstruct negating definitions applied from without. Preparing for her hospital visit, Saran demonstrates the axiom of Sonia Sanchez's poem "Old Words," which is quoted in Frenzella Elaine De Lancey's "Cracking the Skull, Mending the Soul," the second essay in the volume: "We have come to / believe that we are / not. to be we / must be loved or touched and proved to be."

De Lancey's essay on Sonia Sanchez combines a participant-observer study, literary criticism, and psychological theory to discuss the psychological impact of Sanchez's work as a poet and a teacher. De Lancey's conclusions reinforce those of Saran. Sanchez teaches her students to see familiar icons and representations in popular culture from a new perspective and to deconstruct the often none-too-subtle racial meanings imbedded in them. This opening of eyes to racial content and innuendo can at first be experienced as dis/ease, but it soon becomes the basis of psychological reorientation and healthy empowerment. Positive concepts of blackness and of African heritage and identity replace negative stereotypes and the debilitating self-concepts wrought by racism. Linking Sanchez's work with that of Afrocentric psychologists, De Lancey demonstrates that cultural nationalism can be psychologically healing and that the poet and teacher can act as effective healers.

In the third essay, an account of the folk medical practice of a woman ethno-psychiatrist in rural Louisiana, Wonda Lee Fontenot observes the healing aspects of culture and shared understandings of ethnicity and the past from a different perspective. Fontenot reminds us that health and illness are culturally constructed as well as clinically defined. She conducted a participant-observer study with Madame Neau, an elderly practitioner, and follow-up interviews with her son "Doc," who followed his mother in the folk healing profession. Fontenot demonstrates that African-American folk mental health practices in Louisiana counter mainstream ideas of causation and cure and combine African and Christian cosmologies. Ethno-psychiatry is a realm of care where female practitioners predominate. And, as we shall see in essays about midwifery featured in Part Three, the traditional female practitioner is believed to have a special calling or spiritual gift, as well as therapeutic skill. The passing of the therapeutic practice from Madame Neau to her son provided Fontenot with the opportunity to examine ways in which care was transformed in a new generation and by a practitioner of a different sex. In a community where being treated by a Western-trained psychoanalyst can be stigmatizing (socially branding the client as mentally "ill"), practitioners like Madame Neau and her son offer an alternative source of psychological therapy that builds on cultural and spiritual understanding. Seeking such therapy is popularly perceived not as a sign of mental illness, but as active maintenance of mental health.

In "Perceptions of Discrimination," the fourth essay in this section, psychologists Carol M. Cummings and Gretchen E. Lopez and sociologist Adrienne M. Robinson argue—as Madame Neau and Sonia Sanchez might— that the health conditions of African-American women cannot be understood or treated apart from consideration of their life experiences as members of an oppressed and stereotyped minority. Like the previous authors, they maintain that psychological "health" is linked to a positive racial consciousness. Cummings, Robinson, and Lopez argue that effective health policy must be geared not just to individual remedies, but to larger socioeconomic change, for causation of illness is rooted in a traumatic combination of impoverishment and discrimination that compromises black women's physical and psychological well-being. As Saran's essay elucidated, routes to personal health include techniques that combine individual agency and strength with social supports. These include developing a positive image of African-American womanhood and reliance upon the aid and encouragement of women friends, extended family networks, and broader community ties. Cummings, Robinson, and Lopez examine such variables as family responsibility, occupational discrimination, violence, substance abuse, reproductive choices, and lack of health insurance as factors contributing to black women's physical illness and incidences of psychological distress. They show the psychosomatic effects of depression on the function of immune systems and on physical health in general, demonstrating that psychological stress and pain (and its effects, ranging from high blood pressure to alcohol consumption, drug use, or smoking) are linked to high morbidity rates and early mortality. In the final portion of their essay, Cummings, Robinson, and Lopez present findings from a survey of attitudes of black women. The survey results support their argument for psychosocial understandings of women's health and for activist solutions to problems in the provision of health care to African Americans.

In "Older Women of the Project," nurse-sociologist Linda Dumas offers further support for a psychosocial interpretation of illness. Dumas looks specifically at the experiences and attitudes of elderly women of color (primarily African-American and Hispanic) in a Boston-area housing project. She discusses the interplay between the socioeconomic factors of public housing policy and physical and psychological health. She looks particularly at the long-term impact of poverty in conjunction with violence and chronic disability. Like Cummings, Robinson, and Lopez, Dumas chronicles the correlation between depression and diagnosed physical problems. Whereas the former call for greater participation of black women in the making of health policy, Dumas looks at ways in which older women of color have helped to shape the history of a housing project and the ways in which they interpret their own caretaking situations and quality of life. Many of the women she interviews have experienced long lives of hard work. Many have lived to see their children die as a result either of violence or the early onset of disease. Now, in old age, they discount their own disabilities while caring for younger family members who are ill, including mentally retarded and autistic adult children and grandchildren. Dumas argues that for these women, a sense of home and neighborhood and the established support networks of the project as a community are essential for functioning as caretakers and in maintaining the willpower to personally persevere in adverse circumstances.

In a continuation of the theme of psychosocial approaches to the understanding of illness and caretaking, sociologist Shirley A. Hill looks at the experience of stress and at the coping mechanisms utilized by mothers of children with sickle cell disease. Sickle cell disease is an inherited blood disorder found predominantly among African Americans. The disease manifests itself in various forms. Its symptoms are chronic and often painful, with pain caused by the obstruction of the circulation of the blood, resulting in the deprivation of oxygen to body tissues. Like Dumas, Hill uses personal interviews with caretaking mothers to demonstrate that personal coping strategies are related to the availability of social support networks and that the illness of a family member is not an isolated individual affair, but a factor influencing the lives of all family members (particularly caretaking parents and siblings) and extended networks in which the family participates. Hill's interviews also show that a widespread distrust of medical institutions based on prior experiences of discrimination contributed to many mothers' initial denial of the diagnosis of sickle cell disease in their children, as did the fear that greater racial stigma would be attached to the children because of the predominance of the genetic trait among African Americans. Mothers developed "tough love" techniques in rearing children with the disease, emphasizing the need for the children to develop self-reliance and the strength to cope with their illness in consort with racial and class discrimination.

My Guardian Spirits

AMA R. SARAN

October 30, 1989
4:00 a.m.

My Guardian Spirits,

My Beloved Sister-Friends and Brother-Friends, perhaps now I can lose myself in *The Temple of My Familiar*, set a fire for my spirit from the soul-sated litanies she's laid down, fling myself into her sensuous smoke, and wrap myself in her wise words.

I am going to the hospital. Northside. Monday, October 30, 1989, at 6 a.m. At 7:30 I am scheduled for:

1. Repair of an umbilical hernia (or whatever it turns out to be);
2. Removal of my last and much loved ovary; and
3. Exploratory surgery—in search of those pain-producing adhesions.

This is a critical time, primarily because this is an opportunity for my personal and spiritual instruction into healing for my fundamental, life-changing wellness.

I cannot possibly achieve this alone nor do I intend to.
Please know that I would...Welcome;
I would need.........
I would expect you to be with me in this moment:

1. Please remember how much I love the natural gifts that the earth offers up—most of all rose petals, many, many rose petals for my bed.

2. Know I need my familiar—the life and color of Africa to cover the foot of my bed.

3. Bring incense to soak my senses in.

4. Bring good reading—copies of *Vital Signs* for the nurses, assistants, doctors, and visitors to read. Lend me the love poetry of our Brother, Henry Dumas, and short stories on long and well-lived lives of brave black women. Give me Nikky's Wings, Made of Gauze.

5. Bring laughter—being sure to hold my hand, because it will hurt but it does heal.

6. Careful. . . bring what comforts you but think of me also. I am not comforted by religious relics but spiritual sustenance. Gift me with simple prayers, light candles, hold my hand. Please don't be offended—just understand that when I am ill I can't distinguish between communion and the last rites/rights.

7. When visiting, kindly do not speak of my illness as metaphor. I do see it as such and already understand what I'm ridding myself of.

8. Know that this operation *is* a last resort for me. It is not the time to speak of alternatives. This *is* the one. I am grateful for the sister-spirit instruction on where/how/when and who to seek out. I am now using this to heal into a whole. Let's not haggle with Shoulda' and Coulda', keep those two sisters outa' my presence.

9. Bring me music—the sound of your soothing voices and instruments. Bring tapes—old Doo-Wahs, the Soulful Strings, Ferrante and Teicher, Leontyne Price and Clamma Dale.

10. My hair—brush my hair frequently and massage my scalp. I really do believe uncombed hair is a sure sign of dementia.

11. Keep me shining with almond-scented musk oil. Oil my scalp, face, arms, hands, legs, and feet. Note: I've already arranged for my manicure and pedicure before surgery.

12. Please massage me. Particularly my neck and hands and shoulders where I store all my tension and pain. Massage my back, which will ache badly from the cold steel of the surgeon's table.

13. Know this about me. . . I am usually able to "appear" alert. I've been socialized to do so from my birth—a woman's way. Talk to me. . . read. . . sing to me but not *with* me.

14. Feed me well. Water, much water, peppermint or spearmint tea, warm lemon water. Be prepared to replace the solid food they'll insist upon. Pureed soups (potatoes, sister honey, and vegetables), clam chowder, Dick Gregory with juice would be fine.

15. Help me. Help me to walk straight and tall back into the world of wellness. Even when I protest pitifully. It's the only way to fully and quickly regain my strength.
16. Think about me. Inquire but watch the phoning. Abdominal surgery insists that every slamming door, every telephone ring, voice, clinking glass be involuntarily answered by my stomach muscles or their close kin.

I'll be hospitalized for about a week, then home. Come see about me. Help me up and back into the world gently.

> Know that I need you. . . .
> Know that I love you. . . .
> Know that with you I shall be well. . . .

Love and Strength,
Ama R. Saran

Cracking the Skull, Mending the Soul: Sonia Sanchez's Role as Teacher/Healer/Poet

FRENZELLA ELAINE DE LANCEY

S/heroes & Other Matters of Choice
for Sonia Sanchez

Belle of Amherst,
delighted in small meeknesses,
compared herself to a mouse,
pattered about on
tiny feet,
made "necessary" puddings.

Historically incorrect,
constrained by gender,
sewed poetry into neat packets,
concealed talent in dusty drawers,
behind screens and doors.

Virago of Harlem,
transforms blues into bullets,
targets constraints of history, race or gender,
strides abroad, diminutive, disarming,
wording molotov cocktails.

Brandishes tongue/sword,
drawing blood,

26

slaying dragons.
Siren battered against the rocks,
Offering large sacrifices
for her people.
Her tiny self a beacon light.

F. E. De Lancey, 1988

The poet is a creator of social values. The poet, then, even though he/she speaks plainly, is a manipulator of symbols and language images which have been planted by experience in the collective subconscious of a people. Through this manipulation, he/she creates new or intensified meaning and experience, whether to the benefit or the detriment of his/her audience.

—Sonia Sanchez, Ruminations/Reflections
Black Women Writers: 1950–1980

I have tried to be a standard bearer and a guardian against the forces of racism, sexism, homophobia and imperialism that seek to destroy Black people. Progressive people. Christian people. Muslim people. Activist people. People. People. People. I have tried to continue the African woman tradition of excellence.

—Sonia Sanchez, "Moonstone: Paul Robeson Award." April 1990

Introduction

A number of years ago, a science fiction film depicting the heroic actions of humans in space enjoyed phenomenal box office success and became an important part of American popular culture. By the time I initiated my research on Sonia Sanchez and began attending her African-American literature class at Temple University, images from this deliberately mythical film were firmly embedded in the American psyche. In one class Sanchez recalled her twin sons' clamor to see this popular film. A few students in the class, parents themselves, remembering their own children and similar reactions, laughed easily. Younger members of the class, perhaps recalling their own adolescent response to the film, joined in the laughter. Whispering among themselves, students described the talking creatures; the fair princess and the male entourage she enlists to fight against evil in the galaxy; the sagacious mentor who guided his young charge to ultimate success; and the physically distorted characters, particularly those in a key night club scene.

After a few minutes, the seemingly innocuous discussion shifted to the assigned text. At a pivotal moment in her lecture, however, Sanchez referred to the film a second time, presenting a new aspect of its significance. Focusing on the images of the physically distorted denizens of the netherworld—a dark place that the heroine and heroes must enter to confront their final challenge in their mission to save the galaxy—Sanchez noted that they played jazz. Indeed, jazz is the "defining music" for this scene. Having established through dialogue the importance of jazz as African-American music, Sanchez referred again to the fact that the musicians were physically distorted. An uneasy silence enveloped the classroom.

In fact, Sanchez "signified," a rhetorical technique common to African-American discourse and central to her method of instruction. In "Signifying as a Form of Verbal Art" (1973), Claudia Mitchell-Kernan defines signifying as the use of an "alternative message form" achieved when the speaker's message is only part of a larger discourse. Mitchell-Kernan sees signifying as "a kind of art—a clever way of conveying messages" (319). Disrupting the flow of the traditionally direct lecture style, Sanchez makes her points through "indirection and wit." Her style and her art have a particular purpose: to "redress imbalance of power, to clear a space, rhetorically" (311). Signifying, Henry Louis Gates argues in *The Signifying Monkey: A Theory of Afro-American Literary Criticism* (1988), "alters fundamentally the way we 'read the tradition.' " In her "motivated signifying," Sanchez deconstructs the "Western fabulat[ions] of the image of the black" (65). Rereading the mythic construction of the film that makes everyone feel good, Sanchez engenders new consideration of the images. Initially, the effect of this is to make the participants, as one student said, "feel bad." As I shall argue, these moments of cognitive dissonance are temporary. For Sanchez's students, such transitional moments of dis/ease are really the first stages in their movement toward psychological empowerment.

Attempting to protect their psyches, Sanchez's students sometimes struggle visibly. Revealing their initial discomfort through silence or furious whispers, some write surreptitious notes to each other in the margins of their notebooks. Such resistance to Sanchez is simply an act of denial. To use the example of the successful film again: if the African Americans in the room accept Sanchez's assessment of the film, they must also accept that they have, in a sense, been endorsing a heroic journey in which their cultural motifs are signified as negative "other." Initially some do feel they have been subjected to a polemic, no matter how hidden or well intentioned. Further, though many of Sanchez's students are familiar with signifying as a street game, they do not expect it in a college classroom. Its use as a pedagogical tool for exfoliating their misassumptions momentarily threatens their sense of themselves.

Sanchez attributes this teaching strategy to Malcolm X. According to Sanchez, she learned from Malcolm how to make people face themselves by engaging in a number of rhetorical strategies. She is not interested in polemic as a purely rhetorical device, but because of its ability to effect change and help people become aware of their humanity.

"In hidden polemic," Mikhail Bakhtin tells us, "the author's discourse is oriented toward its referential object." Surprised by her rhetorical art, Sanchez's students erroneously position themselves as objects of her signifying, not realizing her assertions about objects are, as Bakhtin points out, constructed in such a way that "the author's [Sanchez's] discourse brings a polemical attack to bear against another speech act, another assertion, on the same topic" (87). Eventually Sanchez's students will come to realize that her attacks are aimed at speech acts or assertions inherent in symbolic portrayals of African Americans. This is borne out by the enormous popularity of the courses she teaches. Nearly thirty minutes before a scheduled class, forty to forty-five students queue up outside the room, where maximum enrollment should be twenty-four. Yet the silence which greets Sanchez's signifying acts occurs because her students are suspended between knowing and not knowing. Recognizing silence as the group's attempt to reconcile painful knowledge with previously held assumptions, Sanchez grasps her forehead, taps it, and speaks into the silence: "It cracks the skull." Coupled with her wry smile, this gesture of commiseration acknowledges and accepts cognitive dissonance as a necessary first phase in the movement toward psychological reorientation.

Poetry, Pedagogy, Psychology, and Afrocentricity

In "The Poet as a Creator of Social Values," an article published in *Black Scholar* (1985), Sanchez emphasizes the importance of cosmology and symbolism. "World view," she contends, is an important constitutive element of the "collective experiences . . . of people who interact within the same environment." This world view "emerges first in the language and symbol[s]" of a people and then is reflected in all of society's institutions. Keenly aware of "the power of symbolism to preserve or destroy social values," Sanchez brings this awareness to her teaching and her poetry. In her poetic system and in her pedagogy, she treats symbols as "arbitrary representations of reality visual or spoken" and, of course, subject to deconstruction. Much of Sanchez's intensity as teacher and poet is based on her belief that the icons, symbols, and axiological principles of Eurocentrism are so deeply engrained that "cracking the skull" is the only effective strategy for combating the Eurocentric construction of knowledge. To a certain extent, Sanchez argues, "black consciousness of the 1960s was eroded in the 70s." The consequences of this erosion further enhance the need for the teacher/healer/poet, and Sanchez is aware of this increasingly important role. "The poet as lyricist," she intuits, "may well occupy center stage in the 1980s" (*Black Scholar* 27). Sanchez astutely recognizes the subtle shift in racism's justification of itself, and, because she understands the power of images, she knows that the psychological aspect of racism must become her focus. Given the pervasive influence of popular culture, "black value setting," in Sanchez's estimation, "may well be a struggle between subliminal seduction of a black moral strength . . . and a new movement to instill positive black family and social values" (*Black Scholar* 28). In a recent interview, she firmly insists that to teach without values is to teach students to be immoral (September 21, 1990). As a pedagogue who also serves as a therapist practicing value-oriented psychotherapy, Sanchez establishes and then follows her own critical path.

By signifying upon the European world view which posits an image of jazz as intrinsically chaotic, Sanchez invites her students to recognize the embedded values in such a portrayal. In "Psychological Aspects of European Cosmology in American Society," psychologist Joseph Baldwin contends that the European world view or cosmology is anti-African because it "projects European supremacy and African inferiority as the natural order" (217). Baldwin defines the Eurocentric mythological construction as one in which the heroic ideal is always "European (i. e., physically, culturally, etc.)" and the hero possesses many nature-mastering characteristics, such as superior intelligence, aggressiveness, fearlessness, and strength. Rarely female, this figure is depicted as "unconquerable, [and] victorious . . ." against evil forces or villains (219).

The individual who must endorse another's cultural symbols, Joseph Campbell contends, is "out of sync" with the self. A growing number of African-American psychologists, Afrocentric in orientation, offer similar views. They argue that the "African survival thrust" is most ably synopsized in Molefi K. Asante's theory expressed in *Afrocentricity* (1980), which demands that Africans in the diaspora should examine the world and its phenomena from an African perspective. Such a perspective, they contend, best sums up "mentally healthy functioning for all Africans." In *African Psychology: Toward Its Reclamation, Reascension, and Revitalization* (1976), Wade Nobles describes insanity among African Americans as being caused, in part, by the "disruption in the natural, harmonious relationship between the spiritual, material, conceptual, affective and connotative aspects of Black psycho-social and geophysical reality" (93).

Under the influence of psychologist Bobby Wright, Afrocentric psychologists have now labeled the "silent rape of a people's collective mind" as "mentacide" (1981). If mentacide is achieved through the perpetuation of alien culture, values, and belief systems, then one is indeed addressing a kind of cultural genocide. Further, as the victim of oppression suffering from psychological misorientation will often embrace the oppressor's images, values, beliefs, and opinions, mentacide serves to modify the behavior of the oppressed for the benefit of the oppressor. When the institutional projection of these images is pervasive, behavior modification can occur. Consequently, much like the students in Sanchez's class, the victims of mentacide begin to endorse and embrace illusions which lead them away from their centers. Psychologist Daudi Ajani ya Azibo further refines the concept of psychological misorientation and mentacide in his article, "African-Centered Theses on Mental Health and a Nosology of Black/African Personality Disorder" (1989). Psychological misorientation (Baldwin 1980a, 1980b, 1982) is the most fundamental state of disorder (Azibo 1982). It can be considered the most "basic Black personality disorder" (Azibo 1982) and occurs when an African "operates without an African-centered belief system." Attempting to live with a cognitive definitional system that is nonblack causes the individual to be misoriented or "out of sync" with her own cosmology. "Misorientation is manifest," Azibo writes, "whenever and to whatever degree alien concepts comprise the cognitive structure" (185).

Like Sanchez and other poets, these psychologists join a continuum initiated by earlier African-American artists and scholars. In their studies of African-American children, Kenneth Clark and his wife, Margaret Clark, used dolls (one black, one white), to demonstrate racism's negative effect upon young African Americans (1947). Their distressing findings influenced the U. S. Supreme Court's decision on the integration of public schools. In *Black Rage* (1968), William Grier and Price Cobbs demonstrated causality between racial oppression and psychological trauma.

Mentacide, then, is the phenomenon Sanchez addresses when she attempts to deconstruct embedded images in her poetry and in her teaching. Because the icons and symbols supporting the axiological principles of Eurocentrism are so deeply embedded, Sanchez uses incisive verbal art, and her being is caught up in the efficacy of her treatment: "The point of me is to treat the souls of Black folk, and others. To be an artist/surgeon and cut out the terrible years of all these slave/years and let Blackness flow healthily, fully" ("Moonstone"). Her aim is to help African Americans achieve a new orientation or mental health, which Azibo, like Nobles, describes as the "achievement in the psychological and behavorial spheres of life of a functioning that (a) is in harmony with and (b) embraces the natural order. . . ." In effect, these psychologists are arguing for individual realignment with the natural cosmology. As scholars and psychologists who study the science of processes and behavior, they, like Sanchez, have added an Afrocentric perspective to their work by attempting to intervene in the mental misorientation of African Americans. In this pursuit, they develop metatheories which address the failure of Eurocentric psychiatry to intervene in the mental illness which African Americans suffer.

Wade Nobles, Daudi Ajani ya Azibo, Joseph Baldwin, N'alm Akbar, Linda Myers, and others are Afrocentric psychologists/scholars attempting to offer solutions based on their study of African Americans. Further, they posit causality between mental illness and oppressive racism. In his further refinement of mentacide, Azibo describes its multi-faceted effect. Mentacide operates on two levels, each equally potent as it renders the sufferer "void of any pro-Black orientations to life," while instilling

> (a) pro-European orientation that commands at surface and deep levels of the psyche an unnatural and unwarranted acceptance and admiration of and allegiance to White persons, and White-dominated society no matter how unjust and inhumane and (b) the relative disparagement of all things African.

> The first type of mentacide alienates the African from him/herself by attaching the psychological Blackness. Therefore, it will be called *alienating mentacide*. Needless to say, alienating mentacide is perpetrated—directly or indirectly—on Africans through practically all facets of European-dominated society, especially 'popular culture.'(186)

Azibo's description conjures up images of people behaving like robots or operating in a "dead-zone." His description parallels one articulated by Malcolm X some years ago: "Just as a tree without roots is dead," Malcolm asserted, "a people without history or cultural roots also becomes a dead people" (25). Sanchez hopes to resurrect these dead people, and, for more than twenty years as teacher/healer/poet, she has addressed the same concern. Her deconstructive techniques are designed to "crack the skull" and help psychologically misoriented African Americans realign themselves with their culture. As teacher/healer/poet, then, Sanchez militates against mentacide, and the urgency of her work is more fully appreciated when one evaluates the psychological situation in which African Americans find themselves. Against such devastating effects as those described by Azibo, Sanchez's confidence that she as an individual teacher/healer/poet can effect such monumental changes represents victorious thought based on her sense of connections with the elders:

> I am the continuation of Black Women who have gone before me and who will come after me. I am Harriet Tubman, Fannie Lou Hamer, Queen Mother Moore, Ella, Ida Wells Barnett, Margaret Walker, Assata Shakur, Gwendolyn Brooks and all the unsung Black Women who have worked in America's kitchens. I am the sister who has been abused by men and loved by men. I am my stepmother, Gerry, a Southern Black Woman who was taught her place and as a consequence was never able to fulfill herself as a human being. ("Moonstone")

By according superhuman and supernatural powers to their enterprise, Sanchez and Afrocentric psychologists also reveal their sense of the enormity of the task. This attribution to the ancestors is also an aspect of Afrocentric psychology. "Almost as if motivated by the ancestral spirit, several Black psychologists began to develop conceptualizations of Black mental health which recognized that natural functioning was the result of being centered in and consistent with oneself" (Nobles 92).

Certainly the movement toward Afrocentric perspective by African-American psychologists validates Sonia Sanchez's historical role as teacher/healer/poet. In fact, both African-American psychologists and poets perceived a serious moral gap in the lack of response from Eurocentered psychiatry. Alarming observations are offered by those few non-African-American psychiatrists and psychologists who admit that Eurocentric psychology and psychiatry have failed many marginalized groups: the elderly and the poor, as well as African Americans. According to Seymour L. Halleck, M.D., in *The Politics of Therapy* (1971), "American psychiatry presently deters social change; it is much more of a repressive social force than it has to be" (38). Halleck sees psychiatrists as reluctant to incorporate this recognition into their practice, and this reluctance has "frequently led them to further the cause of repressiveness." His description of the philosophy and practice of Eurocentric psychiatry and psychiatrists is instructive. He concedes that the "oppression of the poor and the black is one of the tragic realities of American life." Suggesting that this practice is ongoing and partially concealed, Halleck is surprisingly moral in his assessment.

> At first glance the psychiatric profession's record in dealing with these groups looks good: with rare exceptions psychiatrists have emphasized that social discrimination and prejudice—rather than innate weakness or illness—are the main causes of the unhappiness of both groups. However, the profession has also taken an implied negative stand toward these people by ignoring their mental health needs. By failing to uncover, dramatize, or treat the problems of poverty-stricken or minority groups the psychiatrist has made it easier for society to ignore their problems. (110–11)

Halleck published his findings in 1971; yet, nearly twenty years later, African-American psychologists continue to face the same lack of responsiveness from Euro-centered psychology and psychiatry to the mental problems of African Americans. Halleck paints a picture of a professional community suspended between moral and political expediency. If the psychiatrists and psychologists admit that mental illness in African Americans is related to racism and oppression, then they are obliged to empower their patients; yet in empowering their patients, they work against the self-interests of their group (in this case, white America).

Combined with the accepted belief that African Americans experience severe psychological stress, such an extended period of neglect suggests a situation of crisis proportions. Certainly this professional and moral lapse serves, to some extent, as an imperative for the "Black Arts Movement" which dominated during the sixties and seventies. Given the reluctance of non-African-American psychologists and psychiatrists to study the problems of or intervene in mental health problems of the African-American community, the only option for such poets as Sonia Sanchez, Haki Madhubuti, June Jordan, and others was to attempt to militate against the psychological misorientation prevalent in the African-American community.

Halleck maintains that black writers were the only group addressing the impersonal but devastating effect of institutionalized racism. In the August 1977 special issue of the *Journal of Black Psychology*, tributes to that publication's continued commitment to the study of African Americans are conveyed in a series of letters. Among these are letters from the African-American poets Haki Madhubuti and Nikki Giovanni. Giovanni posits a connection between the aims of psychology and those of poetry: "As a layperson whose profession is poetry, I find we are not so different in our professional concerns for not only Black people, but planet earth itself. . . ." She suggests future directions for both disciplines: "Between poetry and psychology perhaps some new views will be presented" (4).

Sanchez as Teacher/Healer/Poet

Once we accept, as do Halleck and others, that a "racist society can impose indirect, but nevertheless powerful, stress upon large groups of citizens" (22) and that poets and writers can intervene to assuage and sometimes heal, we have an appropriate context for evaluating Sanchez's deconstructive techniques and her attempt to address psychological misorientation as teacher/healer/poet. In this role, Sanchez has developed an amazing facility for incorporating cultural, political, and social concerns. Her strength as a community elder is her ability to connect the past and the present in a manner which informs the present and warns about the future. Part of her ability to do this stems from her awareness of what is happening in the world. She reads events with political eyes and brings this insight to her teaching. After teaching about slavery, for example, she may ask the class to tell her how a slave is created, or she may ask the rhetorical question, "Are the masses asses"? In another class Sanchez was teaching from Charles W. Chestnut's *The Wife of His Youth*. Lecturing directly from her notes, Sanchez cited other historians to demonstrate how a slave mentality benefitted the "peculiar institution." She conflated the situation established in slavery with contemporary enslavement. African Americans, she contended, have passed from physical to mental enslavement. At the point of greatest tension in the classroom, Sanchez queried her students, asking them "How did we get to this point?" She stressed the significance of this transition by telling students that the individual who loses the self has lost the war, the struggle. As Sanchez uses historical context and topical allusions, she reinforces the image of herself as community elder. Her validation is found in her longevity as well as in her reputation as an activist, so it is not at all surprising to hear her using terms which suggest struggle and battle. Her favorite exhortation to her students is a single word. "Resist," she urges, "we must resist." Mental enslavement is Sanchez's nemesis, and she goes to any means to combat it.

Sanchez has said that she learned to be stalwart by using the lives of foremothers and forefathers as models. Yet her ability to commiserate with others in their struggle toward psychological freedom is based on her personal experience. Clearly, she accepts that a certain amount of psychological trauma is inherent in this struggle. In her willingness to "crack the skull" even when trauma ensues, Sanchez is reminiscent of Harriet Tubman, who delivered African Americans out of slavery even when they wavered, oftentimes re-enforcing her determination with a gun. From such foremothers as Tubman, Sanchez embraces a legacy which is best described as "Afrocentric womanism." As defined by Alice Walker, a womanist "is committed to survival and wholeness of her people, both male and female" (233). Concern for the self and the people connects womanism to Afrocentricism. Lately, scholars influenced by principles of Afrocentricism have discovered a new paradigm for reading foremothers' lives. Thus we grow more certain that Harriet Tubman, Fannie Lou Hamer, Sojourner Truth, and many unnamed others have always practiced Afrocentric womanism, embracing the modified axiom which defines the first law of nature as "the preservation . . . [of] beings with which one shares a greater biogenetic commonality relative to other beings: the preservation of one's Race" (Azibo 178).

Sanchez clearly views herself as the preserver of her race. Her Afro-centric womanist praxis is informed by the memories of her personal transformation from identity crisis to ideological clarity. In "The Social Construction of Black Feminist Thought," Patricia Hill-Collins notes that "African-American women who adhere to the idea that claims about Black women must be substantiated by Black women's sense of their own experiences and who anchor their knowledge claims in an Afrocentric feminist epistemology have produced a rich tradition of Black feminist thought" (770). Highly personal, empiricist in nature, Sanchez's epistemology informs her actions. Her determination to never again succumb to the psychological misorientation from which she suffered fuels her desire to empower others, helping them to achieve ideological clarity. In what amounts to a mani-festo, she demonstrates how the strength of her convictions are imbued by ancestral legacies:

> I will never again see myself, see other Black women . . . men . . . children secondarily, through the eyes of the oppressor . . . the slave master. I will never see my kinky hair, my big nose, or my big lips as something horrible. I don't want the bluest eyes. I don't want the long straight blonde hair. I maintain that I will never in my life walk secondarily again—or even appear to have any secondary views . . . when I hit the stage, I know that I am just as tough as anyone there. People aren't accustomed to that kind of behavior.

That is a legacy that we've gotten from Malcolm, from Fannie Lou, from Du Bois, and from Ida B. I am aggressive; I will not deny myself. (356)

Her awareness of herself as an elder walking in the footsteps of the ancestor informs her philosophy of "art for art's sake." In an interview with Zala Chandler, Sanchez talks about the freedom of "discovering" the self. This discovery, which took place "in the 1960s—probably the late fifties but definitely manifesting itself in the early sixties—was almost like being reborn (357). Though Sanchez invokes midwifery imagery, suggesting she birthed herself, she also admits that her exposure to Malcolm X's own unparalleled deconstructionist style forced her to think about the embedded images of racism; yet she had to assist in her own orientation, and at times she gives the impression that she created herself. Speaking of her transformative experience, Sanchez uses metaphors of rebirth or conversion. Describing her "discovery," she helps us to appreciate the degree of her psychological misorientation: "For the first time in your life, you did not have to be concerned about your nose, or your lips, or your hair. . . ." Echoing Afrocentric psychologists, Sanchez summarizes the effect of her transformation: "You could be your natural self. What a relief from a peculiar kind of bondage that was there, that we were involved in" (357).

Afrocentric womanist, Sanchez desires the same transformative experience and subsequent freedom for others. She recalls the joy of "seeing people opening up before your eyes, almost like flowers, and coming to the realization that, indeed, they were political" (357). Believing the destiny of the African-American community is also her destiny, Sanchez positions herself as agent of change. "It was beautiful to see people recognize that they had to be political if they were to survive, to live, to 'be.'" For Sanchez, the enterprise of the black poets in the seventies was about empowerment; soon, however, they moved from describing conditions to offering solutions. This parallel between African-American psychologists and African-American artists is clearly evident in Sanchez's assertion that "Poets need to become moral psychologists in the 1980s" because the "struggle between man/woman and the inhumanitarians has escalated into the sophistication of suggestion and behavior modification" (*Black Scholar* 28).

As teacher and poet, Sanchez addresses the "sophistication of suggestion" by deconstructing negative images. As healer, she offers ritual drama and victorious thought to heal and modify behavior. This is the important second half of her pedagogical strategy. Directly related to the first component of Sanchez's pedagogical method of "cracking the skull" and its attendant trauma, this component is designed to heal wounded psyches. Students who register for her classes seem to run an emotional gamut. While rarely hostile to Sanchez, many exhibit open hostility to each other or to the text. Over a period of fifteen weeks, however, a remarkable transformation takes place. Sanchez ends each class by having students join hands and form a circle.

Dona Marimba Richards' brilliant analysis of the importance of African-American spirituality provides a context for understanding Sanchez's use of ritual drama in her class. "African life," according to Richards, is replete with ritual. Her description of ritual focuses on its ability to empower. Through ritual, she writes, the unexplainable is understood, chaos is ordered, trauma is avoided, crises are dealt with and overcome. In Richards' view, ritual drama's importance to the African-American community was demonstrated during their enslavement, as they used ritual drama to assuage the trauma of physical enslavement. Richards describes this ritual drama taking place at special gatherings away from the masters: "We would form a circle, each touching those next to us so as to physically express our spiritual closeness." Holding hands to form this circle, "slaves testified, and shared pain and received affirmation of [their] existence as suffering beings." Through such testimony, enslaved people began "to understand themselves as communal beings. Ritual made them whole again" (217).

By introducing this circle in her class, Sanchez offers a space where her students are free to speak from the heart. In this space, the cognitive dissonance students experience during her lectures is assuaged. Further, those who resist her message can express themselves without censure. Even those students who don't usually speak in class are offered an opportunity to express their feelings. In her use of what I call a "healing circle," Sanchez admits the personal into her classroom. Students are allowed to cry, to speak of anger or joy. The circle is their space. Sanchez's only response to what students have to say, be it critical or other, is "Thank you." In this sense, she is giving voice to the voiceless. Over time, in this space, each student reveals the extent to which he or she is transformed by Sanchez.

Sanchez's pedagogical praxis is informed by the same philosophy that informs her poetic praxis. As she deliberately practices "art for life's sake," Sanchez inverts tradition to reveal and heal. Though the worth of the conventional concept of an impersonal teaching style devoid of value has never been a reality, many educators continue to publicly endorse this pedagogical method. Sanchez, however, openly asserts that one who does not teach values teaches students to be immoral. Certainly this pedagogical philosophy is as daring as her position on the role of the poet. In her theoretical construct, Sanchez divides poetry into two discrete areas: "ethos" and "functionary." According to Sanchez, poetry of ethos is meant to convey personal experience, feelings of love, despair, joy, and frustration arising from very private encounters. What she defines as "functionary" poetry, on the other hand, deals with themes in the social domain: "religion, God, country, social institutions, war, marriage, and death in the distinct context of that society's perception" (*Black Women Writers* 416).

Because functional poetry is offered for life's sake, it must offer truth, and sometimes that truth can be as harsh as the pedagogical technique Sanchez uses in her classroom. As far as African Americans are concerned, Sanchez insists, the fundamental truth to be told in any art form is the "state of the people." For Sanchez this truth is that "America is killing us." Seemingly apocalyptic, this message is balanced with testimonials to communal strength, for Sanchez maintains that "we continue to live and love and struggle and win." As teacher/healer/poet, Sanchez's need to communicate with her audience is crucial because of the nature of her message. Since she wants to convey truth, her statement must have validity (Hill-Collins 770). Thus she contends: "I draw on any experience or image to clarify and magnify this truth for those who must ultimately be about changing the world; not for critics and librarians" (*Black Women Writers* 416).

Concerned about being a responsible artist, not merely a famous one, Sanchez seeks a cautious balance between despair and hope. As in her classroom, she is aware of the need for healing and victorious thought in her poetic praxis. As creator of social values, as one who can effect change, the teacher/healer/poet must also accept responsibility for effecting meaningful change. Rhetoric uttered on stages, from podiums, and in classrooms is ineffectual if it is not informed by a transformative power. In a poem written at the height of the "Black Arts movement," Sanchez worries about irresponsible rhetoric:

> Who's gonna make all
> that beautiful blk
> rhetoric mean something
> like I mean
> who's gonna take the words
> blk
> is beautiful
> and make more of it
> than blk capitalism
> u dig?

If the poet possesses the power of *nommo*, the power of the word, then the poet also has the ability and must assume the responsibility to assist in the passage of the individual from dehumanization to human beingness.

Sanchez may offer this healing element by focusing on certain themes, as in the poem "Old Words," where she comments on both the "alienating mentacide" and its attendant self-denying symptoms:

> We have come to
> believe that we are
> not. to be we
> must be loved or
> touched and proved to be.

In an effort to touch the others, Sanchez is moving toward using her entire being as transformative instrument. She assumes the role of advocate for many, proving that their concerns are important, that, in fact, they do exist. In her public readings she will often wholly assume the persona of the other, sometimes seemingly undergoing a complete transformation as she speaks in the voice of those for whom she serves as advocate. In daring acts of synthesis, Sanchez offers her consciousness, becoming a channel through which the others speak for themselves. Her voice becomes the voice of a slave girl raped by her master, the voice of ancestors. By allowing others to speak, she allows them a hearing. By offering herself as conduit, she continues her role as healer, integrating fragmented selves, past and present.

Works Cited

Asante, M. K. 1980. *Afrocentricity: Theory of Social Change*. Buffalo: Amulefi Publishing Company.

Azibo, Daudi Ajani ya. 1989. "African-centered Theses on Mental Health and a Nosology of Black/African Personality." *Journal of Black Psychology*. 15: 173–214.

Bakhtin, Mikhail. 1971. "Discourse Typology in Prose." In *Readings in Russian Poetics: Formalist and Structuralist Views*. eds. Ladislave Matejka and Krystyna Pomorska. Cambridge: MIT Press.

Baldwin, Joseph. 1985. "Psychological Aspects of European Cosmology in American Society." *Western Journal of Black Studies* 9: 216–23.

Braxton, Joanne and Andree N. Mc Laughlin, eds. 1960. *Wild Women in the Whirlwind, Afra-American Culture and the Contemporary Literary Renaissance*. New Jersey: Rutgers University Press.

Clark, K. B. and Clark, M. P. 1947. "Racial Identification and Preference in Negro Children." In T. M. Newcomb and E. L. Hartley, eds. *Readings in Social Psychology*. (1st ed.) New York: Holt Rinehart & Winston.

Collins, Patricia Hill. 1977. "The Social Construction of Black Feminist Thought." *Signs: Journal of Women In Culture and Society* 4: 745–73.

Gates, Henry Louis, Jr. 1988. *The Signifying Monkey: A Theory of Afro-American Literary Criticism*. New York: Oxford University Press.

Giovanni, Nikki. 1977. Letter. Tributes to the Association. *Journal of Black Psychology* 4:4.

Halleck, Seymour L. 1971. *The Politics of Therapy*. New York: Science.

Mitchell-Kernan, Claudia. 1973. "Signifying as a Form of Verbal Art." In *Mother-Wit from the Laughing Barrel: Readings in the Interpretation of Afro-American Folklore*. ed. Alan Dundes. Englewood Cliffs, N. J.: Prentice-Hall.

Nobles, Wade W. 1986. *African Psychology: Toward Its Reclamation, Reascension, and Revitalization*. Oakland, Calif.: A Black Family Institute Publication.

Richards, Dona Marimba. 1985. *The Implications of African-American Spirituality. African Culture: The Rhythms of Unity*. Westport, Conn.: Greenwood Press. 217–23.

Sanchez, Sonia. 1970. *We a BaddDDD People*. Detroit, Mich.: Broadside Press.

———. 1983. "Ruminations/Reflections." In *Black Women Writers 1950–1980*. New York: Anchor Press. 415–18.

———. 1983. *Crisis and Culture*. New York: Black Liberation Press.

———. 1984. *Homegirls & Handgrenades*. New York: Thunder's Mouth Press.

———. 1985. "The Poet As A Creator of Social Values." *Black Scholar* 16: 20–28.

———. 1987. *Under a Soprano Sky*. New Jersey: African World Press.

———. 1988. *The Paul Robeson Award to Sonia Sanchez: For artistic excellence, political conscience and integrity*. n.p.

———. 1990. Interview. Public Broadcasting System.

Walker, Alice. 1983. *In Search of Our Mothers' Gardens*. San Diego, Calif.: Harcourt, Brace, Jovanovich.

Wright, B. E. 1974. "The Psychopathic Racial Personality." *Black Books Bulletin* 2:25–31.

Malcolm X. 1967. *Malcolm X on Afro-American History*. New York: Pathfinder.

Madame Neau:
The Practice of Ethno-Psychiatry
in Rural Louisiana

Wonda Lee Fontenot

Introduction

Mental health maintenance is a major concern among certain African-American populations in rural French Louisiana. Their folk explanation of mental illness and how to treat it differs from that of mainstream medicine. As a result, many from this community seek the advice and care of an ethno-psychiatrist, a folk medical practitioner.

In this essay, I document the life and folk medicine practice of Madame Neau (pseudonym), an African-American ethno-psychiatrist in St. Elenna Parish in rural southwest Louisiana.[1] I rely on oral interviews with her, as well as with her son, Doc. The folk medical tradition survives among African Americans not only in rural southwest Louisiana, but in other parts of the rural South as well (Snow 1979). The mental health-care provider, an ethno-psychiatrist, is referred to in the community as a "mind reader." A mind reader/ethno-psychiatrist is the functional equivalent of mainstream medicine's psychoanalyst, but the mind reader shares culture and ethnicity with his or her African-American patients (just as the psychoanalyst in most cases shares culture and ethnicity with his/her patients).

For the most part, mainstream medicine defines "health" in terms of pathology—a person free of infection, viruses, or other physical maladies, as determined by clinical tests, is considered "healthy." These diagnoses are primarily based on scientifically-defined results. For communities with folk

41

medicine systems, both mental and physical illness are culturally defined. An unhealthy person is one who is unable to function in his or her role in society and who thus becomes a threat to self and society.

Mind readers, usually women, diagnose causes of illness by divining. Divining is customarily done by means of prayer incantations and a trance-like state. This role is similar to diviners in other cultures of the African diaspora and to shamans in Native-American culture. Mind readers are insiders (members of the community) who treat their patient's illness according to the local culture's concepts of what constitutes illness and what causes illness. Treatments include prayer and lithograph photos of religious saints. The lithograph religious photos are the size of playing cards and are carried by the patient for protection and to bring good fortune.

In this community people believe there are natural and unnatural causes of illness. A "natural" illness occurs as a form of punishment against someone who has sinned or wronged another individual. Examples of such wrongs include lying, stealing, committing incest, and so on. These natural illnesses are acts against God, and the ensuing sickness is based on the Christian belief that God punishes. Lesser examples of natural-cause ailments are those resulting from dressing improperly for inclement weather conditions, resulting in a cold, flu, or the like.

"Unnatural" causes of illness derive from intentional malevolent acts committed against another for the sole purpose of bringing physical harm or misfortune. The results of such acts are more severe than those already mentioned. These malevolent acts are defined within this cultural context as "hoo doo" and "curse." Illness resulting from hoo doo or curse is usually psychological.[2] Hoo doo and curse acts are only effective if the person is familiar with the cultural nuances of the society that practices them. Examples of malevolent acts include openly and verbally wishing bad luck to an individual or performing some magical act, such as sprinkling cornmeal across door paths of potential victims to bring harm. If the victim becomes ill or encounters misfortune, then the hoo doo or curse is seen as the cause.

Going to a mind reader is an ongoing mental health routine for many families in St. Elenna Parish. These cultural attitudes toward health are found mostly among persons about forty years of age and older. This includes at least half of the African-American population in the parish.

According to medical anthropologists George Foster and Barbara Gallatin Anderson, an indigenous ethnic group's definitions of mental health should be studied from a culture-personality perspective. This means it is "necessary to examine mental illness from a psycho-social frame of reference rather than a physiological frame" (1978). The present essay is based on just such a perspective, using participant observation conducted with Madame Neau between 1982 and 1984 and interviews conducted with her son (and daughter-in-law) in 1986–87.

Historical Background

Enslaved Africans came to Louisiana with a knowledge of traditional medicine and religious practices that existed in West Africa. Literature on Louisiana's folk medicine tradition has often mistakenly been equated with the ill-defined ritual practices of Louisiana's Voo doo queen, Marie Leveau, and the supposedly wild orgies and sacrificial rites she held on the bayous. These interpretations provoke uncomplimentary thoughts in readers' minds and portray folk healing customs as bizarre and irrational. Voo doo was openly practiced by Leveau and others in the 1800s. It was at its height around the mid-nineteenth century. In the late 1800s, due to harassment by local authorities, the practice went underground.

Doc, Madame Neau's son who took over her practice after her death, could not specifically affirm that their practices were African or why healing rituals were carried out in a certain manner. He simply said, "this is the way it has always been done." As far as he could remember, his mother, and all those before her in his family who were mind readers, practiced this way. This substantiates African-American theologian and cultural historian Albert Raboteau's (1980) claim: theological explanations are not retained in African-American folk religious traditions, but customs are remembered.

The wearing of a mask to conceal or defy true character is a common practice throughout the cultural history of African Americans. Spirituals are a good example of presenting a hidden message through song—messages not readily discernible to outsiders are easily misinterpreted or ignored by them. Similarities exist in the African-American community's ethno-psychiatric practices, where the practice is conducted in secret. Here, two cosmologies interplay: a Christian perspective and an African one.

Although the new (Christian) theology did not replace the spiritual remembrance of old African theological beliefs, it did offer some protection from the hostile tongues of whites, who condemned the enslaved Africans' folk customs and encouraged conversion. To avoid persecution and ridicule, African Americans camouflaged their religion and healing ways through feigned conformity (Washington 1964, 33). Thus prayer, faith, and the use of lithographed Catholic saints in healing rituals became key "acceptable" elements. This syncretic tradition, defined as beliefs based on the Christian doctrine and manifested in objects based on animistic concepts (Herskovits 1941, 207), became the foundation of traditional folk medical practices in rural southwest Louisiana. The belief in the supernatural survived.

In this African-American community, anyone, regardless of gender or age, may possess the gift of healing and be "called." Unlike the traditional black Baptist belief that God does not call women to pastor churches, women are called by God to this folk tradition. Women mind readers can also be understood by looking at the roles and function of women in the community's church. Especially significant are the roles held by church mothers, steward sisters, and deaconesses, as they are variously called. These women elders, highly respected, are often part of the decision-making process in the church.

Women such as Madame Neau who practice spiritism are also affiliated with the institutional church. Women spiritists as well as women elders are regarded as having sound wisdom. They are, in essence, members of the church's sub-power structure. Most parishioners of the church (including female and male elders and male pastors) have respect for mind readers. All are usually members of the same congregation, and the former view the latter as carrying out an aspect of God's work. Outside of the institutional church, in the realm of folk medicine, female and male spiritists are on equal footing.

Mind readers benefit from womens' high status within the church and, in turn, create womens' high spiritual status. Women mind readers utilize prayer in a very spiritualized/"other worldly" way: they rely on their disassociational state, which intensifies the ritual process. This gives the appearance of divine interception. Thus they are often cited as the "most gifted" (intuitive) congregants, a very necessary skill for mind readers.

In African-American cultures, mysticism is a matriarchal spiritual system. Holy Spirit possessions and similar states are an acceptable, approved, and ongoing form of spiritual expression within the church and the community. Sojourner, a Yoruba priestess, writing in 1982, explained the spiritualism existing among women in African-American religious culture as similar to practices in other African diaspora cultures. She states: "Black theology and folk religion, like traditional African religions, seeks the power or the spirit of God. . . . By attuning yourself to the Spirit . . . you become one with that power. Thus when Black Christians [women] talk about putting themselves in the hands of God, they are generally referring to their . . . ability to tap into a divine source of energy" (1982). This explanation illuminates female mind readers' traditionalism and community support.

Madame Neau's Technique and Environment

African-American folk medicine is widely misunderstood by mainstream observers. Folk practitioners express annoyance and dissatisfaction with standard misconceptions, which often associate folk healing with eccentric behavior or demonic technique. Thus I chose to reveal an "insider's" perspective devoid of preconceived biases. In this community, these folk practitioners and their practices are sacred, Christian pursuits. I was introduced to Madame Neau by a relative of mine. I specifically wanted to observe Madame Neau treating her patients. On several occasions I became a patient myself. I was especially interested in her appearance, location, counseling procedures, and relationship to patients while treating them. I also wanted to know what she did to heal patients, the questions she asked, her state of mind while treating them, and what "implements" she used (e.g., herbs, oils, powders, and so on).

After my initial visits to Madame Neau (1982–84), I returned to record her oral history. I focused on the folk medicine tradition of which she was a part and her life as a mind reader. When I returned in 1986 to Madame Neau's residence, which also served as her work place, I was surprised to find a gloomy house. I was unaware that Madame Neau had died in the summer of 1985. Her home had always been alive with the sound of voices spilling from the living room to the street. Madame Neau regularly saw patients from the wee hours of the morning until the sun set in the late afternoon. This was constant—six days a week. "I never practice on Sunday, that's God's day," she once told me.

A neighbor greeted me as I approached the porch steps of Madame Neau's small, wood-frame, shanty-style home early that morning. Her neighbors were always protective of her. I discovered through conversation with the neighbor that she had died and her son had since replaced her; he would be in later that afternoon. As a result, I obtained much of the information about Madame Neau from her only child and son. He is also a mind reader, who inherited his gift/skill from his mother. This turn of events created an interesting contrast: the participant observation aspect of my research was done with Madame Neau, yet the oral history was provided by her son and daughter-in-law—both "big talkers." Madame Neau, not very talkative, would probably have revealed less. But I did have the opportunity to observe what she did best—counsel.

When next I returned, the small living room which doubles as a doctor's waiting room was packed with patients of both sexes and all ages. I was immediately greeted by an attractive, smartly dressed, brown-skinned woman in her thirties. This was unusual. Madame Neau's normal procedure had been for patients to simply come in, take a seat, and wait their turn. This woman was the wife of Madame Neau's son. I told her my name and purpose and asked if I could see him. She grumbled that her husband was very busy and occupied with a patient. I assured her I wouldn't take very much of his time. She led me to the kitchen and instructed me to wait there.

I waited in the somewhat bare kitchen while she informed "Doc," as she called him, that I wanted to see him. Unexpectedly, Doc came out of the treating room and greeted me. He was about five feet seven with an average build and a dark brown complexion. He wore large diamond rings on all eight fingers. I was somewhat surprised by him, because his appearance was a bit flashy and totally different from his mother's. She was a rather stout, plainly dressed woman, who always wore an apron, although she spent very little, if any, time in the kitchen. She always had someone prepare her meals during her working hours. Wearing an apron was part of the general dress code for women of Madame Neau's era. Many women living in this small rural town came from a farming background, and an apron was conveniently worn to serve as a bucket or basket to pick eggs, fruits, and so forth, as they went about their daily chores. The pockets on the apron held her small change, and her bosom held paper money. Certainly, wearing an apron was comfortable and an acceptable form of dressing. It was functional and symbolic of the ordinariness of Madame Neau's character. Madame Neau was also very reserved and meticulous. On the contrary, Doc was eager and friendly.

I introduced myself and my purpose in the presence of Doc's wife, who was protective of his time and attention. Doc eagerly began to talk: about himself, his mother, and the role of a mind reader. He talked for a solid fifteen minutes before his wife interrupted to remind him that he had patients waiting. He agreed to see me later.

When I returned that afternoon, Doc was seeing his last patient. I was directed by his wife to the bedroom Madame Neau had used as her work space. This was where Doc now counseled and treated. I sat in the patient's chair, facing Doc, just as I had on previous occasions with Madame Neau. The arrangement of the work space was exactly as Madame Neau had left it: two chairs faced each other, with a small table in the center, but the table did not come between the patient and the mind reader. The treating area was in front of a double window, dressed with sheer curtains. This window, which Madame Neau often glanced through, looked out on the street, the sidewalk, her front porch, and those who came and left. With the exception of this special corner of the room and various Catholic statues and saints' lithographs, the room is a typical bedroom. Doc's wife sat in on this first interview and offered her opinions about the mind reading profession.

Oral History Narrative

Doc has a doctoral degree in psychology and is an ordained Protestant minister. After the death of his mother at the age of eighty, Doc relocated to St. Elenna parish, where he continues to provide counseling services for his mother's patients. Madame Neau, a renowned mind reader/ethno-psychiatrist, had been "counseling" or "treating" for approximately sixty-three years. Her patients ranged from the poor to well-known political figures.

Madame Neau was a devout Catholic and a member of the women's auxiliary of the Elks, which was very active in her community. "You must be connected with a church organization to do this kind of work," Doc said. "Doctors [Western] put you under medication and make you tell them problems they don't know about. Where we [mind readers] are gifted through Christ. We don't have to give no medication. Through Christ we can go back in your past and tell you things you didn't know about."[3] Quick to affirm his link with Christianity, he quickly disclaimed connections with fortune tellers: "This is done without looking through a deck of cards, which we don't handle."

The house where he practices is the house in which he grew up. It is in a working-class African-American neighborhood located in a rural town with a population of sixty thousand. Doc, like most folk practitioners, said he was called by God to treat. He has been practicing for eighteen years. Similar to Madame Neau and many folk practitioners in this area, he began practicing at an early age. Doc refers to mind readers as spiritual psychologists, healing counselors, and doctors of human psychology. "Old people," he said, "that have treated people in the olden days call it spiritual psychology, and consider it a gift from God more than anything else."

Doc is unique: he practices the same folk medicine as his mother, even though he holds a doctorate in psychology. Although college-educated, Doc makes it quite clear his ability to treat is inherited and a gift from God. This knowledge preceded college. Madame Neau's harassment by public health officials prompted him to pursue higher education. He obtained a college degree to avoid similar encounters. Even though he is college-educated, he still treats patients with methods that are familiar to and culturally accepted by the community.

Madame Neau saw ten or more patients a day. She treated them mostly with prayer. She prayed silently or mumbled prayers, then went into a trance-like state. This trance-like state is distinctive of mind readers. "While in this state," says Doc, "the Holy Spirit communicates with the mind reader, and through this communication process she or he is made aware of a patient's past, present and future, their problems and/or illness." While still in this trance-like state, the mind reader is able to diagnose an individual's psychological problem. The treatment process and the extent of the treatment are revealed during this period as well. The average treatment session includes listening to patients' complaints, problems, fears, and desires; asking questions; advising; and offering solutions. This is followed by a prayer ritual. Depending on the nature of the problem, a typical session may run from twenty to thirty-five minutes. Some sessions have been known to last an hour, but rarely do they last less than twenty minutes. A person may be seen one or more times for the same problem.

Doc learned much of what he knows about mind reading by observing his mother in sessions and by listening to Madame Neau's lectures about the power of the mind, the power of faith, and the importance of having a relationship with God. The power of the subconscious mind alone can heal, he explained. "Part of healing," he stressed, "has to do with [the mind reader] focusing on an ailment or sore." Reflecting on his mother's teachings, he continued: "The power of the mind is like a person speaking silently to you. You can hear the voice. You go into a stage no ordinary person can understand. They can understand the healing of the physical body, but not the state of mind you are in."

The treatment's success depends on the receptiveness or skepticism of an individual, as well as on the complexity of the problem. Examples of the kinds of ailments Madame Neau treated included persons who felt they were having problems or poor health as a result of curse or hoo doo (e.g., a lingering illness, inability to get ahead financially, multiple deaths in the family in a short period of time, constant disharmony in marriages and families, and the like). Other patients suffered from natural causes, such as headaches, backaches, stomach problems, circulation problems, bronchitis, tiredness, tumors, and warts. She also provided general counseling to persons who wanted help with decisions and career directions. These included traveling advice, choosing a marriage partner, job choice, and infidelity. If the problem required in-depth treatment, Madame Neau would say various saintly novenas. In addition, she used healing oils to anoint the person. These substances, usually applied on the wrist and around the forehead, were oils she had mixed and were similar to those found in occult stores. Patients were also often given a small lithograph photo of a saint, which they carried with them for protection.

As is the case with all mind readers, Madame Neau did not advertise her services. Nor did she have a set fee for her labor. However, she accepted monetary contributions, which ranged from fifty cents to twenty dollars. She was called by God to do this work, and she believed a servant of God ought not charge for God's work: it is charity. Oftentimes her patient's payment was in kind—a bushel of okra, yams, peas, or the like.

Sometimes mind reading needs facilitation. If the patient is one who is particularly "hard to read" or difficult because of uneasiness, uncertainty, or nervousness, then the patient's hand is used as a guide. Madame Neau's methodology was to position and hold the patient's hand, with the palm facing upward in her own. She used her thumb to press certain points in the patient's open palm. Doc asserted this was not to be confused with palm reading. She used the hand merely as a guide, "just as a student uses a book as a guide." It was a means by which she entered the subconscious of the individual. "The contact with the body and the flow of blood," he said, "is to help determine the problem of an individual who might not otherwise be able to be reached or read."

Doc insists that the gift of treating, although a gift from God, is inherited within families from generation to generation. In each generation there is someone who possesses the gift of healing, although this gift is sometimes denied or discouraged by certain families. According to Doc, this denial occurs because some are ashamed to identify with the tradition. They do not understand the spiritual and cultural significance of the practice. Doc remarked that "When an individual denies his or her heritage or refuses to accept the gift [folk medical knowledge], their life becomes one of constant turmoil and misfortune, until they accept their heritage and begin to treat [counsel]." This turmoil is viewed as punishment for refusing to carry on the family's folk medicine tradition. This belief is similar to one related to African-American Baptist black ministers. It is believed that if individuals deny their calling to the ministry, then God punishes: only when individuals give up their worldly ways and become saintly servants of God will their lives become more orderly. The same self-sacrificing and pious character is required of mind readers. Within Madame Neau's family line, stemming back to slavery, each generation's matrilineal predecessors were mind readers. Although mind readers generally are women, most families are eager to have the folk medicine tradition survive, and they usually pass on their knowledge to the child with the greatest interest and spiritual intuitiveness—male or female. Girls, however, are often encouraged or persuaded to take an interest. In Madame Neau's case, she had no daughters and very few nieces, none of whom showed an interest in the tradition. Her son, however, expressed an interest in mind reading from an early age. He shared his calling, via visions and dreams, with his mother. He demonstrated his sincerity by spending a great deal of time developing his spirituality and observing his mother.

Mind readers, Doc believes, fill a void left by technological medicine and irreligious lives. "People," he explained,

> . . . come to mind readers because they cannot express their problem to no one else. We have sickness in the United States that does not have anything to do with medicine. Sickness come[s] to us because persons are not connected with a religion. We encourage the individual to pray and become affiliated with a church regardless of counseling or our help. Being a [folk] doctor of human psychology, we believe in the Word that can take hoo doo off people.

Hoo doo, according to Doc, does not help people, it only condemns them. "We take this word [fear] away from them and we uncross them. And by working against hective work, devil's work . . . we take it off." To accomplish this, some traditional remedies that are used are kept secret. Madame Neau believed that healing was based on faith. The more faith one had, the more help they received from God and the greater their chances were to be cured of illness and disease. The less faith one had, the less help they received from God and the more difficult it was for a mind reader to help them. This is why she often "prescribed" her patients to attend church, regardless of their denominational affiliation.

Critique of Data

Madame Neau was a highly respected and honored member of the community. I interviewed several persons randomly who were once her

patients or whose family members had been. These individuals were recommended to me through family networks of relatives who had utilized the
services of Madame Neau. With them I explored her effectiveness, as well as
their attitudes and perceptions of her. Some of these interviewees were leaders
of the community and others were regular townspeople. Their opinions are
representative of the community.

When I asked Mrs. Marie Santeaux, a former patient, what was it
about Madam Neau that impressed her most, she said, "She wasn't a gossiper.
She could be trusted. She never discussed your problems with other people."
Another patient, Mr. Sam Hosteau, said, ". . . oh she was good! She could
tell you things and most times it was right." Regarding her reputation as
a mind reader, Ms. Lotis Guntrie added that because Madame Neau was
so effective in what she did, many people were hoping that her son was
the reincarnation of his mother. Yet there were doubters. "He doesn't seem
to have the understanding about people like his mamma," continued Ms.
Guntrie. "He's different. . . he lived away for a while and has that book
learning. We'll see how he turns out."

Madame Neau was popular among all classes, sexes, and age groups.
Even among educated African Americans, the idea of going to see a Western-
trained psychoanalyst still carries with it certain stigmas. The most prevalent
stigma is that the person is "coo coo"—the local term for insane. Since no one
wants to be thus labeled, they resort to the more culturally acceptable form of
psychotherapy—treatment by a mind reader/ethno-psychiatrist. For patients,
protection from natural and unnatural illness and the healing that ensues
require certain sacrifices. Thus prayer and affiliation with a local church are
often prescribed as remedies for physical and social ills. Prayer-as-treatment
is not a new healing concept. In most West African cultures, prayer is used
in healing rituals. The belief that one's problems will be solved by "making
prayer a habit" and establishing a relationship with the Almighty is common
in the African-American religious tradition (Mitchell 1986; Evans-Pritchard
1967). Patients had faith in Madame Neau's "gift" of God, and they credit the
folk healer's powerful prayer words with unfailing effect (Oduyoye 1971).

The prayer rituals I witnessed were quite impressive and effective. Her
patients frequently claimed that her prayers had healed them. Mrs. Roselle
Gouteaux stated, "As long as I can remember my family went to see Madam
Neau whenever they wanted to know reasons for unexplainable misfortunes
and illness." Prayer and spiritual advising were the main services people
sought from Madame Neau. Mr. Henri Beggsteau said the healing prayers of
Madame Neau cured his teenage daughter of an ear problem. "My daughter
was in a car accident," he said. "The accident left her with a serious ear
infection which interfered with her hearing," he continued. "I took her to
doctor after doctor, but none of them did any good. I finally took her to see
Madame Neau. We visited her several times. It was her prayer treatments

that finally cured my daughter. She hasn't had problems with that ear since. I am not the only one. I have heard other people say the same thing about her and how good she is."

Questions For Future Study

Religion and magic are closely related to medicine in African and African-American religious traditions. In these traditions people believe that illnesses are the result of natural and unnatural causes. Thus for African Americans in rural St. Elenna Parish, syncretic Christian customs, prayer, faith, and the power of the supernatural became the basis for healing rituals.

This article raises several issues that have not been fully addressed. More comprehensive study is needed to understand the relationship among the early religious conversion experience of the enslaved African, magic syncretism, and religious syncretism (Bastide 1971), and to determine whether in the southern United States this tradition is predominantly matrilineal, as it has been in certain West African societies. The issue of change and continuity is also an important one. What can we determine about the world-view of the community through its healing customs? And, finally, how has the community's world-view changed as a result of outside influences?

Notes

1. In order to protect the identity of persons in my study, St. Elenna Parish and all names of individuals in this study are pseudonyms.
2. Hoodoo and Voo Doo are often used interchangeably within this community context in St. Elenna Parish. In most cases, the term hoodoo is used to describe an act committed against another, e.g., "somebody hoo dooed Mary." Voo Doo on the other hand is used to describe a belief system, e.g., "I don't believe in Voo Doo."
3. This colloquial speech is common to the area. Doc has not changed his speech habits, even though he has a college education.

Works Cited

Bastide, Roger. 1971. *African Civilizations in the New World*. Tr. Peter Green. London: C. Hurst and Company.

Evans-Pritchard, E. E. 1937. *Witchcraft, Oracles and Magic Among the Azande*. Oxford: Clarendon Press.

Foster, George and Barbara Gallatin Anderson. 1978. *Medical Anthropology*. New York: John Wiley and Sons.

Herskovits, Melville J. 1969. *The Myth of the Negro Past*. Boston: Beacon Press.

Mitchell, Ella P. 1986. "Oral Tradition: Legacy of Faith for the Black Church." *Religious Education* 81:93–112.

Oduyoye, Modupe. 1971. *The Vocabulary of Yoruba Religious Discourse*. Ibandan, Nigeria: Daystar Press.

Raboteau, Albert. 1980. *Slave Religion: The "Invisible Institution" in the Antebellum South.* Oxford: Oxford University Press.

Snow, Loudell. 1977. "Popular Medicine in a Black Neighborhood," in *Ethnic Medicine in the Southwest.* ed. Edward H. Spicer. Tucson: University of Arizona Press.

Sojourner, Sabrina. 1982. "From the House of Yemanja: The Goddess Heritage of Black Women," in *The Politics of Womens' Spirituality.* ed. Charlene Spretnak. New York: Doubleday.

Washington, Joseph R., Jr. 1964. *Black Religion: The Negro and Christianity in the United States.* Preface by Martin E. Marty. Boston: Beacon Press.

Perceptions of Discrimination, Psycho-social Functioning, and Physical Symptoms of African-American Women

CAROL M. CUMMINGS, ADRIENNE M. ROBINSON, AND GRETCHEN E. LOPEZ

...For above all, in behalf of the ailing world which sorely needs our defiance, may we as Negroes or women, never accept the notions of our place.

—Lorraine Hansberry

Introduction

The purpose of this essay is to contribute to the understanding that health problems often are endemic to the life experiences of a people. This paper is not meant to be a comprehensive review of the literature on psychosomatic research. Instead we emphasize what we have learned from earlier research on individual reactions and responses (physical and emotional) to conditions of psychological and political oppression. We also attempt to draw connections between the political, social, and economic contexts of black women's lives and "dis-ease" states. This paper aims to promote an integrated understanding of the life and health experiences of African-American females. It is argued that the health status of African-American women is a function of the unique life experiences known by that group as a whole. We hypothesize that the relationship between the quality of life and health problems is mediated by psychological distress, anger, depression, and undeveloped political consciousness. Our analysis implies that the remedy for these conditions is embedded in women's raised consciousness and their movement toward social change.

Current Perspectives

The health of women, especially African-American women, is rarely studied in traditional medical and psychological literature. The few investigations concerned with women often focus on reporting health statistics (Verbrugge 1985), but they do not investigate the causes of health problems. In 1989 psychologists Michelle Fine and S. M. Gordon reviewed and critiqued mainstream psychological research. They argue that to do adequate research on women and women's issues within psychology necessitates that researchers *not* obscure women's data by comparing them to men's data. Such comparisons are inadequate to explain women's lives in their own context. Furthermore, a prominent sociologist notes that black women are rarely if ever studied as a social entity in and of themselves. The typical practice has subsumed the study of black women into research on male-female differences or black-white differences (Allen 1981). This omission persists despite research findings demonstrating that certain forms of oppression have greater effects on specific social groups experiencing additional oppression. For example, social scientists R. C. Kessler and H. W. Neighbors (1986) found low income to be a greater factor in psychological distress for blacks than for whites. This was explained as the "synergistic effects of both poverty and discrimination in heightening subjective distress." Since black women typically experience the effects of poverty, in addition to race and gender discrimination, it is critical that we recognize the unique consequences of this triple oppression in terms of their mental and physical well-being. As Fine and Gordon point out, it is necessary for researchers to understand that gender relations are shaped by different power inequalities and that gender always braids with social class, race/ethnicity, age, disability, and sexual orientation.

Some investigators focusing on issues of race and gender emphasize that social groups must be understood within their own social, economic, and political contexts. For example, scholars have pointed to the need for black women's own interpretations of their experiences and theories which "explicitly incorporate ethnic and gender identities as a unity" (McComb 1988; Allen 1981). H. G. McComb's work takes a strong position: alleviating the psychological distress in black women's lives must involve continuous discovering who "we" are without the hindrance of mainstream assumptions or "telling them what they are." McComb argues that effectively aiding African-American women with psychotherapy means understanding and appreciating the internal psychological constructions of African-American womanhood. Research which lacks this perspective is less likely to discover and utilize key interventions, including strong community ties, extended family networks, and reliance on other black women (Stack 1970).

Psycho-social Conditions of Black Women

Black women encounter a number of mental and physical problems as a consequence of their racial, historical, cultural, and structural positions in American society. A report by A. E. Headen and S. W. Headen shows black women head over 53 percent of all black households. In 1981 the median income of female-headed black families was $7,506 yearly. In those families where the female head of household worked full-time and year-round, annual income was $13,380. In married black households where both partners were in the paid labor force, the median income was only $25,040 (Headen and Headen 1985). As we approach the twenty-first century, it is clear that economic conditions are not changing for the better. Poverty is increasing among women and children—a phenomenon that has been termed the "feminization of poverty"—and poor families are disproportionately headed by women of color. The lack of economic resources among black women is expected to play a large role in their psycho-social functioning. Given the hardships faced by this group, it can be expected that psychological distress will contribute to health problems.

African-American women have always had to work in the public sphere as well as the domestic (Belgrave 1988). Multiple oppression (primarily on the bases of race, class, and gender) has pushed black women to take jobs with the lowest wages, longer hours, little or no autonomy, minimal or no benefits (such as insurance or vacations), and no authority over other workers (Chappell 1980; Allen 1983). Work historian Sharlene Biber-Hesse (1982) argues that multiple oppression places many black women in difficult (labor intensive), stressful, and boring jobs. Choice is a non-factor in accepting such work, since more than half of black families are headed by single women who are the sole breadwinners. Research has demonstrated that such jobs contribute to women's felt level of "distress." This problem is compounded as women (more so than men) perceive their jobs as making competing demands on already over-taxed personal resources (Lowe and Northcott 1988). This picture of social and economic hardship becomes even more dreary when the focus turns to women of color who also face language barriers, disability, and old age (Allen 1981; Harel 1986; Taylor et al. 1982).

In general women of color are more likely to be undereducated, underpaid, underemployed, divorced, separated, and in poor physical health than any other social group in the United States. For unemployed women, government social welfare assistance barely permits survival. Indeed, it presents barriers to social mobility by prohibiting full-time employment, continued education, and marriage/cohabitation. The traumatic economic conditions suffered by the majority of black women have a full-blown impact on their mental and physical health. As pointed out by social commentator Felix Greene (1972), their stressful living conditions can be likened to those of a colonized people within an imperialist nation. Black women are denied access to resources and power through a social system of race discrimination that also exploits their labor.

Black Women's Health Concerns

The disadvantages associated with being black, poor, and deprived of vital resources not only impair social mobility. They also contribute generously to "excess deaths" among black Americans (D. H. H. S. 1984). The term refers to the number of deaths in a population that would be expected (the normal amount); in the United States the "normal amount" is based upon the white population's death rate. Blacks' excess deaths are the number of deaths disproportionately over and above white deaths. Political scholars and commentators have equated these conditions with "genocide"—motivated by political and cultural imperialism favoring white, Western, rational, Protestant patriarchy (Marable 1983; Davis 1983). Thus genocide—the deliberate destruction of a racial, political, or cultural group—is a direct result of black women's and black people's status as exploitable internal colonies.

According to Byllye Avery, director of the Black Women's Health Project in Atlanta, Georgia, one manifestation of genocide is violence: the principal health problem of African-American women. Violence has multiple meanings and takes on various forms. It has shaped the history of African Americans since the institution of slavery began. Violence has robbed the black woman of her "generations," which she bore only to have them torn from her and sold into slavery. It necessitated her submission to sexual abuse and beatings at the hands of slave masters. It kept black families economically unstable and dependent upon the "good will" of a morally bankrupt government and employment system. Historically and currently violence takes the form of undernutrition, inadequate clothing, homelessness and overcrowding, and restrictive social welfare policy. Violence also shapes black women's social relations both inside and outside their own households, involving other family members and acquaintances. This causes feelings of alienation and marginality among black women, making responses to treatment or therapy more difficult. At a recent conference (February 1990), Avery stated that 80–90 percent of black women participants in self-help groups reported recent experience of physical or psychological abuse within their own homes (Nursing Conference, Ann Arbor, University of Michigan 1990). Additionally, black women become victims of violence at the hands of authorities and legal systems which refuse protection to women of color from domestic violence, incest, rape, sexual harassment, gender and race discrimination, lynching, and police brutality. Not surprisingly, studies show that high levels of fear exist among U. S. females, who dread rape and other crimes common for city dwellers. Finally, women's studies literature is replete with examples of women's restricted opportunities to define their own lives, because of fear of victimization (Gordon et al. 1980). For example, in Alice Walker's 1982 novel *The Color Purple*, the main character, Celie, is threatened with physical abuse by her husband when she attempts to make friends, write or receive letters from her sister, and start her own business.

Health statistics and reports show that black women, most of whom have low incomes, suffer inordinately from malnutrition, psycho-social deprivation, hypertension (Willie et al. 1973), and a myriad of other illnesses. Research on alcoholism—a growing problem in black communities—shows the death rate for women of color and white women from cirrhosis of the liver has increased significantly in a twenty-five year period (1950–75): 36 percent for whites and 162 percent for women of color! Alcoholism is associated with violence, accidents, and child abuse, and is also a symptom of stress occurring among blacks. Social scientists Rudov and Santangelo (1978) argue that the higher incidence of cirrhosis among women of color could be due to nutritional deficiencies rather than to patterns of alcohol consumption. Since black women have poorer health and nutrition, as well as more stress from the outset, they are more susceptible to cirrhosis of the liver when they do drink.

Chemical dependence on such drugs as heroin, ICE, and crack-cocaine among black women has become a pernicious factor in the maintenance of good health. Besides the direct negative impacts of drug use on individual women's minds and bodies, there are also consequences for future generations of African Americans. Recent reports show that the use of such drugs as crack-cocaine is often related to other behaviors, contributing to the spreading of the illness across the population and through generations. Crack and heroin users become addicts, for example, and then are compelled to engage in sexual promiscuity in order to have continued access to the drug. This behavior contributes to prostitution and places women at high risk for AIDS and other sexually transmitted diseases. Moreover, children born to these women are likely to suffer both physical and mental retardation through AIDS or drug addiction at birth. In birth- and pregnancy-related problems, women of color experience a higher incidence of complications and maternal deaths. Rates of infant and maternal death among people of color in the United States are higher than in many developing countries. And the number of low-birth-weight babies (those weighing less than five pounds at birth) is increasing in spite of a decrease in the incidence of black teen pregnancies. Social scientist Charlotte Muller points out that as health care consumers, women of color will continue to have special problems because they face especially restricted economic opportunities and lack of insurance coverage, as well as political blocks to such services as abortion (Muller 1986).

Finally, the combined effects of such factors as stress, white oppression, loneliness, alienation, and frustration form what social scientist Elsie Smith has called the "syndrome for suicide death." According to Smith, both suicide and alcoholism may reflect the "social depression" of black women. She claims that the psychological cost of their "abject resourcelessness" is a profound social depression characterized by a sense of powerlessness, self-doubt, and hopelessness (Smith 1981). We contend that social depression leads to a failure to thrive which manifests in disease and ill health.

Black Mental Health and Psychological Distress

There is a direct correlation between poverty, increased morbidity, and early mortality. There continues to be a significant disparity in morbidity and mortality between African Americans and whites (Jones 1986). According to the National Center for Health Statistics (D. H. H. S. 1984), the risk of dying is 50 percent greater for blacks than whites in infancy or from heart disease, stroke, cancer, homicide, accidents, cirrhosis, or diabetes. Lower-income blacks are also at greater risk for hypertension than are higher-income blacks and whites. Blacks are also more likely to reside in crowded environments with higher crime rates (Fleming et al. 1987).

Psychosomatic Influences: A Review of the Literature

In 1987 a review of the medical literature on psychological distress and immune deficiencies showed that immune dysfunction is the underlying cause of ill health and that the notion of psychological states fostering illness is "as old as medicine" (Baker 1987). Evidence for this relationship is scattered throughout medical literature on psychosomatic disease. For example, longitudinal studies show that "depressed" male workers in a Cleveland factory showed twice the number of expected deaths from cancer in a seventeen-year follow-up study. This relationship superseded the respondent's age, smoking or drinking behavior, occupation, and family history of cancer (Shekelle et al. 1981). Similarly, among women awaiting the results of breast biopsies, those who rarely expressed anger were found to have malignancies more often than women who manifested their fears and resentment (Greer and Morris 1975). Among those giving three-month follow-up interviews, 80 percent of those who expressed feelings of hopelessness died within five years. This is in marked contrast to a 10 percent mortality rate among those who expressed denial or a "fighting spirit" (Greer et al. 1979). Although these studies do not specifically address the experiences of oppressed groups, they do present evidence that emotions, environmental stresses, and the impacts of life-events do affect the functioning of the immune system; they play a role in illness from onset to outcome. Furthermore, "there may . . . be a general pattern in which acute stimulating stress alerts the immune system whereas chronic, frustrating stress ultimately impairs it" (Baker 1987, 2).

In some studies African Americans experienced a sharp rise in blood pressure in response to anger- and anxiety-provoking laboratory experiments (Anderson 1989; Light 1981). These studies generally used male subjects, and thus the meaning of the findings for females is unclear. Such research relies heavily on the development of such personality assessment tools as "Type A"—which is characterized as hostile, rushed demeanor, and self-engendered behaviors—and "John Henryism"—which is unrelenting perseverance toward goals in the face of tremendous obstacles (Friedman et al. 1987; James et al. 1984). These researchers studied such personality factors as hostility, anger expression, socio-ecological stress, and anger-coping styles (Harburg et al. 1973; Johnson et al. 1987). With the possible exception of Type A, these kinds of measures are important precursors of cardiovascular responses, disease, and mortality, even more so for blacks than for whites.

Research including black women subjects reveals important gender and racial differences. Psychologist Norman Anderson (1987) reports that blood pressure elevations among black and white women with a parental history of hypertension show black women slower to recover normal blood pressure levels following a stressful situation in the laboratory. Black subjects showed greater rise in blood pressure during a stressful mathematics task. They also showed greater anxiety, guilt, fear, and restlessness and decreased alertness, happiness, and relaxation. These observations are compounded by considerable evidence showing that women experience anger chronically, and at high levels, and this may be due to treatment perceived as unjust (Johnson et al. 1987; James et al. 1984). Other studies show that in general people's physical symptoms are exacerbated by their reluctance to discuss personal problems (Cumes-Rayner 1989). These findings combine to paint a potentially grim picture of black women's mental and emotional well-being.

The Survey Instrument and Method

The Stress and Health Survey for Women of Color is an instrument designed to assess emotional and physical health and political thinking among women of color. All respondents attended the Women of Color Conference at the University of Michigan in the spring of 1989. The questionnaire was constructed to survey their quality of life. Thus relationships with family, friends, and co-workers, complex roles in everyday life, and emotional responses to negative situations within those roles were targeted. The questionnaire also measured emotional intensity in an important life role, identification with social groups, and trait anger (general tendency to experience anger). Negative coping responses to stress through cigarette and alcohol use were also examined.

One hundred and eight respondents were surveyed. They were asked to identify their own ethnicity. The sample consisted of African-American women (N=76), Latinas (N=4), Asian-American (N=2) and Anglo-American (N=13) females, and one Greek woman. Ten persons did not identify themselves ethnically. We analyzed the data from the 76 black respondents only. Most had achieved some college education (60 percent). The remainder had earned a college degree or more. The majority of our sample (69.7 percent) did not consider themselves feminists, although 65 percent of the sample did identify with women as a social group. The average income ranged from $12,000 to $24,000 per year. The majority of family incomes ranged from $19,000 to $44,000 annually.

Most respondents were between twenty-seven and forty-two years of age. About 45 percent were married, 22 percent divorced, 27 percent never-married, 8 percent separated, and 2 percent widowed. Most (78 percent) had at least one child, and the mean number of children was 2.21. The average household size was two persons, including the respondent. Thirty-eight percent of the sample lived alone. Most respondents had at least one other person in the household dependent on them for financial and emotional support.

Measures

Six scales were used to measure psycho-social functioning. Those included the Trait Anger subscale of the State-Trait Anger/Anxiety Scale; Rosenberg Self-Esteem measure; Problematic Life Circumstances Scale (PLC); Emotional Intensity Scale (EI); and a Group Identification measure (GI). The four latter scales were constructed for the purpose of assessing psycho-social functioning, which is defined as the willingness to feel and demonstrate emotions and actions taken in the interest of self-improvement.

The PLC scale asked all respondents to rate the degree of difficulty in the circumstances and relationships in their daily lives. The scale ranged from 1 (hardly any problems) to 5 (many problems). They assessed relationships with co-workers, family members, children, and friends; finances; satisfying emotional needs; work efficiency on the job and at home; and ability to express feelings in general and anger in particular.

The emotional intensity scale (EI) assessed emotional intensity "when things go wrong" in an important life role. Respondents listed five important life roles. Within their two most important roles they reported the level of emotional intensity they experienced when things went wrong in that role. The EI scale ranged from 1 (I feel fine) to 5 (extremely upset; emotional; angry; scared/confused). Two separate intensity scale ratings were utilized.

The group identification (GI) scale measured the degree to which respondents believed their lives were affected by what happens to various other social groups, including women, men, blacks, Latinos, Asian Americans,

American Indians, whites, middle-class, working-class, women of color, and Third World women. This measure assessed the degree to which respondents feel consciously connected to other groups. We hypothesized that high scores on GI indicate awareness of other groups' circumstances being similar to one's own and affecting one's fate. High scores may also indicate greater self-efficacy and less hopelessness because of the sense of feeling solidarity with others.

Results

Three hypotheses were tested. First, perceived gender or race discrimination (or both) is a source of psychological distress exacerbating health problems. Second, measures of psycho-social functioning are related to the number of health problems, that is, poor functioning indicates more health problems. The third hypothesis measures relationships among the psychosocial scales and responses such as depression, abuse, high blood pressure, and health problems in general. Age and perception of discrimination are also factored in as variables.

In testing the first hypothesis, correlations among measures of perceived discrimination showed that respondents reporting gender discrimination in their workplace identified more with blacks as a social group, had more problems with co-workers and finances, and felt that people at work made contradictory demands on them. The perception of both gender and race discrimination was correlated with drinking less alcohol but also with having higher systolic blood pressure (see Table 1). Similarly, respondents perceiving race discrimination at work identified with blacks as a social group, had problems with co-workers and finances, and experienced contradictory demands at work. They also reported feeling less satisfied with themselves, had higher systolic blood pressures, and drank more alcohol. Those reporting gender discrimination also reported more vaginal infections, aching joints, and "trouble breathing" in the past twelve months. Difficulty in breathing is also associated with perceived race discrimination. These relationships indicate that women of color experiencing either race or gender discrimination are likely to experience both types of prejudice. Perceiving oneself as discriminated against is associated with identifying with other oppressed groups. This perception is linked to coping behaviors and health complaints.

In testing the second hypothesis, respondents', scores on psychosocial scales were assessed and correlated with their total health problems (see Tables 1 and 2). Respondents' health problems showed significant relationships with the PLC scale scores. Thus the more problematic routine life-events, interpersonal relations, and finances, the greater the number of health problems. Those respondents who reported being emotionally abused in the past year also reported more health problems. Also, having intense feelings "when things go wrong" in an important life role increased one's health problems. Finally, respondents who identified less with social groups (GI) reported more health problems.

To test the third hypothesis we evaluated correlations among psycho-social scales measuring depression, abuse, high blood pressure, and other health problems, as well as age and perceived discrimination. Results showed that experiencing depression and emotional abuse within the year is related to higher Trait Anger scores. This finding complements the literature on depression which links anger with psycho-social stress. Being older (forty-one to fifty-seven years of age in this predominantly young sample) yielded

Table 1

Measures of Association Between Variables
(Correlations)

Variable Name	Correlation	Probability (*) less than .05
PERCEPTION OF DISCRIMINATION		
Gender * Race	.692	*
Systolic Blood Pressure	.350	*
Drink Beer	−.278	*
Problems with Co-workers	.286	*
Problems with Finances	.309	*
Contradictory Demands	.416	*
Gender Discrimination Personal	.441	*
Race Discrimination Personal	.396	*
PERCEPTION OF DISCRIMINATION		
Race * ID with Blacks	.307	*
Systolic Blood Pressure	.466	*
Drink Beer	.324	*
Frequently "things go wrong"	.268	*
Problems with Finances	.269	*
Problems with Co-workers	.328	*
Contradictory Demands	.295	*
Gender Discrimination Personal	.269	*
Race Discrimination Personal	.573	*
GENDER AND RACE DISCRIMINATION ON HEALTH PROBLEMS		
Gender * Vaginal Infections	.191	*
Aching Joints	.255	*
Trouble Breathing	.216	*
Race * Trouble Breathing	.232	*

higher self-esteem, but greater depression, higher blood pressure, and more frequent reporting of discrimination at work. This finding complements the literature on aging and indicates that life experiences for women of color too often result in acceptance of a harsh reality and chronic physical disability (see Table 3).

Discussion

The data support our hypotheses. Black women who report gender and race discrimination at the workplace are more likely to experience decreased psycho-social functioning in terms of depression and anger. Depression impacts psychosocial functioning through the experience of anger which may be inappropriately expressed. It is also related to problematic life circumstances, emotional intensity, and middle age, which can encompass a certain weariness and resignation to harsh daily circumstances. These findings indicate that financial and interpersonal difficulties experienced by women of color contribute to feelings of anger and depression. These, in turn, impede their willingness and ability to cope with life's stresses.

The data also contribute to understanding the complexities of black women's health experiences. Those reporting gender discrimination identified with a wide spectrum of social groups. Respondents who answered

Table 2

Analysis of Variance

Perception of Discrimination on Total Number of Health Problems

Gender Discrimination (all responses—"yes or no" on Health Problems Significant)	
Variable Name	Probability level
Financial Problems	.000
Emotional Abuse	.000
Emotional Intensity Scale 1	.040
Gender Discrimination "yes"	
Less Identification with Social Groups	.040
Race Discrimination (all responses—"yes or no" on Health Problems)	
Financial Problems	.000
Emotional Abuse	.000
Emotional Intensity Scale 1	.11 (marginal)
Race Discrimination "no"	
Less Identification with Social Groups	.042

"Yes" to gender or race discrimination at work but identifed with few social groups had experienced a greater number of health problems in the past year. This implies that identification with other social groups is one of the keys to promoting mental and physical well-being among women of color. In other words, consciousness of commonalities and similarities (common ground) among social groups and their experiences helps women cope with their daily "multiple oppression." Raised awareness might ideally promote group action and social change ameliorating life circumstances for women of color.

We must be realistic and not underestimate the powerfully stressful contexts of our lives. The cumulative effects of stressful life events such as poverty, unemployment, divorce, physical and psychological abuse, and other forms of violence profoundly impact black women in the United States. This is often ignored. Efforts aimed at preventing mental and physical illness in black populations that are often caused by traumatic living conditions too frequently overlook these primary contextual realities. We contend that revolutionary changes are necessary in the larger social and economic institutions which effectively disadvantage women of color. This perspective is not new, but it is consistent with protest philosophy of the 1960s and 1970s. We echo the basic notions of that era: African-American women are reproducers of a social order which necessitates their subordination and exploitation. It is therefore imperative that black women and other women of color become more active and more socially conscious in order to replace a passive and

Table 3

Analysis of Variance
N=76

Independent Variables	Psychosocial Functioning and Age	
Depression	Trait Anger	P = .000
Emotional Abuse	Trait Anger	.070
Age Group (older age)	Self-Esteem	.090
Health Problems	Problem Scale (PLC)	.080
Depression	Problem Scale (PLC)	.020
Depression	Emotional Intensity 1	.010
Emotional Intensity 1	Emotional Intensity 2	.020
Depression	ID with Social Groups	.083
Perception of Gender Discrimination	ID with Social Groups	.054
Depression	Age Group	.013
Perception of Race Discrimination	Age Group	.014
High Blood Pressure	Age Group	.011

seemingly apathetic health service system. A new health movement designed to increase their empowerment and health is the necessary "first step" toward social parity.

Works Cited

Allen, W. 1981. "The Social and Economic Statuses of Black Women in the United States." *Phylon* 42 (1): 26–40.

"Hypertension Detection and Follow-up Program Cooperative Group: Race, Education and Prevalence of Hypertension." 1977. *American Journal of Epidemiology* 106: 351–61.

Anderson, N. B., 1989. "Racial Differences in Stress-induced Cardiovascular Reactivity and Hypertension: Current Status and Substantive Issues." *Psychological Bulletin* 105: 89–105.

———, R. B. Williams, et al. 1987. "Parental History of Hypertension and Cardiovascular Responses in Young Black Women." *Journal of Psychosomatic Research* 31: 723–29.

Baker, G. H. B. 1987. "Psychological Factors in Immunity." *Journal of Psychosomatic Research* 31: 1–10.

Belgrave, L. L. 1988. "The Effects of Race Differences in Work History, Work Attitudes, Economic Resources, and Health on Women's Retirement." *Research on Aging* 10 (3): 383–98.

Biber-Hesse, Sharlene. 1986. "The Black Woman Worker: A Minority Group's Perspective on Women at Work." *Sage* 3 (1): 26–34.

Chappell, N. L., and B. J. Havens. 1980. "Old and Female: Testing the Double Jeopardy Hypothesis." *Sociological Quarterly* 21 (2): 157–71.

Cumes-Rayner, D. P. and J. Price. 1989. "Understanding Hypertensive Behavior—I. Preference Not to Disclose." *Journal of Psychosomatic Research* 33: 63–74.

Davis, Angela. 1983. *Women, Race and Class.* New York: Vintage Books.

Department of Health and Human Services (DHHS) 1984. *Report of the Secretary's Task Force on Black and Minority Health.* Volume I Executive Summary.

Fine, M., and S. M. Gordon. 1989. "Feminist Transformations of /Despite Psychology." In M. Crawford and M. Gentry. *Gender and Thought: Psychological Perspectives.* New York: Springer-Verlag. 146–74.

Fleming, I., A. Baum, L. M. Davidson, E. Rectanus, and E. McArdle. 1987. "Chronic Stress as a Factor in Psychological Reactivity to Challenge." *Health Psychology* 6: 221–38.

Friedman, H. S., and S. Booth-Kewley. 1987. "Personality, Type A Behavior, and Coronary Heart Disease: The Role of Emotional Expression." *Journal of Personality and Social Psychology* 53 (4): 783–92.

Gordon, M. T., S. Riger, R. K. LeBailly, and L. Heath. 1980. "Crime, Women, and the Quality of Urban Life." *Signs* 5 (3): 144–60.

Greene, F., 1972. "But We Are Not Imperialists!" In *The Enemy.* New York: Harper and Row.

Greer, H. S. and T. Morris. 1975. "Psychological Attributes of Women who Develop Breast Cancer." *Journal of Psychosomatic Research* 19: 147–53.

Greer, S., T. Morris, K. W. Pettingale. 1979. "Psychological Response to Breast Cancer: Effect on Outcome." *Lancet* ii: 785–87.

Harburg, E., J. Erfurt, L. Hauenstein, C. Chape, W. Schull, and M. Schork. 1973. "Socioecological Stress, Suppressed Hostility, Skin Color, and Black-White Blood Pressure: Detroit." *Journal of Chronic Diseases* 26: 595–611.

Harel, Z. 1986. "Older Americans Act–Related Homebound Aged: What Difference Does Racial Background Make?" *Journal of Gerontological Social Work* 9 (4): 133–43.

———, M. Jackson, G. Deimling, and L. Noelker. 1983. "Racial Differences in Well-Being among Aged and Disabled Public Housing Residents." *Journal of Housing for the Elderly* 1 (1): 45–62.

Headen, A. E., and S. W. Headen. 1985. "General Health Conditions and Medical Insurance Issues Concerning Black Women." *Review of Black Political Economy* 14: 183–98.

James, S., A. Z. LaCroix, D. G. Kleinbaum, and D. S. Strogatz. 1984. "John Henryism and Blood Pressure Differences among Black Men: II. The Role of Occupational Stressors." *Journal of Behavioral Medicine* 7: 259–75.

Johnson, E. H., N. J. Schork, and C. D. Spielberger. 1987. "Emotional and Familial Determinants of Elevated Blood Pressure in Black and White Adolescent Females." *Journal of Psychosomatic Research* 31: 731–41.

Jones, E. I. 1986. "Preventing Disease and Promoting Health in the Minority Community." *Journal of the National Medical Association* 78: 18–24.

Kessler, R. C., and H. W. Neighbors. 1986. "A New Perspective on the Relationships among Race, Social Class, and Psychological Distress." *Journal of Health and Social Behavior* 27: 107–15.

Light, K. C. 1981. "Cardiovascular Responses to Effortful Active Coping: Implications for the Role of Stress in Hypertension Development." *Psychophysiology* 18 (3): 216–25.

Lowe, G. S., and H. C. Northcott. 1988. "The Impact of Working Conditions, Social Roles, and Personal Characteristics on Gender Differences in Distress." *Work and Occupations* 15 (1): 55–77.

Marable, Manning. 1983. *How Capitalism Underdeveloped Black America*. Boston: South End Press.

McComb, H. G. 1986. "The Application of an Individual/Collective Model to the Psychology of Black Women." *Women and Therapy* 5: 67–80.

Muller, Charlotte. 1986. "Health and Health Care of Employed Women and Home-makers: Family Factors." *Women and Health* 11(1): 7–45.

Rudov and Santangelo. 1978. "Health Status of Minorities and Low-Income Groups." *DHEW Publication (HRA) 79-627*. U. S. Department of Health, Education, and Welfare, Office of Health Resources Opportunity.

Shekelle, R. B., W. J. Raynor, A. M. Ostfeld, D. C. Garron, et al. 1981. "Psychological Depression and 17-year Risk of Death from Cancer." *Psychosomatic Medicine* 43: 117–25.

Smith, Elsie. 1981. "Mental Health and Service Delivery Systems for Black Women." *Journal of Black Studies* 12 (2): 126–41.

Stack, Carol. 1970. *All Our Kin*. New York: Harper and Row.

Taylor, R. J., J. S. Jackson, and A. D. Quick. 1982. "The Frequency of Social Support among Black Americans: Preliminary Finding from the National Survey of Black Americans." *Urban Research Review* 8: 1–4.

Verbrugge, Lois M. 1985. "Gender and Health: An Update on Hypotheses and Evidence." *Journal of Health and Social Behavior* 26: 156–82.

Willie, C. V. 1974. "The Black Family and Social Class." *American Journal of Orthopsychiatry* 44: 50–60.

Older Women of the Project: The Socio-medical Consequences of Urban Change

LINDA DUMAS

Well, I count each day. I don't let my mind—my mind doesn't really focus on what it will be like when I get real old. Maybe I don't think like everybody, but I count each day. Take each day at a time. Yes, I do. See I been used to, as I say, bein' the man and the lady in the house, so I never had time to think about when I can't do anymore.

—Woman of the Project

Introduction

This essay is about older women and the socio-medical consequences of community disruption. They are the women of what was a notoriously violent, poverty-ridden Boston housing project built in the 1950s and redeveloped in 1988. It is their story, a story that integrates perspectives about their health, their coping in face of gentrification, and their inner strength that through the years has carried them through many different dimensions. They are survivors. They were survivors at thirty years old; they remain survivors at eighty. In their conversations, basic themes emerge concerning "a good life that changed."

In 1985 I went into the housing project to begin a longitudinal study on the elderly minority men and women who lived there. It was to be a chronicle of their socio-medical status as they entered what was for most of them the most significant social change in their lives, the gentrification of their community and the loss of what was the familiar context of "home." In March 1988 the first of forty-seven very low-income, primarily black, older men and women moved from their homes in the project to their new home, "the senior building" in the redeveloped community.

My work is a chronicle of their story, an intensive case study of how they felt, what they saw around them, and the status of their health over time. Its value will not rest with the objectivity of the data. Rather, the richness of the data and the ethnographic detail about the lives of these older people will be complemented by data about their health, social, functional, and psychological status. The picture will be a multidimensional one. It will begin with a snapshot and will conclude as an album, a chronicle of lives over times of change. The data are, and will continue to be, testimony to their personal strength and to their potential for adaptation when continuity and social order are disrupted by events over which they had little or no control.

As the project of the 1950s moves through the transitional process to a luxurious apartment complex of the 1990s, developers and residents alike hope it will become a symbol of community in the next decade. If it works, it will symbolize racial and economic integration by showing that the poor and the well-to-do can live side by side. If it works, many urban developers and the Boston Housing Authority feel that the problems of the ghetto and its underclass are on the way to resolution. Others feel that it cannot work and that the new development is doomed to failure as a band-aid approach to the underlying problem of structural inequality.

Women were an integral piece of the project's history. Mary Kennedy, an historian, writes of the earliest history of the project during the mid-fifties, and she argues cogently against the commonly held assumption that the project was a symbol of a nationwide public housing policy that failed. Public housing was set up to fail, and public housing should not be laid to rest as private developers set out to renovate the slums and ghettoes of the nation. She writes that if it were not for the women, there would be no community today. History has ignored the power of the women in public housing and has blamed them, rather than the housing authority, for its decline (Kennedy et al. 1987). It was a community made by women and sustained by women through the worst of social times, the sixties and seventies.

The earliest tenants of this public housing project, black and white women, set out to achieve what was denied to them. They gained bus service to the isolated peninsula, a church, and a school. The community was built through the tireless efforts of the Mothers' association, a group of women activists who wanted better lives for their children (op cit. 12). It was not a community that failed; it was a community that survived against the greatest odds.

Poverty in Old Age

Poverty in old age is increasingly concentrated among black women living alone. "A stunning 68 percent of black women living alone subsists on less than $2,000 annually, the figure for males is only slightly lower, 57.4 percent" (Manning 1975, 105).

The aging of our population is among one of the most significant demographic trends in this century. According to the U. S. Census, there are 6.8 million people over the age of sixty-five. In the twenty-first century, one in eight Americans will be over age sixty-four (McKinlay and Tennstedt 1986).

This phenomenon of extended old age raises serious concerns. First, what will be the quality of life for the elderly? As people live longer, not all will lead quality lives. Many more will live in poverty and poor health, as additional years are spent in chronic illness and disability. Women will make up the dominant proportion of this group. For aged minority men and women, the picture for the twenty-first century is bleak. For women it is even more depressing. Many women have combined non-paid labor in the home with lifetimes of under-employment in the paid work force. Low-paying jobs or jobs without benefits have primed them for poverty in old age.

> And did you work after you came here?
>
> Oh yes I did. I worked in . . . for four years when I first came here.
>
> What kind of work?
>
> A linen service. I didn't, you know, have the education to do no office work so I did that for four years . . . machines, pressin' and foldin'. Yes, I worked there for four years when I first came here. I wasn't able to do too much after I had those special girls because I had to be home.

Today, in her sixties, this woman continues to care for her two severely retarded adult daughters, "those special girls." And another woman, who cares for an autistic grandchild: "I'm satisfied with my life 'cause I worked hard in my life. An so, what I'm doin now, I appreciate it because this is nothing. . . . I worked hard. I worked in the laundry, Chinese laundry. I worked in the fields. I worked in the tobacco, and I always worked hard. . . . I picked cotton. Shucked peanuts. Potatoes on the ground."

Jacquelyne Jackson (1971, 1975, 1978, 1980), a social gerontologist with expertise on black older women, points out that minorities should be studied in light of their multicultural and racial distinctions, between each other as well as between themselves and whites. She argues that ethnicity and race are most likely mediating factors in the problems of aging and health, but the data are scarce and theories about minority elders remain underdeveloped.

Jackson makes a salient point: intra- and interracial differences should be examined as well as intraracial gender distinctions. In general, my data

(Dumas 1985, 1988–1989) have illustrated that minorities share in the general national profiles of mortality and morbidity patterns, but they experience the problems inherent in these patterns disproportionately from their white counterparts. The mediating factors include life styles, stressors, socioeconomic deprivation, racism, and such cultural factors as nutritional practices. However, it should be emphasized again that data on minority elders are scarce, and in most cases black and Hispanic elders are not isolated from general findings on larger elderly groups.

Socio-medical and Ethnographic
Aspects of Aging: Forced Relocation

The concepts basic to this longitudinal study are the problem of poverty in old age, the problem of gentrification, and the problem of community loss. All the socio-medical data collected will reflect changes in the older cohort over a ten-year period (1986–96).

Since the 1970s, literature has developed addressing the problems imposed on low-income, urban minority elders by gentrification, redevelopment, and forced relocations. Researchers point to the deleterious effects of displacement on the mortality and morbidity of the old (Henig 1981; Eckert and Haug 1984). The phenomenon of gentrification most often affects the most vulnerable of age groups, the elderly poor. Increasingly, the elderly poor are Hispanic and black women. They are the people most likely to occupy a neighborhood for many years, and thus they are the most likely targets of forced relocations when rents rise and the composition of the neighborhood changes.

Researchers have found that important variables in forced relocation of urban elderly are social networks, health status prior to relocation (Eckert and Haug 1984), and a sense of control over one's environment (Upshur et al. 1981). Further, we know that growing old in America is not the same for everyone and that lower-class blacks and ethnic minorities are at a distinct disadvantage compared to their middle-class, white counterparts (McNeely and Colen 1983).

This small cohort lacks representativeness, but this is compensated for by the depth of the ongoing inquiry. The study of individuals at home is fruitful because they are seen in interaction with their everyday environments rather than in the more commonly selected context, the clinical setting.

Some interesting gender distinctions emerged which relate primarily to family and caretaking. One-third of the women in the cohort have grandchildren or handicapped dependents to care for. Six of the women cared for retarded adult children. Many of the women, even at an older age, were still heads of families and fulfilled roles of primary caretaking for children or grandchildren. This is a theme that has been consistent over the years. As the women talk about their lives in the project, the number of references to dead children is striking.

The children of many of the elders either died as young adults from heart disease or stroke or died from violence. Several of the elders and many of the families had lives affected by violent death, homicide, and suicide. Life in the project was not, and is still not, easy. Each year young adults or people in their middle years succumb to crimes of violence, dying at the hands of others with guns or inadvertently by their own, with drugs. Premature death occurs with increasing frequency, and each year one or more elders is preceded in death by a son or daughter. One elder lost a thirty-year-old daughter to AIDS. Three years later, she cares for the grandchildren. The connectedness of these women and their families persists in the best and in the worst of times.

The Demographics of the Cohort

The demographic profile, thirty-two women and fifteen men, illustrates the predominance of women of color, predominantly black and Hispanic. There are three white women. The women in the senior building are widowed or separated and live alone. The older women who reside in the midst of the community live with families and are primary caretakers of children. Their language is English, income is below the poverty level, and only three have high school diplomas.

There is a health center not far from the community. Medical coverage for all is good, with Medicare and/or Medicaid supplement. Forty-two of the elders are literate and are able to read and write at a functional level. This is surprising considering their early years in the South and their limited education.

Ten percent of the cohort is eighty-one years and older. Fifty-five percent are in the young-old group, sixty-two to sixty-eight. The oldest is a Caucasian woman who is ninety-one.

Utilization behaviors are good, with a majority going for regular health care. Access is sometimes difficult, as the community sits on an isolated peninsula. The neighborhood health center remains in the new community. Many of the men and women have a dual utilization pattern, seeking health promotive care at the health center and specialty care in the city at the large teaching hospitals. This is unsurprising.

Health Outcomes: Have they Changed?

As expected, the health and psycho-social data for this work were inconclusive. The baseline years were 1986–87. The move occurred in early 1988, and the cohort will be revisited again in 1990. Health outcomes such as mental illness, alcoholism, depression, functional status, utilization behaviors, and mortality/morbidity profiles were not appreciably higher in the second year; nor did they differ significantly from national norms.

The following morbidity profile reflects rank by prevalence: heart disease, hypertension, diabetes, pulmonary diseases, and arthritis.

There are no distinctions between race or gender, but it is a small cohort. Cardiovascular diseases, angina, congestive heart failure, and the problem of diabetes rank high together, and poorly controlled hypertension is a significant problem—as it is nationally. Stroke related to cardiovascular disease, in particular hypertension, and cancer are other medical problems. Pulmonary problems relate to asthma and chronic obstructive lung disease.

Many elders are quite disabled by arthritis, and it is an underestimated problem. Significant problems in other areas relate to marginal nutritional status, poor dentition, and poor vision. These problems are not unique to minority elders, but they are seen with greater prevalence in lower socio-economic groups which have more people of color. In my opinion, it is class or socioeconomic status, rather than race, which differentiates the mortality and morbidity problems of older adults. Race in the United States, while a contributor to class status, is often treated as a proxy for class.

Oral health and vision are overlooked parameters of health and illness in older adults, and only now are people beginning to pay attention to relationships between frailty (functional status), marginal nutrition, and poor dentition.

Glaucoma, cataracts, and blindness from poorly controlled diabetes reinforce the need for promotive health teaching in a group milieu. It is, however, very difficult to change long-term behavioral patterns. When addressing vision that is irrevocably lost, functional status should be the focus for intervention, focusing on safety issues and assistive devices. Five of the elders, all women, were frail and homebound.

Mental illness, alcoholism, and depression were assessed, and there were no significant gender distinctions. Approximately 20 percent of the cohort was alcoholic, 20 percent exhibited depressive symptoms, and the number of perceived mental health problems was significant.

Self-rated health by women was fair to good, and their attitudes were reflected in their communication. It is difficult to make gender distinctions here, as most of the cohort are women. Four men have died since the study began. There are now only eleven men left in the cohort. Three women have died, leaving twenty-nine.

> Do you feel that your health has changed in the past two years? For the better or for the worse?

> Yes, it changed, gettin' older all the time, not getting any younger. I'm eighty-four years old.

Are you better than you were two years ago or worse?

No, I'm worse, cause I can't see.

How do you feel about your health?

Not too good.

In what way?

I have high blood pressure. I have the gout and I've got a lot of little problems. But other than that I get around.

And from T—

I always been a fighter. I fought back. All the things they told me I was fighting back. They said I wouldn't walk too much anymore, but I walk. I used to walk, if I could, a mile every day. I used to walk down to the bank which is a mile from here. I'd walk down there and I'd walk back here even though I had to sit on the curbstone and rest. I learned to get on the bus again, because I couldn't get up on it. I'd go out there and I'd see someone and the bus would come and I'd say "Give me a boost." So I'd pull myself up.

There was significant correlation between alcoholism, number of physical problems, and depression. Half of the alcoholics were depressed. And all had a high prevalence of diagnosed physical problems.

There were no significant correlations between alcoholism and living arrangement, and most of the alcoholics lived with family members. There was no significant correlation between alcoholism and gender. The interesting finding relates to social supports. With the exception of one alcoholic, all had a close or intimate friend, and each had children visiting at least weekly. They did not present with social isolation, and it may be that in communities where drinking has a high prevalence over time, alcoholism may be endemic.

Over half of the cohort said they had a "major life crisis" in the past year. The common reason noted was "fear of the future." Depression was much more of a problem in the second year follow-up and will be carefully evaluated in future data collection. Many felt that the stressors of moving and community change had taken a toll on their health.

I try not to let _____ worry me. I gotta live somewhere. I feel, well, if I can get in the senior citizens, they're going to put me somewhere. I'm not going to be in here, the old building. Wherever they put me and it's nice, I'll go along. I have to go along. I'm nervous at times. I let one thing stay on my mind. Change. I can't sleep. You know. And sometimes I worry 'bout, really worry 'bout; I'm losin' weight like this.

Social Supports

All but two of the older adults had daily contact with others, and all but ten got out of doors each day. Interestingly, thirty-six of the forty-seven older adults were satisfied with current housing. They liked where they lived. Those who were not satisfied tended to live with families in the larger community rather than in the senior buildings. The majority were seen by their children on a daily or regular basis; only one woman had not seen her son in thirty years.

The formal and informal supports were strong, in particular the informal supports located in the old community. Antipoverty agencies had been part of the community for twenty years, and one particular agency, run by the Sisters of Notre Dame, was especially supportive of the older adults. Gender differences were noted in the use of some of these agencies and services, with the women assuming a more active role. There were few activities on an everyday basis, and it is doubtful the women would socialize in activities which are structured for them.

Who do you depend on most here?

Well, for one thing we all love the Sisters. They go out of their way for to help you, out they way to pitch in for you. They go places, they take us places. It's beautiful. It's not right what they is doin' to the Sisters. The Sisters deserve to stay right where they are now. Because it's not fair toward them [that they were forced out] 'cause they loved a whole lot, especially by the older people . . . in general by all the people, but especially the older people, you know.

The women are close to the Sisters, and the Sisters are a significant informal support system that is being taken away. The developers have forced out the neighborhood supports and installed formal supports, such as a large, bureaucratic, elder services. Formal supports cannot and do not provide the warmth, the intimacy that informal supports such as family and friends bring to older people. Informal supports are meant to complement, not exclude one another.

In summary, this longitudinal study of a small group of very low-income, urban minority elders presents an opportunity to get to know the cohort and to chronicle the health and social changes occurring in their lives over time. This is an opportunity to fill in some of the literature gaps that exist in the study of minority, very poor, older adults from a housing project.

The health data are, for the most part, inconclusive. They present a profile of both men and women, but predominantly women, and will become more meaningful over time as they compare with national profiles. The data in these first few years serve as baselines and are unsurprising with respect to either the types of health problems, the prevalence of health problems, gender differences, or the emergence of new symptoms. I anticipate that 1990 will reflect some health changes. It will be interesting in time to compare this cohort to a counterpart cohort, the market-rate elder tenants who will be moving into the senior building, mostly higher-income, non-minority women.

What was more striking than the health data were the interviews. The interviews provided a rich account of their lives in the old project. The earlier, "good days" of the fifties did not last long. The most striking features of their accounts were the unexpected details of their suffering in the midst of the escalating community violence of the past few decades.

The women have not been asked for their opinions. They have not had much to say about the emergence of the new community or about the kinds of services they wanted. Their needs have been decided for them, and although some have vigorously "fought back," most have resigned themselves to a loss of the familiar. The older women do not, as a group, hold much power in their later years. The decades of social upheaval and violence in the project following the fifties diminished their energies, and the early anger has dissipated. The men have never spoken out, and this has not changed.

However, an important observation is reflected with certainty again and again: the juxtaposition of strength, integrity, and quiet courage with the powerlessness the older women have endured for much of their lives. Their power as women is a personal one; it is reflected in their perceptions of survival through the hardest of times. This time of social disruption and life change may prove to be just as important a life event.

Before concluding this essay on the women of the project, I would like to offer a few comments on the concepts of loss, change, and community disruption in the lives of the older adults.

The Problem of Community Loss

An important aim of the research was and continues to be the measurement of the impact of change on a group of older people who have lived for many years in what outsiders call a ghetto. This cohort calls it home.

Few sociologists have captured the essence of loss suffered from community destruction. Despite the fact that none of them has focused directly on older people, their work has relevance here. As Young and Wilmott (1957) put it: "Planners of redevelopment put faith in buildings, in brick and mortar. All that is necessary to community spirits, it is assumed, is a community center. There is more to community than that. A sense of connectedness, a sense of loyalty . . . connecting people of one house-hold to people of another" (198–99). Marc Fried (1963) wrote about the effects of post-relocation, loss reactions. He suggested that spatial identity and group identity are the critical components of continuity and that the loss of either or both may lead to severe grief: "Both are bases for a sense of ongoing, or sameness or connectedness. The feelings of being at home and of belonging to a place are integrally linked to a specific place. The sense of spatial identity is fundamental to human functioning" (156).

The important point is that community spirit or ethos represents human sharing. It is a sense of communality with other people. It is, quite simply, the knowledge that one is not alone. It is a rare person who can live without a presence of community. It means many things to different people. When one loses a home through displacement, one also loses a way of life. The social, cultural, and health consequences can be devastating.

Works Cited

Dumas, Linda. 1985. "Assessing the Home Care Needs of Columbia Point Older Adults." Community Service Fellowship, the Gerontology Institute, University of Massachusetts, Boston. Unpublished manuscript.

———. 1988. "Life on the Margin: An Intensive Care Study of Community Disruption and its Socio-medical Consequences on the Old." Ph.D. diss., Boston University.

———. 1989. "One year follow-up study on the Columbia Point Elders." Unpublished manuscript.

Eckert, J. Kevin and Ruth E. Dunkel. 1984. "Need for Services by the Elderly Experiencing Urban Change." *Gerontologist* 24(3): 257–60.

Eckert, J. Kevin and Marie Haug. 1984. "The Impact of Forced Residential Relocation on the Health of the Elderly Hotel Dweller." *Journal of Gerontology* 39(6):753–55.

Fried, Marc. 1963. "Grieving for a Lost Home." *The Urban Condition.* Leonard J. Duhl, ed. New York: Basic Books.

Henig, Jeffrey. 1981. "Gentrification and Displacement of the Elderly: An Empirical Analysis." *Gerontologist* 21(1): 67–75.

Jackson, Jacquelyne. 1971. "Negro Aged: Toward Needed Research in Social Gerontology." *Gerontologist* (Spring), Part II: 52–75.

———, ed. 1975. *Aging Black Women: Selected Readings for NCBA.* Washington D.C.: College and University Press.

———. 1980. *Minorities and Aging.* Belmont, California: Wadsworth.

———, and Bertram Walls. 1978. "Myths and Realities about Blacks." *Readings in Gerontology.* 2nd ed. Molly Brown, ed. St. Louis: Mosby.

Kennedy, Marie, Charlotte Ryan, and Jeanne Winner. 1987. "The Best Laid Plans . . . The Early History of Boston's Columbia Point Public Housing." Columbia Point Oral History Project, Center for Community Planning, College of Public and Community Service, University of Massachusetts at Boston.

Manning, James D., Jr. 1975. *Aging in American Society.* Ann Arbor: University of Michigan, Wayne State University Institute of Gerontology.

McKinlay, John B. 1975. "The Help Seeking Behavior of the Poor." Kosa and Zola, eds. *Poverty and Health.* Cambridge: Harvard University Health.

———, and Sharon L. Tennstedt. 1986. *Social Networks and the Care of Frail Elders.* Final Report, NIA National Institute on Aging. Grant No. AGO 3869 (February).

McNeely, R. L. and John L. Colen, eds. 1983. *Aging in Minority Groups*. San Francisco: Sage Publications.

Myerhoff, Barbara. 1979. *Number Our Days*. New York: Dutton.

Upshur, Carole C., Elaine Werby, and Gayle Epp. 1981. "Social Service Programs Essential for Mixed Income Housing Developments." *Journal of Housing* (May): 262–69.

Young, Michael and Peter Willmott. 1957. *Family and Kinship in East London*. Great Britain: Routledge and Kegan Paul.

Cognitive Coping Strategies among the Mothers of Children with Sickle Cell Disease

SHIRLEY A. HILL

Introduction: Stress, Social Support, and Coping

Research on the relationship between stress, social support, and coping has grown substantially in recent years. This has been fueled by a growing interest in the social-psychological and familial aspects of the experience of illness. Stress has been broadly defined as "virtually every form of disturbance of equilibrium" (Shontz 1975, 133). Yet critics of the event-initiated model of stress are careful to note that a complete state of equilibrium rarely if ever exists prior to the emergence of a particular stressor (Mestrovac and Glassner 1983; Walker 1985). Most stress theorists assume a direct inverse correlation between stress and the availability of social support (Jacobsen 1986); they assume that social support enhances the coping process and reduces stress (Shapiro 1989).

Having a family member diagnosed as chronically ill is a stress-inducing event; furthermore, providing long-term care for a chronically ill person threatens the stability and functioning of the family (Hill 1954; Chodoff et al. 1964; Kessler and McLeod 1984; Kazak and Marvin 1984; Koch 1985). Conversely, the way in which the family experiences, perceives, and responds to the illness can affect the social-psychological adjustment of the sick family member as well as the course and outcome of the disease (Shapiro 1983). Some early theorists viewed the modern family as structurally and functionally ill-equipped to deal with the vicissitudes of long-term illnesses

(Parsons and Fox 1952). Others emphasized that the ability to manage stressful events was mediated by the family's resources and its definition of the event as threatening (Hill 1954). In recent research the latter position, which views families as generally capable of adjusting to changes imposed by external events, has prevailed.

This study examines the responses of black mothers to the diagnosis of sickle cell disease in their children. Interviews with these mothers reveal that the diagnosis of this chronic disease is stress-inducing and that the women develop a variety of coping strategies in response to that stress. Coping has been defined as "the things people do in their own behalf to avoid or minimize the stress that would otherwise result from problematic conditions of life" (Pearlin and Aneshensel 1986, 418). Active-cognitive coping is "managing one's own appraisal of the situation" (Billings and Moos 1981). This research addresses a use of language I call "cognitive coping." This refers to the ways in which supposedly objective, scientific definitions of disease are altered by those experiencing it so that the disease becomes less threatening and more manageable. In this framework the mothers are active participants in the diagnostic and treatment processes. Through their own internal, interpretive processes, they construct meanings which affect their acceptance of the diagnosis, responses to symptoms, home and medical care, and future reproductive decisions.

Sickle Cell Disease

Sickle cell disease (SCD), a category of inherited blood disorders marked by the presence of sickle cell hemoglobin (HbS), is a painful and incurable disease found predominantly among blacks. Sickle cell hemoglobin causes red blood cells to assume the shape of a "sickle," thereby obstructing the flow of blood through the vessels, depriving the body tissues of oxygen, and precipitating what is generally referred to as a "pain attack" (Pollard 1986). The three most common SCDs are: 1) sickle cell anemia (a condition in which all of the hemoglobin in the blood is HbS and there is no normal hemoglobin); 2) sickle cell hemoglobin C (commonly known as S-C disease, as the patient inherits a sickle cell gene from one parent and a hemoglobin C gene from the other); and 3) sickle cell thalassemia (commonly known as S-thal disease, as the patient inherits a sickle cell gene from one parent and a thalassemia gene from the other). SCD is distinguished from sickle cell trait, which does not result in sickled cells in the bloodstream and is generally considered harmless.

First reported in 1910, SCD's medical implications were not widely examined until the late 1960s (Rosner et al. 1982), and research on the psycho-social aspects did not begin until 1974 (Whitten and Bertles 1989). The sickle cell trait is found in one out of every ten to twelve blacks in the United States. One in every 144 black couples has the potential for having a child with SCD (Whitten and Nishiura 1985). The symptoms of SCD generally appear in early infancy, between the ages of six and twelve months, but sometimes as late as puberty. These symptoms include poor appetite, paleness, fatigue, yellowness in the whites of the eyes, frequent colds and infections, and bodily pain. In addition to the most frequent consequence of having the disease—periodic pain attacks—a child with SCD may experience a wide variety of physical problems. Some of these include frequent urination and bedwetting; increased susceptibility to colds, strep throat, and pneumonia; gall stones; delayed puberty; destruction of bone (especially hip-joint bone); damaged bodily organs; stroke; and early death (Whitten and Nishiura 1985; France-Dawson 1986).

The Study

This study, drawn from in-progress research, is based on interviews with twenty mothers whose children have been diagnosed as having SCD. The mothers participating in this study have children who are patients at Children's Mercy Hospital located in Kansas City, Missouri. This hospital is a regional center for SCD which provides routine and emergency medical care for approximately 120 patients under the age of twenty-one. Mothers (or caretakers) of children receiving medical care at the hospital were sent letters explaining the purpose of the study and requesting an interview. Interviewees responded by returning a self-addressed postcard included in the letter or by telephoning. This study, essentially qualitative and descriptive, relied on data collection consisting of a series of open-ended questions designed to probe several aspects of the illness experience. These included: extent of knowledge about SCD prior to the diagnosis; family history of SCD; the diagnosis experience; parental reactions to the diagnosis; the provision of home and medical care; and respondents' assessment of the impact of SCD on the child and the family.

Personal, in-depth interviews, sixty- to ninety-minutes long and tran-scribed verbatim, were conducted with mothers who agreed to participate in the study. Interviewees, including one grandmother and one great aunt, ranged in age from twenty-four to seventy-two years old, with an average age of 36.5. Six of the twenty interviewees were currently married; the others were either single (six), separated (three), or divorced (five). Three of the six married mothers were married to the biological fathers of the SCD child. The majority (sixteen of the twenty) had at least a high school education, and eleven were employed outside of the home. Their children (twenty-three in all, as some had more than one child with SCD) ranged in age from four to twenty-one years old, with an average age of 10.7 years. Most (sixteen) were diagnosed with sickle cell anemia, five with S-C disease and the remaining two with S-thal disease. Diagnosis occurred between the ages of birth and seven years old: the average age of diagnosis was eighteen months old.

Stages of Response

Research literature examining how parents respond to their children's diagnosis of chronic illness generally describe a "stage theory adaptation." These stages of emotional response are: initial shock and denial, followed by grief, and culminating in acceptance (Fortier and Wanlass 1984).

Initially, mothers of children with SCD deny the accuracy of the diagnosis. This is a widely documented pattern of coping. Many of the mothers had never heard of the disease prior to their child's diagnosis, and even those with some prior knowledge seldom understood the consequences of having SCD or the trait. Denial generally gives way to acceptance. Yet this study found that denial, a persistent and strong element of doubt, pervades the entire illness experience. Underlying the process of denial are: mystification of the disease's origins; selective inattention to the physical symptoms of disease; distrust of medical authorities and defining one's own children as being unlike others they have seen who have SCD.

Mystification of the disease's origins results from the family members' inability to determine exactly which family members have the sickle cell trait. Most mothers agree intellectually that passing the disease on to a child requires both parents having the sickle cell trait, yet they often suggest that their family is an exception. Mothers' attempts to trace the disease's origins through members on both sides of the family represent one of the few examples of familial rather than individual responses to a diagnosis. These mothers have consulted with members on both sides of the family in their efforts to discover the disease's origin. For example, one grandmother who has custody of a ten-year-old grandson with SCD, began the interview explaining that she has extensive knowledge about the disease. In fact, she educated others about it. However, she has difficulty tracing the origin of the disease in her own family: "Well, how can I say this—I don't know. I don't know how it came about, from where, or what happened. I don't have the trait. Of course, I don't know what my ex-husband had or has, but my daughter [mother of the grandson with SCD] doesn't have it and neither do I. I wouldn't know what my ex-son-in-law's parents had, but my ex-son-in-law doesn't have it either." This grandmother's response clearly mystifies the origin of the disease and effectively exonerates the immediate family of responsibility for passing it on to the child. Another mother, also convinced that no one in her family had the sickle cell trait, managed to deny the diagnosis for nearly two years: "I was like, 'Oh, well, it couldn't possibly be. She couldn't possibly have anything like that.' So I didn't check this out; I didn't! I just didn't go back." Alarmed when her daughter experienced symptoms, this mother sought medical care and accepted the diagnosis. Intellectually, she acknowledges that she has the trait and her daughter has the disease. Yet, a shadow of doubt remains, because she does not understand exactly how she inherited it: "I was shocked. I was shocked to death to have thalassemia, and never heard of it, everybody is still in shock. My parents are like, 'what is this thalassemia stuff?' [and] 'where'd you get something like that from?' So they've never been tested still; we still don't know anyone else in the family that has it. No one else."

Previous research found that fathers use denial as a coping strategy more often than mothers (Barbarin, Hughes, Chesler 1985) and that this pattern of denial among fathers is especially true in the case of SCD (Travis 1976). Although this study is based on the responses of mothers only, it reveals fathers' tendencies to deny their share of responsibility for passing the disease on to their children. Many of these fathers denied they had the trait and refused to be tested for it. Some mothers who fail to trace the origins of the disease resolve the etiology by attributing it to the child's father. This assignation of blame stands unchallenged, as the fathers tend to be uninvolved in the family. Blaming the father's side of the family has consequences for future reproductive decisions. For example, one mother of eight explained her lack of concern about having additional children with SCD. She believed she did not have the trait and felt that since her other children had a different father there was no chance of passing the disease on to them: "It's not a possibility that I would [pass the trait on]. I don't have the trait, I don't have anything, how could another child have sickle cell if the father and his people didn't have a history of it? I don't worry about things like that."

The diagnosis of SCD is a political as well as a medical issue. Black Americans, historically victimized by racism, may fear that the diagnosis of SCD will become another reason for discrimination (France-Dawson 1986; Sullivan 1987). One mother ignored her daughter's symptoms of SCD for two years. She believed the diagnosis, made when the child was three years old, was racially-motivated:

> Well, I was always taking her back and forth to the hospital for checkups and stuff, she just had colds and stuff like that. But when she got five years old . . . she came running home from school one day crying that something in her head [was hurting]. So when I really accepted it, she was five. They had first said it when she was three, but I said no way! Because they were just going crazy with sickle cell, every time a black child came in there, they'd say sickle cell.

Mothers who persistently deny (or doubt) the diagnosis often do so by comparing their child to others who have the disease. For example, one mother with two SCD children has been coping with the disease for thirteen years. Yet, she still sometimes doubts the diagnosis: "I work [at the hospital] and I'm thinking of others who have SCD and saying, 'they [my children] are nothing like that.' Are they [the doctors] sure, you know, that they diagnosed it right? But each year I go back for the physical, and each time they check it and it comes out the same."

Persistent denial may also be attributed to disease-specific characteristics of SCD. These vary considerably in course and severity. However, there is no clear link between severity of symptoms and maternal persistence in denial. One forty-five-year-old mother has provided care for her nineteen-year-old daughter with SCD for more than fifteen years. She sometimes doubts her daughter's disease, despite the fact that she had a stroke at age three, is partially paralyzed, and requires blood transfusions every six weeks. This persistent denial, even among mothers who adhere to medical regimens, illustrates that denial and acceptance are not discrete response categories but often coexist. Denial is the coping strategy which underlies maternal efforts to minimize the nature and extent of the symptoms and disability; it enables them to emphasize the child's ability to lead a normal life.

Responses: "Naming" the Disease

Parents who care for chronically ill children "name" or label the child's sickness. This labeling affects how they respond to the symptoms of the sickness. The pain, generally unverifiable in SCD, leaves little physical evidence to reveal the nature and extent of discomfort. These mothers respond variously to the symptoms. They might administer an analgesic (or a vitamin as a placebo) or rush the child to the hospital for emergency medical care. Their responses are shaped by their subjective appraisals of the disease and the pain it elicits. One mother reported considerable frustration in determining how much pain her fourteen-year-old daughter experienced. Asked how she knew when her daughter was in severe pain, she used previous experience as a gauge:

> Well, she lets the whole neighborhood know she's in pain. It seems she only gets sick in the middle of the night, she starts screaming and hollering [and] I can't understand a person being in that much pain, it's hard for me to accept that she's not just screaming unnecessarily. So she always let you know. But this last time she didn't run a fever, so I really didn't know if she was in a crisis, because always before she had a fever.

Another mother ignored her young daughter's pain for practical reasons. She did not want to make her daughter too emotionally dependent on her or accrue unpayable medical bills:

> How can I say this? At one time she'd come and say her stomach hurt and I'd say there was nothing wrong. She gets pains in her stomach that are just out of this world. I just give her that little bit of comfort and kind of take

it away, so she won't depend on me to be there all the time when she has this pain. I guess I put [it] in my mind that I refuse to go to the hospital every time she gets a pain. I just refuse to take her all of the time. Also, too, I didn't have insurance.

Normalization aimed at diminishing the illness's stigma and creating a sense of control is a major coping strategy among those confronting chronic illnesses and disabilities (Birenbaum 1971; Voysey 1972; Krulik 1980). Among mothers of children with SCD, normalization includes emphasizing the child's normal looks and unhampered ability to engage in other activities. Some mothers made a special point of having their children available for the interview. Others desired that I meet the child with SCD, confident that I could not identify the child as one having the disease. One mother, responding to people who pitied her five-year-old son with SCD, said: "And people keep saying, 'Oh, he's got sickle cell.' And I say, 'Yeah, he's got sickle cell. Does he look any different to you? Is there anything wrong with him? Look at him! Would you know he has sickle cell?' "

Mothers emphasized the strengths and determination of their children and expressed pride in their children's coping abilities and hopefulness regarding their children's abilities to achieve their goals despite their illness. They were confident that their children's physical difficulties would not prevent participation in normal activities. One mother, asked if the pain kept her ten-year-old son from very many activities, responded: "No, because he's a real strong little boy. He's real strong. I have seen that little boy [when] he was in so much pain! If the ball is laying over [there] and he's in pain and he's full of medication—still in pain and crying—he pulls himself until he gets to [it]. That's determination. To me, he's no different from anybody else, because he can cope with pain." Another mother describes her six-year-old daughter similarly: "Oh, yeah, she's real intelligent. And she's real strong willed. If she wants to do something, she's going do it. And I don't think having SCD is going to stop her at all. I think she's just gonna be able to ride that right out. If she's having a crisis, she'll be able to handle it and keep going. I don't think she'll have any problem at all."

At times, mothers' psychological adaptations redefined the disease: rather than being a misfortune, it promoted personal growth or actually improved their children's futures. One thirty-one-year-old mother reported: "I used to think it was real bad. I don't think it's so bad anymore. Because I'm a real religious person, I don't take it as being bad. I just figure I have to deal with it, and it's no different than other things we have to deal with. It actually makes you strong. Something I have to work harder at. Maybe God was seeing how patient I am." Another mother said of her four-year-old son that the disease might motivate him to get an education rather than be oriented toward sports: "Well, I'm kind of glad to know that maybe he won't be a star athlete—that way he'll use his brain. He wants to be an engineer. Since his foot is kind of curved, I won't have to worry about him thinking sports all the time. Yeah, I think he'll be fine. As far as the disease affecting him when he gets older, I don't think it will."

Conclusion

The mothers participating in this study are socio-demographically similar to the majority of black women in the United States: they have low to moderate education levels, became mothers at a relatively young age, and are single mothers primarily responsible for childrearing. The majority no longer have significant contacts with the child's biological father, yet they receive a great deal of social and emotional support from extended family ties. When asked who has been most supportive and helpful to them since the diagnosis of SCD, most respond by saying "my mother." In 25 percent of the cases, the grandmother had primary responsibility for the child during some period, and two mothers relied completely upon their own mothers to make decisions about the medical treatment and care of their children.

The diagnosis of SCD precipitates considerable psychological distress for mothers. Most of them initially fear early childhood death; however, as they become more familiar with the consequences of the disease for their children, they gradually develop effective coping strategies. Only two of the twenty children represented in this study had life-threatening cases of SCD, marked by strokes, surgeries, and paralysis. For most mothers, SCD meant frequent aches, pains, and infections—symptoms which resulted in emergency medical treatment and/or hospitalization between two to four times a year. Mothers followed recommended medical regimens, but developed their own coping strategies to make the disease more manageable. Clearly, the responses of these mothers were influenced by race- and class-based patterns of childrearing, and they must be viewed within that context. Research indicates that blacks (Stack 1974) and members of the lower socioeconomic classes (Kohn 1989) are much less likely to indulge or pamper their children. Pride is placed on children developing their own strengths and learning to cope with hardship, including both the hardships of illness and of racial and class discrimination.

The responses of the mothers are also shaped by decades of official neglect of the medical and social implications of SCD. Prior to having a child diagnosed with SCD, few of these mothers had been informed that they had the sickle cell trait or understood the potential reproductive consequences of having the trait. Several had difficulty obtaining an accurate diagnosis, as physicians lacked familiarity with the disease. Most, especially those diagnosed more than five years ago, were given very little information about the disease and virtually no instructions for caring for their children. Only recently have educational and support services become more available for the parents of children with SCD.

Works Cited

Barbarin, Oscar, Diane Hughes, and Mark Chesler. 1985. "Stress, Coping, and Marital Functioning among Parents of Children with Cancer." *Journal of Marriage and the Family* 47:473–80.

Billings, Andrew G., and Rudolf H. Moos. 1981. "The Role of Coping Responses and Social Resources in Attenuating the Stress of Life Events." *Journal of Behavioral Medicine* 4:139–57.

Birenbaum, Arnold. 1971. "The Mentally Retarded Child in the Home and the Family Cycle." *Journal of Health and Social Behavior* 12:55–65.

Chodoff, Paul, Stanford B. Friedman, David Hamburg. 1964. "Stress Coping Behavior: Observations in Parents of Children with Malignant Disease." *American Journal of Psychiatry* 120:743–49.

Fortier, Laurie M., and Richard L. Wanlass. 1984. "Family Crisis Following the Diagnosis of a Handicapped Child." *Family Relations* 33:13–24.

France-Dawson, Merry. 1986. "Sickle Cell Disease: Implications for Nursing Care." *Journal of Advanced Nursing* 11:729–37.

Hill, Reuben. 1954. "Social Stress on the Family." *Social Casework* 39:139–56.

Jacobsen, David E. 1986. "Types and Timing of Social Support." *Journal of Health and Social Behavior* 27:250–64.

Kazak, Anne E., and Robert S. Marvin. 1984. "Differences, Difficulties and Adaptation: Stress and Social Networks in Families with a Handicapped Child." *Family Relations* 33: 67–77.

Kessler, R. C., and J. D. McLeod. 1984. "Sex Differences in Vulnerability to Understanding Life Events." *American Sociological Review* 49:620–31.

Koch, Alberta. 1985. "If Only It Could Be Me: The Families of Pediatric Cancer Patients." *Family Relations* 34:63–70.

Kohn, M. L. 1959. "Social Class and Parental Values." *American Journal of Sociology.* 65:337–51.

Krulik, T. 1980. "Successful 'Normalizing' Tactics of Parents of Chronically Ill Children." *Journal of Advanced Nursing* 5:573–78.

Mestrovac, Stjepan, and Barry Glassner. 1983. "A Durkheimian Hypothesis on Stress." *Social Science and Medicine* 17:1315–27.

Nagel, Ronald L., Mary E. Fabry, and D. K. Kaul. 1984. "New Insights on Sickle Cell Anemia." *Diagnostic Medicine* May: 26–33.

Parsons, Talcott, and Renee Fox. 1952. "Illness, Therapy and the Modern Urban American Family." *Journal of Social Issues* 13:31–44.

Pearlin, Leonard I., and Carol S. Aneshensel. 1986. "Coping and Social Supports: Their Functions and Applications." *Applications of Social Science to Clinical Medicine and Health Policy.* Aiken and Mechanic, eds. New Brunswick, N.J.: Rutgers University Press, 417–37.

Pollard, Cathy. 1986. "Sickle Cell Anemia: A Review." *Physician Assistant* October: 76–84.

Rosner, Fred, Lynn St. Clair, Gungor Karayalcin, and Basic Tatsis. 1982. "A Decade of Experience with a Sickle Cell Program." *New York Journal of Medicine* 82: 1546–54.

Shapiro, Johanna. 1983. "Family Reactions and Coping Strategies in Response to the Physically Ill or Handicapped Child: A Review." *Social Science and Medicine* 17:913–31.

———. 1989. "Stress, Depression, and Support Group Participation in Mothers of Developmentally Disabled Children." *Family Relations* 38:169–73.

Shontz, F. C. 1975. *The Psychological Aspects of Physical Illness and Disability.* New York: Macmillan.

Stack, Carol. 1974. *All Our Kin: Strategies for Survival in a Black Community.* New York: Harper & Row.

Sullivan, Louis. 1987. "The Risks of Sickle-Cell Trait: Caution and Common Sense. *The New England Journal of Medicine* September: 830–31.

Travis, Georgia. 1976. "Sickle Cell Anemia." *Chronic Illness in Children: Its Impact on the Family.* Stanford, Calif.: Stanford University Press, 432–54.

Voysey, Margaret. 1972. "Impression Management by Parents with Disabled Children." *Journal of Health and Social Behavior* 13:80–89.

Walker, Alexis. 1985. "Reconceptualizing Family Stress." *Journal of Marriage and the Family* 47:827–37.

Whitten, Charles F., and John F. Bertles. 1989. *Sickle Cell Disease.* New York: New York Academy of Sciences.

Whitten, Charles F., and E. Nishiura. 1985. *Sickle Cell Anemia: Issues in the Care of Children with Chronic Illness.* Hobbs and Perrin, eds. San Francisco and London: Jossey-Bass Publishers, 236–60.

PART 2

TRADITIONAL MEDICINE AND HOLISTIC CONCEPTS OF HEALTH: QUESTIONS OF CULTURE AND POLITICS

Introduction

Part Two explores ideas of traditional medicine among Southeast-Asian, Mexican-American, and Native-American women. The authors of the four essays in this section ask us to recognize that dominant Anglo-European cultural beliefs represent just one of many systems of thought and that the growing cultural diversity of American society demands that practitioners take into account traditional belief systems in order to offer quality health care to ethnic minority populations.

At the same time that the authors call for recognition of culture as a factor in medicine, they point to the danger of becoming so immersed in ideas of cultural difference that the political and socioeconomic origins of illness (discussed in Part One) are overlooked. They also raise the issue of whether the introduction of a new cultural relativism will serve the interests of people of color who seek to become active agents in the formation of health policy or if their concerns will be diffused by the assimilationist attitudes of white health care providers, administrators, scholars, and theorists who begin to take culture into account but remain in control of policy, interpretation, and the structure of practice.

The first two essays—by public health specialist Barbara Frye and feminist political theorist Françoise Vergès—look at traditional theories of health and illness as alternatives to Western beliefs. They argue that U. S. health practitioners need to understand traditional cosmologies of illness in order to effectively treat and communicate with ethnic patients.

Frye looks at the health needs of Southeast-Asian refugees (primarily Cambodians) resident in the United States. Traumatized by past horrors experienced in war and the political repression, death, and disease that came in its aftermath, these Indochinese immigrants manifest high rates of suicide, depression, post-traumatic stress syndrome, and SUNDS (Sudden Unexpected Nocturnal Death Syndrome)—a malady wherein sufferers, primarily male, die prematurely in their sleep. As in other cultures, Southeast-Asian women assume the primary role of caretaking within their families and communities. They practice health care according to traditional belief systems based on the principles of equilibrium and balance. These principles are extended to ideas about proper interaction with the environment, the intake of food, and the interpersonal dynamics of family relations, work, and rest. Frye explains dualistic concepts of "hot" and "cold" conditions, as well as foods and theories that relate physical illness and depression to states of disequilibrium.

Like the African Americans who consult ethno-psychiatrists in the Louisiana town featured in Wonda Lee Fontenot's essay in Part One, the Cambodian refugees Frye describes here believe that disease is rooted in spiritual causes. In the past they turned to traditional healers (kru khmer) in their villages for interpretation. In the United States, they combine visits to Western physicians with traditional remedies and practices within the home.

Frye examines barriers that Cambodian refugees face in utilizing the American health care system, and urges health practitioners treating Cambodians to recognize that scientific medicine can be complementary to traditional practices. As in Shirley Hill's essay on mothers of children with sickle cell disease featured in Part One, Frye depended on interviews with adult women in families to determine women's attitudes toward and management of illness. Like Hill, she demonstrates that women's definitions of illness and coping incorporate psycho-social and cultural as well as somatic causes. And as was the case in Hill's study, the women Frye interviewed voiced a great deal of stoicism and belief in individual strength, group support, and personal accountability.

Frye argues that Western medical providers and hospital administrators should respect the Indochinese emphasis on family solidarity and provide support services for refugee women that recognize the stress they experience as primary caretakers within their homes.

In the next essay, Françoise Vergès offers an interpretation of *curanderismo*, Mexican-American folk medicine, which is, like health practices in the Cambodian refugee community, part of the larger symbolic system that guides traditional world views of members of the Mexican-American community. Vergès describes the dualistic hot-cold philosophy that underlies traditional Mexican-American health beliefs—a philosophy similar to that which Frye described as operational in Cambodian health care practices. Using French feminist theory, Vergès then examines *curanderismo* as a discourse, deconstructing gender elements in its praxis, and critiquing ways in which it has been interpreted by Western social scientists in the past. She argues that the emphasis on culture in interpretation often leads us away from systemic consideration of the political realities of health, including the power dynamics that guide Western dualistic notions of "modern" and "traditional" and First and Third worlds.

In the third essay, Denise Drevdahl adds to this debate about cultural interpretations by arguing that knowledge of cultural difference is critical to the provision of quality patient care in a multicultural society. A nurse and community health specialist, Drevdahl conducted a small survey study of Native-American women using an urban clinic in Denver, Colorado. Though these women came from different ethnic backgrounds and traditions (Apache, Navajo, Sioux, and Ute), there was consistency in the ways they defined well-being. Rather than preserving strict dualisms between mind and body, these women conflated emotional and physical factors, offering a holistic model of health that emphasized unity of thought and feeling and an ideal of exuberance.

Drevdahl takes a "women's culture" approach in developing a thesis for her study. She looks to discover ways in which women define and organize their world and relations with one another separate from people of other cultures and from their relationships with men within their own culture. She combines these concerns with social-scientific statistical methods. Like the Cambodian women whom Frye interviewed, the Native-American women Drevdahl spoke with told of diversified health practices that combined traditional ways of healing and remedies with Western medicine. Drevdahl concludes that Western health care providers should learn to work in conjunction with traditional healers and to respect the Native-American search for a restoration of balance between human beings and the environment.

The feeling of multiple consciousness, of occupying more than one world, articulated by the Native-American women Drevdahl interviewed is echoed in Gregoria Rodriguez's personal narrative. Rodriguez, a doctoral student in the Department of Preventive Medicine and Community Health at the University of Texas Medical Branch, writes of her journey to a border town to interview Hispanic-American women about their health. The exercise soon turned from the academic to the personal, as the familiarity of the town's culture brought back memories of Rodriguez's own upbringing and revived questions she struggled with as a woman in a Hispanic community and as an Hispanic woman seeking a career in a scientific field.

Rodriguez's poignant essay speaks to the sensibilities of women of color who become health practitioners and health scientists, who straddle the worlds of institutionized medicine and public health and the ethnic communities in which they were raised. Like Vergès, Rodriguez recognizes the power dynamics involved when medical practitioners or health officials are granted authority by virtue of their professional positions to label the illnesses and behaviors of others. Rodriguez also underlines the facts already testified to by the authors in Part One—women's health and illness are inextricably tied to their status as women within their culture, to their lives as workers and family caretakers, and to their positions as women and racial minorities within a socioeconomic system that affords them little privilege.

Health Care Decision Making among Cambodian Refugee Women

BARBARA FRYE

Introduction

Since 1975 almost one million Indochinese refugees have entered the United States. The majority of them have come from Southeast-Asia. The first wave of Southeast-Asian refugees, mostly Vietnamese, were generally well educated. In 1979 the second wave of Southeast-Asian refugees arrived. They were a heterogeneous, highly traumatized population from the war-torn villages and camps of rural Asia. Among the most traumatized have been the people of Cambodia, the Khmer. There are now 140,000 Khmer refugees in the United States, with the largest concentration residing in the Southern California basin (Holley 1986; Montero 1979; *Refugee Reports* 1985). The Khmer are among the least educated of the Indochinese immigrants, and they suffer the greatest amounts of physical and psychological illness (Meinhardt et al. 1984).

Hidden away in a jungle environment that protected them from outside interference for thousands of years, the Khmer people created some of the world's finest sculpture in the temples at Angkor Wat. Fed by the silt-carrying Mekong, the land of Cambodia was the rice basin of Indochina. Life followed the rhythm of the rice harvest and the non-violent teachings of Theravada Buddhism. Yet, historically, Cambodia has been caught in a cross fire of wars between Vietnam and Thailand.

A neutral country in the Vietnam War until the Viet Cong used its borders as sanctuaries, Cambodia came to the attention of the world when its

93

fertile rice fields were cratered by secret American B-52 bombings. Cambodia was then plunged into civil war, resulting in a reign of terror under Pol Pot's Khmer Rouge forces in 1975. In 1979 the Vietnamese communist forces overcame the Khmer Rouge, and they continue to dominate the country today. The consequences of this prolonged war included holocaust, mass arrests, and detentions in which half the country's population died of starvation or massacre. There was almost total destruction of the educated class, including physicians. There was mass refugee migration to the Thailand border, and from there many refugees continued on to the United States (Anderson 1981; Becker 1986; Chanda 1986; Chandler 1972; Edmonds 1970; Ponchaud 1977; Shawcross 1979; Song 1979).

Suicide, clinical depression, somatization, post-traumatic stress syndrome, and sudden unexpected nocturnal death syndrome (SUNDS) are among the conditions faced by the refugees (Baron et al. 1983; Blanchard et al. 1986; Boehnlein 1987; Kinzie et al. 1984; Lin et al. 1985; Meinhardt et al. 1984; Mollica et al. 1987; Nicassio and Pate 1984; Nolan et al. 1988).

Khmer Beliefs About Health and Illness

In the Khmer world view, medicine and religion blend. Causation of illness is attributed to both natural and spiritual causes.

NATURAL CAUSES

The central principle of health in the traditional Cambodian belief system is equilibrium. This principle of equilibrium extends to interaction with the environment, the intake of food, emotional states, interpersonal relations, and the pace of work and rest. For example, the Khmer perceive that exposure to high winds is an unbalancing and potentially illness-producing force. One Khmer woman commented, "The Khmer people, they are very worried for the wind. They always think about the wind." Imbalance in food intake is another potential source of disequilibrium. Culturally-defined "hot" foods exacerbate "hot" or overly active physiological states, whereas "cold" foods exacerbate "cold" or weakened states. Hypertension is culturally defined as a "hot" state. In this state, such "hot" foods as meat, salt, alcohol, and highly spiced dishes should be avoided and such "cold" foods as fruits and vegetables should be consumed. The purpose of this oppositional food therapy is to bring the body back into equilibrium. Conversely, "hot" foods are used to strengthen the weakened body in a "cold" condition. Childbirth, for example, is a culturally-defined "cold" state and is treated with liberal amounts of "hot" food (Fishman et al. 1988; Kemp 1985; Kulig 1988; Marcucci 1986).

Disequilibrium is also attributed to excessive work or deep states of anger or grief. Such disturbances of balance are perceived to affect the body holistically and result in "wind illness." Mild states of wind illness, such as a headache, are treated with dermabrasive techniques. One example is *kos khyal* or "coin rubbing," massaging the skin with tiger balm ointment and then rubbing the skin with a hot coin. Other practices include pinching the skin and placing a lighted candle in a small bottle on the forehead, resulting in raised, reddened welts. The purpose of these practices is to bring the "bad wind" in the body to the surface of the skin so it can be excreted (Kemp 1985; Marcucci 1986; Martin 1983).

A more serious manifestation of wind illness is *kchall koo*, a state in which the bad wind becomes "frozen wind." This is believed to be the result of extreme states of exhaustion, emotional distress, or spirit possession. Frozen wind is considered life-threatening because it causes the blood to cease circulating. The affected person demonstrates a catatonic state comparable to that seen in severe depression. Treatment is emergency acupuncture. Family members are expected to pray, chant, and embrace the sick person to prevent further development of the catatonic state (Duncan 1987; Marcucci 1986).

SPIRITUAL CAUSES

In traditional Khmer thinking, the world is populated by a variety of spirits. The guardian spirits of the village are the *neak ta*. Failure to treat these generally benevolent spirits with proper respect can enrage them. They have the power to release the soul from the body. The soul can then wander, haunting family members and creating havoc. *Neak ta* also cause gastrointestinal problems, fevers, nightmares, and emotional lability, as well as sudden death from cardiac arrest or trauma. These spirits can enter the body as a result of breaking a taboo or through witchcraft. *Thmop* is the power of black magic, and the *arak* spirit resides in hateful people. Ancestral spirits can haunt the family if there is immoral behavior being practiced by family members (Duncan 1987; Frye 1986; Kemp 1985; Marcucci 1986; Martin 1983; Ong in Bowlan and Bruno 1985).

Traditional Healers

Since the fourteenth century, Cambodia has been primarily a Buddhist country. The practice of Buddhism was fused through time with the earlier practice of animism and with the subsequent introduction of Islam and Christianity (Chandler 1972; Ebihara 1968; Edmonds 1970; Ponchaud 1977; Song 1979; *Refugee Reports* 1984).

Traditional Cambodian healers are called *kru khmer*. In pre-revolutionary Cambodia, an aspiring kru khmer was trained under the Buddhist monks in a temple for at least three years. Then he served an apprenticeship under an experienced kru for specialization in herbal medicine, preparation of amulets and talismans, black magic, or meditation. The role of kru khmer is limited to males (Hiegel 1982; Marcucci 1986). At present, in the Cambodian refugee camps in Thailand, the kru khmer work collaboratively with scientifically trained internists and psychiatrists in treating physical and emotional problems. There is very little reported use of kru khmer in America, the elderly ones having died during the holocaust and the Khmer youth lacking interest in preparing for this role. Although American physicians are sought as care providers, traditional remedies continue to be used frequently in Khmer homes (Frye 1989).

The Khmer in the American Health Care System

Khmer refugees in America have not actively sought entrance into the American health care system. This reticence to seek care has been attributed to depression, lack of English language skills, and a cultural norm which precludes questioning (Blanchard 1986; Boehnlein 1987; Kemp 1985; Muecke 1983b; Rosenberg and Givens 1986). At the same time, American health care providers lack understanding of the Khmer concepts of disease causation and the dynamics of health care decision making in the Khmer family.

In Khmer thinking, scientific medicine is complementary to but does not replace traditional medicine. In addition to accepting a pluralistic approach to the treatment of illness, the Khmer culture discourages questioning or confrontation with authority figures (Kinzie et al. 1987). Muecke (1983a, 435) states that: "Authority figures should not be questioned or opposed directly so as not to offend or embarrass them openly. They may, however, be discreetly disobeyed 'behind their backs.'" In accordance with cultural norms, the Khmer patient may be indirect in communication with health care providers.

Purpose of the Study

This study examined the process of health care decision making within the Khmer refugee family as explained by the highest ranking woman in the household. Specifically it compared the women's cultural explanations of health and illness with reported treatments of illness. A close congruence was found between belief and behavior. Health care decision making patterns demonstrated an individual and matriarchal pattern.

Method

Data was collected through open-ended, in-home interviews in the Khmer language. Thirty consenting informants were selected, using a convenience sample of thirty families known to the translator—a middle-aged woman with children who had served as the medical translator in the local county health department. She is highly regarded by the Khmer women in the community as an informal leader.

Three in-home interviews were conducted with each informant. In the first interview, information was gathered on cultural health beliefs about six age categories: infants, children, adolescents, women, men, and elders. Categories of information included beliefs about disease causation; illnesses to which the Khmer of each age category were perceived to be susceptible; the cultural treatment and avoidance behaviors associated with illnesses for the specific age group; and which family member managed given illnesses. One month later, in a second interview, information was gathered on all illness episodes currently afflicting the family and all recalled episodes during the six months prior to the first interview. In the third and final interview, conducted one month after the second interview, information was gathered on all current illnesses and recalled illnesses within the preceding month. Data was also collected on beliefs about cultural health promotion behaviors. A total of 226 illness episodes involving 157 family members of the thirty informants were tracked.

Findings

The thirty informants in the study considered themselves to be the primary female managers of the households. The median family size was 5.5 persons. The population of these households was young, with 56 percent of the participants aged eighteen years or less.

HEALTH CARE DECISION MAKING

The majority of informants reported that they sought care which provided a comfortable cultural fit, either through the use of traditional home remedies or through seeking a physician who offered them language and cultural comfort. Most of the informants reported driving at least sixty miles to seek culturally acceptable care.

In spite of being surrounded by a large number of primary and tertiary care facilities within a five-mile radius, the women did not perceive these facilities as comfortable or accessible. Language difficulties, the need for interpretation by younger, linguistically more fluent family members, and the lack of cultural sensitivity by health care personnel were some reasons verbalized for avoiding the health care facilities within close proximity to their homes. All the women reported having access to automobile transportation through their social network, and thus they had an opportunity to choose the care they received. The majority of women did not depend upon their husbands to drive them or their children to medical care locations.

In most cases concerning children, the mother was described as the decision maker. The father had a central role in decision making when there were long-term, chronic problems with children. An individual pattern of decision making was described for adults seeking health care.

Management of Illnesses

The Babies

The illnesses that the women identified as commonly afflicting babies were generally the same ones they reported as having been diagnosed by the physicians whose care they sought. Commonly perceived and subsequently occurring illnesses in infants were fever, diarrhea, and upper respiratory infection. These illnesses in infants were generally perceived to be caused by the traditional sources of imbalance—exposure to environmental forces (especially high velocity winds) spoiled food, or "sour breast milk." Spiritual explanations were also given. A frequent explanation for the onset of convulsions in a febrile infant was that an evil ancestral spirit was seeking revenge against an offending or immoral family member. One woman qualified this by stating, "Babies don't get convulsions so much in America because there are fewer evil spirits here than in Cambodia." When subsequently questioned about causes of actual reported illnesses, however, the women mixed cultural explanations of causation—i.e., sources of imbalance or vindication by evil spirits—with scientific explanations—specifically, germ theory. This finding suggests a transition in the belief structure and an effort to merge the explanations of both cultures.

Culturally recommended treatments were almost exclusively traditional remedies, but the reported management of the actual illnesses was a blend of traditional and scientific treatments. Cultural treatment for an infant with a fever, a "hot" state, included wrapping him or her in cold towels, coin rubbing, and Khmer herbal tea. However, actual treatment for babies in the study who developed fever was almost exclusively the use of antipyretic drugs, such as Tylenol. One nine-month-old infant developed febrile convulsions with measles. He was rushed to the nearest emergency room, where he was packed in ice and treated with Tylenol. His mother described the experience as follows: "Chanla was in a very 'hot' state. The doctor was wise to give him a 'cold' treatment. But the Tylenol also made him balanced."

Diarrhea was identified as a "cold" condition precipitated by "sour breast milk" or spoiled food. The culturally recommended treatments for diarrhea included coin rubbing, rice soup, herbal tea, boiled guava leaves, and cessation of breastfeeding. However, in this study the most common treatment for diarrhea was a mixture of traditional and scientific methods. Scientific treatments included medically prescribed antidiarrheal drugs and physician encouragement to resume breastfeeding. Prior to seeking scientific care for their babies, however, the women frequently used coin rubbing. As one woman explained, "coin rubbing is necessary before going to the doctor. If the baby has no coin on his skin before he gets Western medicine he will die."

Cultural avoidance behaviors, i.e., what not to do when ill, are protective behaviors which are practiced when illness occurs. In this study there was a pragmatic acceptance of blending scientific treatment and cultural remedies. However, disease causation was still culturally defined, and traditional avoidance behaviors were used, such as avoiding warm clothing for a febrile infant in a "hot" state or avoiding breastfeeding when the milk was considered to be "sour."

The vulnerability of babies, the seriousness of their illnesses, and their susceptibility to death were common threads throughout the interviews. During the interviews, the women consistently avoided using the actual word "death" in reference to babies, yet they talked around the issue continuously, expressing their concern for the "weakness" of babies and the high probability of losing the infants. When queried about this behavior, a number of informants explained that if they used the word "death" when they were talking directly about specific babies, this would incur the attention and wrath of evil spirits against these babies.

This sense of the vulnerability of the Khmer infant and the maternal protective response is further exemplified in the story of Apsara. Born very prematurely, Apsara was immediately admitted to the neonatal intensive care unit, where she battled with severe respiratory distress syndrome. The American doctor forthrightly explained the seriousness of the baby's condition to her worried mother. The Khmer community disapproved of the doctor's approach, believing that such discussion of impending death would not only incur the attention of evil spirits, and thus endanger the infant's life, but would also create a state of disequilibrium for the mother in the postpartum period. They reasoned it would be better for mother and child alike if the doctor kept quiet about the seriousness of the baby's condition. Convinced that her baby had no chance of living, the young mother named her baby girl Apsara. The origin of this name lies in Khmer mythology. It embodies the concept of Khmer femininity, gracefulness, gentleness, and seductiveness. It was the name traditionally carried by the lead dancer in the temples of Angkor Wat. It is considered the most beautiful name a girl can bear. Lying on her postpartum bed, the mother explained, "I have nothing I can give her now. I cannot even give her the gift of my milk. But I can give her the most beautiful name so that when she dies she will carry it with her into the next incarnation. Then she will know that I love her." Apsara, however, has not had to carry her name into the next incarnation. Before the completion of the study, she was reunited with her mother and making steady progress in health and development.

The Children

The illnesses which were perceived to affect children generally corresponded with those that were reported by the women as diagnosed by physicians. The most common illnesses were fevers, upper respiratory infections, and measles. Chronic disabling conditions were fairly common, but they were not perceived by the informants as conditions to which Khmer children were susceptible. The illnesses of children were considered serious, but death was not such a common theme as it was with infants. The exception was measles—a disease which was reported frequently among the children in the study. It was feared as a potential cause of death and described as a curse wrought by evil spirits. Yet it was also considered a "normal" childhood event to which all children were highly susceptible. One perceived sequela of measles was the development of food allergies. In order to prevent these allergies, the custom is to introduce many different kinds of food to the infant prior to the age of susceptibility to developing the measles. As one mother stated, "Measles causes the child to get rashes from food. This happens because he did not get enough kind of foods when he was a baby."

There was close agreement between perceived cause and treatment of illness, both reflecting the traditional concept of imbalance. Imbalance resulting from exposure to weather changes, especially high winds, was perceived to create the condition of "bad wind." This condition was especially manifested in the child with a fever or an upper respiratory infection. The culturally recommended treatment for this imbalance was to release the bad wind through coin rubbing. The actual treatments the women used, however, were a mixture of traditional balancing remedies and scientific medications, including Tylenol, antibiotics, and cough medicines. As with the infants, the women emphasized the importance of coin rubbing before the child visited the physician, as the scientific medicine was considered strong and potentially life-threatening.

Reported avoidance behaviors mirrored the culturally recommended avoidance behaviors, suggesting the importance of verified ways of maintaining control over the disease process. For instance, a child with fever or upper respiratory infection was not allowed to exit the house. If it was absolutely necessary to leave, the child was completely bundled against the winds to avoid their contaminating effect. Another example of an avoidance behavior was preventing a child with measles from having contact with a menstruating woman. It is a cultural belief that a menstruating woman has a toxic effect upon a child, and measles would exacerbate the illness. "When a woman has her blood, she knows she is able to make children with measles get very sick and even die. It would be very dangerous for her to be near the sick child," stated one informant.

The Adolescents

The illnesses which were perceived as most commonly afflicting male and female adolescents were not the illnesses that were actually reported as occurring. The commonly reported illnesses were upper respiratory infections and chronic physical and psychiatric disabilities. The major problems perceived by the informants as affecting adolescents were menstrual disorders and "bad" behavior. Menstrual disorders were described in traditional terms as a weakness of body and blood. Irregular menses, especially if the girl missed her period for more than six months at a stretch, were considered an ominous sign of impending death. In order to insure regular periods, the traditional treatment was to regularly drink Khmer herbal tea in which an iron nail had been boiled—an interesting cultural link between regular menstrual periods and the intake of iron. The traditional treatment for dysmenorrhea, placing heated stones on the abdomen, has been replaced by heating pads. As painful menses is considered a "cold" condition, one culturally sanctioned treatment was to offer the girl heated wine. This "hot" treatment was given to restore balance and promote adequate menstrual flow. Foods to be avoided included seafood, fish sauce, and sour food.

"Bad behavior"—defined as substance abuse, sexual promiscuity, disobedience, or "acting too separate from the family"—was perceived to be a social problem primarily caused by adolescents' exposure to American culture. According to one woman, "Teenagers are bad in America. We did not have this problem before in our country. In Cambodia, we make a marriage for them and so we don't have a problem." However, should a teenager become unruly, the cultural recommendation for parental management included gentleness, avoidance of confrontation, and keeping the family and adolescent out of the legal system. "If the teenager disobeys," commented one woman, ". . . we talk sweet to him. If he does not listen, then we don't talk anymore about the problem. Mostly he needs love and we don't want to hurt his spirit." She continued by saying, "We would never call the police—never! If he is a bad child, we will call the monk to talk to him or some of the men."

Emotional problems in Khmer youth are generally presented psychosomatically rather than in acting out behavior (Messer and Rasmussen 1986). It is not uncommon for an emotionally stressed adolescent to present symptoms of abdominal pain or chronic headaches for which no organic cause can be found. One informant stated that she knows many adolescents who have headaches. She attributed these headaches to "sadness." Depression is a problem of major concern, particularly as manifested by intentional drug overdose among adolescent Khmer girls (Blanchard et al. 1986; Nolan et al. 1988).

The informants frequently stated that adolescents had no problems as long as they had full stomachs. This belief suggests continuing anxiety about the food deprivation and starvation experienced during the holocaust in Cambodia. It also suggests either a lack of knowledge or a denial of the cross-cultural issues faced by the Khmer adolescent who attends school in the American cultural milieu and returns home to the cultural milieu of Cambodia.

Traditional causation was attributed to almost all illnesses, with the exception of chronic physical and psychiatric conditions. The occurrence of these conditions was attributed to the environmental conditions of the holocaust. Among the chronic problems experienced by the adolescents in this study were recurrent headaches, neuropsychological impairment secondary to brain damage, and post-traumatic stress syndrome. Weeping bitterly, one woman described her hyperactive, brain-damaged teenage son.

> The Khmer Rouge take him away from me. He was a little child. I don't understand. He couldn't work too hard in the rice field. The soldiers were angry with him. They hold his head in the water in the rice field so he can't breathe. They hold my arms so I can't help him. Finally his friends beg the soldiers to stop. His face looked very bad when he came out of the water. Now he talks out of his head.

This teenager is receiving special education and psychological care. His mother sought scientific care, as did the other women in the study whose adolescents had chronic physical and psychiatric problems.

The Women

The informants perceived women to be highly susceptible to reproductive and gynecological disorders. The disorders included menstrual problems, vaginal infections, and complications of childbirth. Causes of these problems were reported to be a mixture of scientific and traditional reasons. Women were described as being very vulnerable and at high risk for death from complications of reproduction.

Menstrual disorders were attributed to physical weakness and violation of taboos. Menstrual taboos included eating meat, seafood, fish sauce, or sour food, or taking cold showers during menses. Another frequently reported problem was vaginal infection, a "hot" condition. The majority of informants linked vaginal infection with lack of cleanliness, "too much" sexual activity with the husband, or sexual promiscuity on the part of the husband. The informants were not able to quantify how much sexual activity was "too much." One informant stated that vaginal infection resulted from the uterus opening up during the birthing process, allowing evil spirits to enter.

The most important reproductive problem described was the crisis of *toa*. *Toa* is a cultural disease classification which does not equate to a scientific disease entity. Basically it is a state of physical collapse and failure to regain strength after childbirth, an excessive "cold" imbalance. Childbirth itself is considered a cold state, but toa is an extreme cold state in which death will surely occur if the culturally appropriate balancing activities do not occur. As such, it is intensely feared by Cambodian women. Toa can be caused by having a very weak body; resuming heavy work too soon after delivery; having sexual relations before the third postpartum month; eating taboo foods during pregnancy or in the postpartum period; or by emotional stress during or after childbirth. The women emphasized the importance of an unpleasant emotional climate as a causative factor for toa. If the birthing environment was not pleasant and the mother was not handled gently during labor, she would die. The birthing milieu was proposed as the major reason why so many women died in childbirth during the holocaust in Cambodia. To avoid toa, the laboring and postpartum woman must be sheltered from any distressing news, including information on the stillbirth or perinatal death of her infant.

Taboo foods during pregnancy include fruits, unboiled vegetables, sour foods, seafood, bamboo shoots, watermelon, jack fruit, and any foods to which the woman had shown a previous allergic reaction. If a woman proved allergic to a specific food during pregnancy, preparations would be made to treat early signs of toa should these signs occur postpartum. The allergenic food, for example, a banana, would be burned to a charcoal state and preserved. If signs of toa occurred postpartum, the ashes of the banana would be boiled down in water for three consecutive boils. The third concentrate would then be ingested by the woman. One elderly woman described another traditional treatment for toa, one which, she said, the young Khmer women scoff at. She observed, however, that the young women of today are too unwise to appreciate the benefit of this treatment, described as follows: A piece of the bed post from the marital bed would be soaked in soy sauce, then boiled down three times into a concentrate, and the ailing woman would drink the concentrate.

In discussing toa, one informant stated, "It is very strange that American women eat cold foods after childbirth, and even eat ice. They aren't afraid of toa and they don't get toa. How can this be?" During the postpartum period, the new mother must eat "hot" foods to restore balance and prevent toa. These foods include fish and meat, black pepper, salt, ginger, cooked vegetables, hot herbal teas, and liberal amounts of rice wine. In addition, she must be kept warm through the practice of "mother roasting." This is the practice whereby the Khmer postpartum woman is restored to a balanced state by placing a charcoal burner under her bed (Kemp 1985; Ong in Bowlan and Bruno 1985). In the United States this practice is sometimes continued with the use of small electrical space heaters (Frye 1989). In this study, the perceived treatments and avoidance behaviors for pregnancy and childbirth matched very consistently with the reported practices, suggesting the strength of the cultural beliefs surrounding childbearing.

Although the informants did not perceive women as susceptible to chronic degenerative diseases, such diseases were in fact quite frequently reported in this study population of relatively young women. Major problems included hypertension, diabetes, chronic gastric pain, chronic neurological pain from shrapnel and gunshot wounds, and stroke in one forty-year-old diabetic grand multipara. However, these young to middle-age Khmer women did not perceive themselves to be highly susceptible to the effects of stress. An exception was the sister of one of the informants. The behavior of the sister included hallucinations, withdrawal, and severe startle reaction. The sister, Samban, would frequently sit on the floor, rocking back and forth, asking for news about her children. The informant explained, "The Khmer Rouge shot her husband and two of her children in front of her. She cannot forget seeing them die. The other two children were taken away. She has never seen them since that time." The informant further explained, "Samban is very sad but Khmer women are not like this. We are strong."

The Men

The women perceived that stress was a major problem among men. The informants stated that Khmer women have primary responsibility for the management and recovery from stress among the men. Attributed to rumination about the sufferings during the holocaust, stress was described as "thinking too much." This state implied an imbalanced mental state, a condition out of harmony with the teachings of Buddhism. The women perceived that among the men "thinking too much" resulted in insomnia, headaches, substance abuse and violence—including attempts at suicide and potential violence toward women and children.

Identifying themselves as stress-bearers for the men, the informants described their roles as counselor and manager. When a man is "thinking too much," the woman must "talk sweet to him," the informants explained. The woman's role as counselor was defined as advising the man to ignore sad thoughts, abstain from alcohol, and spend time in prayer and meditation. If he needed spiritual help from a religious leader, such as a Buddhist monk or a Christian pastor, it was her responsibility to insure that he sought this assistance. The informants described the manager role as follows: The woman must not nag the man; she must dispose of any alcohol in the house; she must never leave him alone; and she must make him laugh. Making the man laugh was perceived to promote a state of mental balance—and her responsibility was to laugh and make him laugh, even if she did not feel like laughing.

The most frequently reported physical problems among the men were illnesses of a chronic nature, such as hypertension, gastric ulcers, headaches, and chronic pain from gunshot wounds. These illnesses were treated with coin rubbing, stress-reduction techniques administered by the women, and scientific medications. The informants perceived that these physical problems were also caused by "thinking too much."

The Elders

The elderly Khmer had the highest incidence of illness episodes per person. Acute illnesses, stress among both elderly males and females, and chronic degenerative diseases—including arthritis, hypertension, sensory losses, heart disease, diabetes, and cancer—were the problems both perceived and subsequently reported. The cultural explanations of imbalance and "thinking too much" were cited as the causative factors. With degenerative diseases among the elderly, treatments were scientific, but avoidance behaviors reflected the search for balance through avoiding excessive work, emotional distress, and "thinking too much." In spite of scientific interventions and attempts at harmony, the treatment of these conditions among the elderly was generally perceived as unsuccessful.

Promotion of Health

The women were consistent in their responses that the most important, controllable, health-promoting behavior for Khmer people of all ages was the intake of adequate amounts of food. The quality of food was not as important as the amount of food. This finding suggests that the informants are still haunted by their starvation experiences in Cambodia. The second most important health-promoting behavior was the avoidance of exposure to weather changes, especially to high winds. This finding fits with the cultural emphasis on balance and the perceived need to avoid dangerous environmental forces which could result in "bad wind."

Discussion

The Khmer have great respect for their traditional practices—which evolve out of the belief system and provide a sense of control over illness, the environment, and an alien culture. In the process of acculturation, the Khmer will most likely blend these traditional practices with American ways regardless of any advice to the contrary. Thus it is recommended that the helping professionals support this merging of cultures unless obvious harm is occurring. Professionals can be a bridge to the American culture in interpreting the need of the Khmer people to maintain traditional practices which promote equilibrium.

Parallel to the theme of equilibrium is the Buddhist principle of individual accountability. This principle extends to maintenance of smooth interpersonal relationships through generosity and non-confrontational communication. It also extends to the multiple ways in which health care decision making is done. The findings of this study indicate that individual decision making occurred among the adults, whereas health care decisions for the children and adolescents were handled by the mother—except when the problems were of a chronic or behavioral nature. These patterns of accountability and decision making within the family need to be incorporated into counseling and health education strategies used with this population.

Khmer children, like the children of Jewish concentration camp survivors, are growing up in a world radically different from that of their parents. Cultural gaps may exist between first-generation refugee parents and their growing children. The adolescents especially are caught between two cultures. The findings of this study suggest that Cambodian parents do not perceive adolescence to be a difficult passage, as do American parents. The findings also indicate that when behavioral problems occur, the American culture is perceived as the cause of the problems. The professional needs to be aware that Khmer adolescents may be experiencing loneliness and stress as they attempt to deal with fluctuating cultural expectations.

The interviews with the Cambodian refugee women suggest that women play a key role in the Khmer family in promoting the health of the children and in supporting the men emotionally when they "think too much." Given the Buddhist affirmation of selflessness, the women may attempt to support the mental health of family members to the exhaustion of their own. Thus there is a need for health education strategies which promote the value of the Cambodian woman beyond her role as the family's mental health maintainer. In addition, there should be recognition that the Khmer customs of childbirth are based upon themes of gentleness, protection, family involvement, and unity. It is especially important that professionals encourage the continuation of these practices, which enhance family solidarity.

Works Cited

Anderson, J. 1981. *The Cambodian File*. Garden City, N. Y.: Doubleday.

Baron, R., et al. 1983, December 2. "Sudden Death among Southeast Asian Refugees: An Unexplained Phenomena." *Journal of the American Medical Association* 250: 2947–51.

Becker, E. 1986. *When the War Was Over*. New York: Simon and Schuster.

Blanchard, P., et al. 1986, December 12. "Isoniazid Overdose in the Cambodian

Population of Olmsted County, Minnesota." *Journal of the American Medical Association* 256: 3131–33.

Boehnlein, J. 1987, July. "Clinical Relevance of Grief and Mourning among Cambodian Refugees." *Social Science and Medicine* 25: 765–72.

Boehnlein, J., et al. 1985, August. "One Year Follow-up of Post Traumatic Stress Disorder among Survivors of Cambodian Concentration Camps." *American Journal of Psychiatry* 142: 956–59.

Bowlan, J., and E. Bruno. 1985, Spring. *Cambodian Women's Project: Proceedings from the Conference on Cambodian Mental Health.* New York: American Friends Service Committee.

Chanda, N. 1986. *Brother Enemy.* New York: Harcourt Brace.

Chandler, D. 1972. *The Land and People of Cambodia.* Philadelphia: Lippincott.

Duncan, J. 1987. "Cambodian Refugee Use of Indigenous and Western Healers to Prevent or Alleviate Mental Illness." Ph.D. diss., University of Washington.

Ebihara, M. 1968, "Svay: A Khmer Village in Cambodia." Ph.D. diss., Columbia University.

Edmonds, I. 1970. *The Khmer of Cambodia.* Indianapolis: Bobbs-Merrill.

Fishman, C., et al. 1988, November. "Warm Bodies, Cool Milk: Conflicts in Postpartum Food Choice for Indochinese Women in California." *Social Science and Medicine* 26:1125–32.

Frye, B. 1986. "Health Beliefs of Selected Southeast Asian Cultures." M. P. H. manuscript, Loma Linda University.

———. "The Process of Health Care Decision Making among Khmer Immigrants." Ph.D. diss., Loma Linda University, 1989.

Hiegel, J. 1982. "Cooperating with Traditional Healers." *World Health Forum* 3: 231–35.

Holley, D. 1986, October 27. "Refugees Build a Haven in Long Beach." *Los Angeles Times* 1–4.

Kemp, C. 1985. "Cambodian Refugee Health Care Beliefs and Practices." *Journal of Community Health Nursing* 2: 41–52.

Kinzie, J., et al. 1984. "Post Traumatic Stress Disorder among Survivors of Cambodian Concentration Camps." *American Journal of Psychiatry* 141:645–50.

Kinzie, J., et al. 1987, August. "Antidepressant Blood Levels in Southeast Asians: Clinical and Cultural Implications." *Journal of Nervous and Mental Disease* 175: 480–85.

Kulig, J. 1988, June. "Childbearing Cambodian Refugee Women." *Canadian Nurse* 84:46–47.

Lin, E., et al. 1985. "An Exploration of Somatization among Asian Refugees and Immigrants in Primary Care." *American Journal of Public Health* 75:1080, 1084.

Marcucci, J. "Khmer Refugees in Dallas: Medical Decisions in the Context of Pluralism." Ph.D. dissertation, Southern Methodist University, 1986.

Martin, M. 1983, June. "Elements de Médecine Traditionnelle Khmere." *Seksa Khmer* 135–71.

Meinhardt, K., et al. 1984. *Santa Clara County Health Department Asian Health Assessment Project.* San Jose, Calif.: Santa Clara County Health Department, Division of Mental Health Services.

Messer, M., and N. Rasmussen 1986, August. "Southeast Asian Children in America: The Impact of Change." *Pediatrics* 78:323–29.

Mollica, R., et al. 1987, December. "The Psychological Impact of War Trauma and Torture on Southeast Asian Refugees." *American Journal of Psychiatry* 144: 1567–72.

Montero, D. 1979. *Vietnamese Americans: Patterns of Resettlement and Socioeconomic Adaptation in the United States.* Boulder, Colo.: Westview Press.

Muecke, M. 1983a. "Caring for Southeast Asian Refugee Patients in the USA." *American Journal of Public Health* 73: 431-438.

———. 1983b. "In Search of Healers: Southeast Asia Refugees in the American Health Care System." *Western Journal of Medicine (special issue): Cross Cultural Medicine* 139:31–36.

Nicassio, Paul, and J. Pate 1984. "An Analysis of Problems of Resettlement of the Indochinese Refugees in the United States." *Social Psychiatry* 19:135–41.

Nolan, C., et al. 1988, April. "Intentional Isoniazid Overdosage in Young Southeast Asian Refugee Women." *Chest* 93:803–06.

Ponchaud, F. 1977. *Cambodia: Year Zero.* New York: Holt, Rinehart and Winston.

Refugee Reports. 1985. Office of Refugee Resettlement, U. S. Department of Health and Human Services. 5:23–24.

———. 1984. *Refugees from Cambodia: A Look at History, Culture, and the Refugee Crisis.* Washington, D. C.: United States Catholic Conference.

Rosenberg, J., and S. Givens 1986, March. "Teaching Child Health Care to Khmer Mothers." *Journal of Community Health Nursing* 3: 157–68.

Shawcross, W. 1979. *Quality of Mercy.* New York: Simon and Schuster.

Song, C. 1979. *The Origin of the Cambodian-Vietnamese Border Conflict.* Falls Church, Va.: Cambodia Affairs Institute.

Mind and Body: Revising Approaches to the Analysis of *Curanderismo*

FRANÇOISE VERGÈS

> The mind is governed by the spirit of the body. If the body feels
> something the mind is affected. Deliria depends [on] how you were born
> and the people surrounding you. People envy you and therefore you
> are sad. [You] start thinking it is true what they were thinking—Mind
> is like rubber—
>
> (Ari Kiev, *Curanderismo, Mexican-American Folk Psychiatry*)

Introduction

This vision of health and illness by a *curandero* (a Mexican-American healer)[1] presents us with a conceptualization of body and mind where both are intimately interconnected and affected by the outer environment. The body—flesh, matter—possesses a spirit which alters the states of the mind, and these three forces seem at play. Within any sociocultural group, the notions of health and illness, and the ways these notions are constructed, depend upon the group's representation of the world and of life and death; their system of beliefs and values; and their reactions to the environment. Because "one suffers in/according to one's culture" (Sicard and Pottier 1987, 101), and because this culture is affected by changes in social structures and mentalities, these notions cannot be seen as static definitions, but rather as dynamic concepts constantly undergoing alterations. *Curanderismo* (Mexican-American folk medicine) thus presents us with a conceptual vista that informs us about the Mexican-American community's larger symbolic system.

I will first describe curanderismo and then examine the dynamics of gender within its vista, inquiring whether curanderismo discourse, albeit eclectic and syncretic, is ultimately logocentric and masculine. Is it, for example, a phallocentric discourse (to use the concept defined by the French philosopher Jacques Derrida)[2]—one that gives primacy to the spoken word and the phallus through a unitary drive toward a single goal and rests on dualist oppositions after the fashion of Western thought?

Curanderismo: Symbolism, Cosmology, and Western Perspectives

The stance adopted by the researcher in human sciences rests upon an epistemology that Michel Foucault has described as paradoxical, for "Not only are the human sciences able to do without a concept of man, they are unable to pass through it, for they always address themselves to that which constitutes his outer limits" (1971, 399). Scientific methods, assumptions, and discourse can obscure rather than illuminate questions of life and consciousness (Stoller 1986, 62). According to this scheme, the researcher must also "behave as if he has no judgment, as if his experiences were inconsequential, as if the contradiction between his origins and his vocation did not exist—Moreover, he will imagine that he has no politics, and he will consider that a virtue" (Diamond 1974, 94).

Researchers of Mexican-American medicine who are faithful to these rules have indiscriminately used the concepts of "modern/traditional" or "scientific/non-scientific" in their writings. It is worthwhile to remember that the modern/traditional opposition was introduced by Western scholars who, when studying Third World countries in the period following World War II, felt the necessity to create a new paradigm that would explain the differences between highly industrialized and colonized nations. "Development" came to be understood in terms of technological realizations which were the product of a capitalist system. As the post-World War II period was also the core of U. S. imperialism's consolidation throughout the world, it was important from an imperialist viewpoint that these differences be explained in cultural rather than in political terms. Hence, the notion of "modern societies" (i.e., Western, industrialized, and urban societies with an insistence on rationality and individualism) was set in opposition to that of "traditional societies" (i.e., rural, tribal, clannish societies, supposed to be stable and unaltered through time, and characterized by the refusal to change, irrationality, and the primacy of the group over the individual) (Andezian 1987). In fact, traditional society was seen as an artifact that served as a negative image of modern society.

The former was everything that the latter was not. In line with this culturally determined model, some scholars of Mexican-American folk medicine insisted on noting the "unusual, be it charming or bizarre" (Roeder 1982, 229). Others adopted stereotypical generalizations. For example, Kiev wrote that:

> An inclination to be suggestive, to react to minimal stimuli with irrational outbreaks, to stress the dramatic and the histrionic, and even in children, to accept mendacity [the state of being given to deception or falsehood, traits frequently attributed to Mexican Americans] are, according to Fenichel,[3] expressions of an individual's readiness to reactivate infantile types of objects relationships. (1968, 63)

An ahistorical, nonmaterialist approach reinforces the cultural determinism that pervades most of the studies which regard curanderismo as pre-scientific psychology. For instance, Mexican Americans are often said to avoid mental health institutions because of a stubborn attachment to folk beliefs (Kiev 1968; Madsen 1964; Saunders 1954). Chicano scholars have refuted this view and criticized its implications (Andrade 1978; Arredondo-Holden 1978; Baron 1979; Blea 1981; Rose 1978). The Chicano scholar Nick C. Vaca has stated that: "It seems certain that the major reason for the triumph of cultural determinism in the 1950's was ideological. For only by viewing the causality of the social ills of the Mexican-American as stemming from within himself—his cultural baggage—all complicity was removed from American society" (quoted in Roeder 1968, 244).

Vaca advocated an alternative "structural-environmental determinant approach which stipulated that the causes of the Mexican-American's social problems could be traced to the economic and social structure of American society and its oppressive nature" (Roeder 1982, 245).

What could this approach mean for the interpretation of curanderismo? For Chicanos, there has been first and foremost the necessity to reevaluate these practices and to demonstrate that folk medicine was the result of syncretism between Aztec and medieval European beliefs brought by the Spanish (Ortiz de Montellano 1976, 1979; Garcia 1979). But among Chicano scholars, the study of curanderos' practices has usually been done either in contrast to Anglo mental health institutions or as a celebration of precolonial theories and practices which demonstrated a significant non-Western-based body of knowledge. Curanderismo also needs to be studied from a Chicano point of view, as a system with its own rituals, symbols, dynamics, and language. Studies have offered contradictory statements regarding the use of folk medicine. While some have concluded that folk medicine is still largely used by Mexican-American families regardless of educational level, employment status, or primary language (Marsh and Hentges 1988, 257), others have indicated that utilization of curanderos is not that widespread (Farge 1975, 1977; Garza 1981; Padilla, Carlos and Keefe 1976). Nonetheless, the reality of different approaches to health and illness has convinced some physicians that a "position of awareness of patients' beliefs and open discussions of these beliefs" in order to "avoid conflicts and injurious outcomes" is needed, for the goal is to "treat the actual disease and the patient's perception of illness" (Marsh and Hentges 1988, 261–62).

For others, the healer's role could be adaptive (Clark 1959; Kiev 1968), and s/he could be seen as easing the entrance of the "traditional" Mexican into the "modern" Anglo world. In this view, curanderos and curanderas could become appendices to Western medicine and serve as mediators, as "cultural-brokers," between Mexican Americans and Anglo capitalist society, insofar as this mediation would enhance the incorporation of the former into the latter. When the social control function of folk medicine is underscored by scholars and health care professionals, we must be aware that "Western medicine also has social control functions, and the norms that it upholds are Western middle and upper class, primarily Anglo norms" (Scrimshaw and Burleigh 1978, 33). These norms are also masculine.[4]

The subtext of this apparently epistemic literacy presents a narrative that reveals a project of assimilation, an erasure of differences, rather than an interweaving of different methodologies. Indeed, we are presented with the coexistence of supposedly antithetical systems—scientific versus non-scientific, magical versus empirical—where it is assumed that one system must prevail (in this case, Western medicine). By incorporating new paradigms, the symbolic capitalism of the West is enhanced. The accumulation of new knowledge does not threaten its foundations, because the elements of these sciences are simply rearranged within the parameters of the Western, logocentric (centered on one discourse, one concept), phallocentric, and dualistic system. Indeed, the acceptance of healing networks demonstrates the flexibility of capitalism as long as these rules are abided. If nonprofessional healing remains on the fringes and is economically nonthreatening; if it preaches spiritual but not political cures; and if it plays a role in relieving tensions and anxieties that could otherwise overwhelm the functioning of society, it is deemed acceptable.

The economic interests that are at stake should not be underestimated. When curanderismo is associated with a form of spiritual "talking-cure," the fact that an important pharmacopoeia exists is obscured. Numerous scholars have confirmed that Amerindians' knowledge of curative plants has proved invaluable for Western medicine's advances in curative drugs (cocaine being the best known example). Yet the economic benefits produced by the commodification of this knowledge have never reached the national populations of the Americas.[5] In a way, this points to another facet of cultural determinism, namely the protection of the economic interests of drug companies and medical institutions. Some scholars, however, have offered an alternative to cooptation or rejection. They argue that Western "health

quotes parents pleading with administrators to recognize that not only were their children being deprived the emotional sustenance of family life, but that the family needed their help in harvest and hunting seasons, times of illness and death. The children were also being denied the kinds of inter-generational apprenticeships important to maintaining the cultural continuity of their communities. Indian parents found themselves largely powerless when their children fell ill at school; students were often exposed to communicable diseases—including measles, influenza, tuberculosis, and trachoma—that their bodies were ill-prepared to fight.

Historian Priscilla Ferguson Clement uses archival sources to examine another kind of institutional control during the same period of history (1870–1918). She scrutinizes the attitudes of the operators and volunteers of white medical charities who extended care to ill African-American women in sample northern and southern cities. Drawing documentation from case histories of several hundred women who were placed in the care of a city mission in Philadelphia and the Associated Charities of Charleston, Clement concludes that there were both similarities and differences in the ways that northern and southern institutions responded to black clients.

In the North as in the South, racial discrimination prevailed. In 1890 almost half of private and public hospitals in Philadelphia refused to admit black patients; those that did maintained segregated wards for blacks and whites. Access to hospital care in Charleston, where seventy percent of the population was black, was even more restricted. Black mortality rates, meanwhile, were higher than white mortality rates in both cities. Black women in both cities were more likely to receive outpatient care from dispensaries than inpatient hospital care. They also could turn to charities that provided assistance, food, and clothing, but few chose to do so, for a number of reasons. Screening procedures required that black clients have recommendations from whites and display "proper" deferential behavior toward their white benefactresses; such overt prejudice was less prevalent in Philadelphia. Still, the majority of black women preferred, if possible, to rely on family, church, and benevolent societies within the black community for succor in times of illness and economic distress rather than turn to any type of white-controlled infrastructure.

This same spirit of community self-reliance in the provision of health care is demonstrated in essays about midwifery by Sheila P. Davis and Cora A. Ingram, and by Gloria Waite. While few black physicians and nurses were available as practitioners to black clients in urban areas of the North and South in the early twentieth century, and while resources for black hospitals were scarce, lay midwifery remained a community tradition in rural areas.

Nursing specialists Davis and Ingram conducted a qualitative survey with midwives and individuals who received care from midwives in Alabama. Using findings from questionnaires and follow-up telephone interviews, Davis and Ingram detail elderly black midwives' philosophies about their profession and the high degree of respect accorded to them within their communities. As in Mary Petersen's experience among Native Americans, African-American midwives learned from assisting older women caretakers during prenatal and postpartum care and during childbearing. Black midwives were socially empowered by their skill and recognized as community authorities in the area of female health care, pregnancy, fertility, and childrearing. Their role was also seen as important because of the high value placed on motherhood and on the birth and care of black children. In the last portion of their study, Davis and Ingram trace the development of laws restricting lay midwifery and the modern movement toward certification and clinically trained nurse-midwives, changes that have marginalized and demeaned elderly black midwives and the values and philosophies of care that they represent.

Gloria Waite also addresses the history of lay midwifery among African Americans. She profiles the work of the Traditional Childbearing Group, Inc., of Boston, whose goal is to combine modern midwife-attended home birthing with traditional values and practices. Like traditional lay midwives, Traditional Childbearing Group, Inc., practitioners offer a full range of services designed to promote maternal and child health, including nutrition, breastfeeding, and child care and parenting skills. Founders were motivated by the secondary provision of health care to African Americans and by the exclusion of black women from medical practitioning. Waite places the recent history of the Traditional Childbearing Group, Inc., in the context of the legal history of midwifery and in the historical contexts of separate institution-building within the African-American community, the black family, and the feminization of poverty. The Traditional Childbearing Group, Inc., addresses these issues, seeks to reverse the effects of racism and discrimination, and represents a return to the kinds of community-based values that Davis and Ingram emphasized in their essay: spirituality, family, self-help, home birth, the safety of black women and children, and the empowerment of black providers and of black mothers who have control over their own childbearing experiences.

Part Three concludes with Caroline Westbrook Arnold's study of breastfeeding among African-American (primarily Haitian), Hispanic, and Asian immigrants. Just as there has been a movement in childbirth practices away from natural and social meanings toward technological and scientific controls, and away from home and community settings toward institution-alization, so breastfeeding has given way to bottle-and-formula feedings, natural methods to mechanistic ones controlled by the interests of large corporations. Arnold describes the detrimental effect on minority children of the trend away from breastfeeding. Children of color suffer higher in-fant mortality rates and lower birthweights than Anglo-American children. Nursing supplies infants with essential nutrition and immunities, as well as an emotional bond. It also benefits the health of the mother by minimizing postpartum depression, helping reduce the size of the uterus, and delaying the resumption of ovulation. After demonstrating the health benefits of a return to breastfeeding, Arnold discusses the promotion of breastfeeding and the ways in which it has been limited by institutional policies, the bias of physicians, and the financial interests of formula-distribution companies. Arnold stresses the importance of social support networks for mothers to counteract these barriers. In addition, she describes traditional health philosophies that inform ideas of illness among Latin-American, Haitian, and Southeast-Asian immigrants to the United States.

Mary Petersen:
A Life of Healing and Renewal

JOANNE B. MULCAHY WITH MARY PETERSEN

And when we speak we are afraid
our words will not be heard
not welcomed
but when we are silent we are still afraid.

—Audre Lorde

Introduction

Kodiak Island lies in the heart of the Gulf of Alaska almost two hundred and fifty miles southwest of Anchorage. The rich waters surrounding the island and its central location have made Kodiak a crossroads for trade and cultural exchange since the early days of exploration. Beginning with Russian contact in the late eighteenth century, the indigenous Alutiiq people have adopted aspects of Russian, European, and American cultures into their hunting and fishing culture, often through force by the colonizing group. Today, the island's Native population lives poised between the modernity of Kodiak's lucrative fishing industry and the maintenance of traditional ways. From new bilingual programs to recreating traditional dances, Native people are now reclaiming aspects of their cultural identity lost or suppressed during the past two centuries.[1]

When I moved to Kodiak in 1979, I knew little about the cultural or natural landscape I would encounter. I was soon spending hours in the Alaska

148

collection at the local library, gleaning what I could from the diaries of the Russian fur traders and missionaries who had colonized much of southwestern Alaska. They recorded a romantic and exciting history of clashes between the human and natural worlds and between cultural groups vying for economic resources. I was struck by the absence of women from both archival sources and more recent popular literature. Later, when I began working as the Program Coordinator for the Kodiak Women's Resource Center (KWRC), I traveled to the six Native villages which ring the island and had the opportunity to meet many Native women whose ancestors had lived on Kodiak for centuries. I visited with them in their homes, picked berries and grass for basketmaking, and sometimes helped them escape a cycle of violence wrought by the cultural changes of the last century. Their stories of life on the island stood in marked contrast to what I had been reading. Their focus was the everyday world of giving birth, raising families, and subsistence living. They also chronicled the importance of women's practice as healers in roles which had continued until well into the 1960s, a version of medical history which differed substantially from the written literature. I collected oral histories from women all over Kodiak between 1979 and 1981 and when I returned on field trips every two years throughout the 1980s. I began to piece together other versions of history which traced the continuity in women's roles as healers and their strength in facing social problems. Of all of the remarkable women that I came to know, the memory of Mary Petersen Simeonoff stayed with me.

I met Mary in the summer of 1980. In my position at the KWRC, I was responsible for the arrangement of safe homes for women in danger from domestic violence. One night, through efforts coordinated with the Kodiak Area Native Association (KANA), a woman in her fifties from the village of Akhiok was flown in, silent and afraid. I still recall my amazement that such a young-looking woman had endured the hardships she described with so few visible scars. I could envision the life she was escaping: nights spent , cowering, sometimes beneath the bed, other times under the floorboards of the house, to escape the wrath and beatings—and even once the knife—of a man transformed by alcohol, an otherwise good husband. She would try to hide in a treeless terrain where there were no hiding places, a small village where everyone knew the circumstances of her life. She would wait—for daybreak, for him to sober up—so that she could go and make breakfast, ready the kids for school, and prepare for her own long morning as a kindergarten teacher. Afternoons she worked at the clinic as the community health aide, a position that links villages throughout Alaska with the centralized health care system. As dusk approached, so did the familiar feelings of dread and anticipation of another night of violence and fear.

Mary left Kodiak for the shelter in Anchorage, and I often pondered her fate. Several years later, in 1985, I was looking for a Mary Petersen whom I had been advised to seek out for her knowledge of traditional healing. I was amazed to discover the Mary Simeonoff that I knew from Akhiok, now using her maiden name. Living in Anchorage, she had begun a new life after leaving the village. Later, a friend told me that she had stayed on as a volunteer in the shelter for battered women in Anchorage, aiding women from all over the state.

Mary is one of a growing number of Native women who have left violent homes, sometimes even their villages, to begin life again. Domestic violence is certainly not restricted to Native homes or to villages, but it is a particularly unwelcome and frequent companion to modernization and cultural change in Alaska. Some aspects of Mary's story are part of a typical pattern of women escaping domestic violence. Like many women, she has felt the effects of alcoholism as well as violence, and, more recently, the suicide of a son.[2] However, she is also a noteworthy example of personal courage and cultural tenacity. She displayed unequalled strength in her ability to relocate and begin her life again, creating a powerful role model for her children and other Alaskan women.

Mary now serves as a bridge between cultures. While her story is unique, she is also important as a representative of women's roles and traditional life on Kodiak. Her family followed a subsistence lifestyle during her early years, moving seasonally to hunt and fish. As a bearer of traditional knowledge, her skills are wide-ranging. She was a midwife with extensive knowledge of herbs and healing methods. She knows the Alutiiq language, basketweaving, and the songs, stories, and celebrations of the Russian Orthodox Church. Living through periods of intense cultural change, Mary integrated traditional life with working for wages in the canneries, as a teacher, and as a community health aide. Living now in a trailer in Anchorage, she maintains a subsistence lifestyle to the degree that she can, returning to the village to fish in the summer. Mary's maintenance of her Native heritage is evident throughout her life, from traditional foodways and basketmaking to her patterns of speech.[3] It is precisely these aspects of traditional culture to which the younger generation of Natives is now turning for strength and example in patterning their lives.

Mary Petersen's life is the success story of a woman strong enough to escape a cycle of violence that encircled her for years. There is yet a bittersweet quality to her story. She lives now on the edges of longing, waiting for the summer fishing seasons and the ritual world of Russian Christmas when she can return to the village. Mary is an exile, wrenched from the land and her culture by alcohol and violence and the wreckage of cultural destruction. Her story offers a view of village life in transition and chronicles one woman's quest to create cultural meaning from a shattered past. Mary's story deserves wide recognition for what she can tell us about women healers in Kodiak history, cultural change in Native-Alaskan life, and the resilience of the human spirit.

Early Memories and Traditional Life

Mary Petersen was born in 1927 near Akhiok, a village on the southern tip of Kodiak Island. As she describes her home, it was at Red River or "Ayakulik" between a settlement called Carmel and the present-day village of Karluk. Originally she had eighteen brothers and sisters, but the toll of disease and hardship gradually reduced their number to eight. They lived in the early years with her grandparents, who had a fox and mink farm, and then moved with the fishing and hunting seasons. Her father fished in Karluk in the summers, and she moved back and forth between Akhiok and Ayakulik until she began school in Karluk when she was six. Some of her strongest and happiest memories recreate life in the villages, particularly events surrounding the Russian Orthodox holidays. The religious rituals and sense of community fostered by the Church connected the diverse places of Mary's childhood. The calendar divides into summers at fishcamps and the central celebration of light in the winter darkness, Christmas "starring." This Slavonic folk tradition is named for the large, brightly decorated and tinsel laden stars villagers carry as they travel from house to house celebrating in prayer and song. "Starring," referred to in Western Alaska as "Selaviq" (from the Rusian, "Slavit," "praise or glory"), illustrates the common integration of Russian and indigenous traditions on Kodiak and in other areas of Alaska.[4] Christmas celebrations are enmeshed in Mary's memories of life in the villages of Karluk and Akhiok.

> In Karluk, we'd go "starring" all over
>   and then walk clear way over and cold!
> We never used to wear pants.
> We'd wear dresses and long socks,
>   and we'd go starring.
> I'd just follow the star from house to house.
> I just like the way they sing, you know,
> I just loved hearing them singing,
>   trying to learn,
>   trying to remember.

Mary also recalls the finale to the season's festivities, the "devil dance," which inaugurated the new year on the night of January 14th as the ghost of the old year was banished by the "devils." Her memories of these ritual events create a rich tapestry of Native life in the villages well after the U. S. purchase of Alaska in 1867. Despite attempts by the government to eradicate the Native language and culture, Mary's stories—part of an ongoing oral traditional—attest to the tenacity of many cultural practices well into the twentieth century. Moving from the public arena of ritual, her stories of everyday, private life open another whole arena of memory, one shaped by and expressive of women's reality.

"Helping" and Traditional Healing

A central and enduring metaphor for women's lives on Kodiak emerges from Mary's stories of healing and of "helping" other women through her practice as a midwife. Women throughout the island articulate enormous respect for the village midwife and her role as an everyday healer. These reflections carry the threads of historical memory back to the earliest women healers, who provided a general knowledge of herbs and medicinal plants.[5] Midwives continued to practice in the Kodiak villages well into the 1960s, long after it was assumed the practice had died out. As with childbirth in many other traditional cultures, midwives provided prenatal care in the steambath ("banya" from the Russian for "bath"), repositioned the fetus through massage, eased women through the process of birth, and stayed with a woman for a week or more beyond the birth to provide care and support.[6] Women's stories of the midwives take shape around several recurring images, epecially that of the "knowing" midwife "helping" women through the birth ritual.

Becoming a midwife was a natural transition for Mary from her early days of simply being with the old people, "helping" in whatever ways she could. From her first recall, she knew that she wanted to be a nurse and just "be among the old people because they used to tell stories." "Helping" was later formalized into working as a midwife and community health aide. Her understanding of many herbal treatments and cures was bound to a belief in the good health and superior knowledge of the elders.

> *Ever since I could remember,*
> *I was taking care of old people,*
> *helping them spill their spit cans.*
> *Even if they're not sick,*
> *I like to be around them*
> *and HELP them.*
> *Just be among them.*
> *Everybody learned from each other,*
> *from the elder people.*
> *They would tell them what to do,*
> *and try to keep each other fed good, you know.*
> *If anybody got sick,*
> *the older people would tell them what to do.*
> *They used vinegar and water,*
> *soak a piece of rag*
> *and wrap it around their feet for fever.*
> *Or they would use potatoes,*
> *put it in a rag,*
> *put it on the bottom of the feet.*
> *When they use those potatoes,*

they turn real black.
That means it's pulling the fever down real fast.
If they don't get black,
  then it's not working.
If they stay white,
  they know they're gonna lose that person.

Mary learned to use chamomile and a variety of other herbs that are common throughout the island. But the strongest "medicine from the land" that she remembers is the fern-like plant that grows amidst the blackberry bushes up in the hills, the one they call "mogulnik" on the north end of the island.[7] The plant is a strong symbol in Mary's mind, opening a floodgate of memories about the older healers she learned from. When she returns to the village now, she goes up on the mountain to find this medicine, which cured her when doctors told her she had tuberculosis. Affirming the many stories about the superiority of Native healing, Mary insisted that the medical doctors did not know how she had been cured. "The next time they checked on it," she said, "it was gone. I guess because I BELIEVE in it." As a symbol, it recreates all that is good about life in the village, connecting past and future.

Back in them days,
  they had to look to the land just to survive.
  they probably tried everything.
And the OLD PEOPLE,
  they just knew what to do.
There's ALL kind of medicine in the LAND
  that we don't use now that's real important.
This one, it looked like a fern . . .
  this tea . . .
Some of them call it, "chaihuwok."
  it smells real good and has tiny white flowers . . .
It smells so good,
  so good!
That's what I remember.

These memories are congruent with those of other villagers—the use of "medicine from the land," stories of using potatoes and vinegar to draw out fever, the triumph of traditional healing over Western medicine. However, Mary's understanding of healing bridges two worlds. She relates stories about Katya, a "blind old lady" from Karluk who cured her of an eye ailment when she was a child. Following her advice, Mary's father cleaned her eyes first with a newborn boy's urine and then with salt water from the ocean. "That ocean water must have have been good," she said, "that and the urine. I was thinking it's sterile, you know, and clean." She displays an awareness of Western scientific thinking in noting the presumed sterility of the urine.

Similarly, she explains that people were seldom sick in the old days because they ate the moldy dried fish they saved for winter. "When I found out that penicillin was made out of mold, I was thinking no wonder they never got sick!" However, Mary also firmly adheres to the traditional side of healing, to belief and faith, and to an intuitive "knowing." This is evident in her faith in the blind old lady, the medicine "from the land," and, especially, in her strong memories of Oleanna Ashouwak.[8]

> *She was REALLY something!*
> *She just KNEW!*
> *She helped the midwives, too.*
> *I guess she just liked taking care of people.*
> *She felt it was her job to do.*
> *I guess the Elders in Kaguyak trained her.*
> *She was really something.*

In describing her own ways of "helping" people, Mary stressed the intuitive part of knowledge and a respect for learning from lived experience. She described the early days when the chief would call the whole community to decide on a midwife if there weren't enough women practicing. The degree of formal initiation varied in the villages; for Mary, it was a relatively informal process. She became a midwife in 1947 when she was twenty years old. She stressed that "nobody really showed me anything, but I just KNEW what to do because I had so many brothers and sisters." She had watched other midwives deliver children, and, even where apprenticeship patterns are more formalized, Mary believes that certain aspects of healing cannot be learned. This belief in "knowing" as an intuitive, often religiously inspired knowledge, is central to the oral tradition about women healers on Kodiak. It is evident in Mary's memory of her first birth, where she reveals belief to be pivotal:

> *First time by myself, I happened to be home alone*
> *when one of the girls was ready to have her baby.*
> *I guess it was one of my sisters.*
> *So, I delivered her baby,*
> *and it was like I had been doing it for a longtime.*
> *I just KNEW, you know,*
> *knew what to do,*
> *Like there was somebody with me*
> *but using my hands and my mind.*
> *No fear,*
> *or worry*
> *or excitement.*
> *Only after the baby was born,*
> *when I got everything done,*
> *got the mother settled and drinking tea,*

then I started shaking and sweating ALL OVER!
When I think about it,
  it was like coming out of a trance,
  like it wasn't me.
I always think that God was using my hands to help this lady.

Mary's stories of births were, like narratives from all over the island, accounts of creating a warm atmosphere for a woman, a place of privacy and comfort. She reinforced the view held throughout the island that banyas were essential. The only problem she had in bearing eighteen children was during one pregnancy, when they could not get wood for the banya. Women she helped started coming to the banyas on a weekly basis at about five months. "If it's too small, then the heat might make you start bleeding." She used heat to detect both pregnancy and the position of the fetus, saying that "without hot packing, you can't press down and feel it too easy." Oleanna had also taught her how to feel for the heartbeat, checking consistently throughout the pregnancy. When a woman was ready to deliver, a sheet was hung on the window to alert the midwife to come. If too many people knew a woman was in labor, she related, "you'll labor long because they're sitting, worrying, wondering." During delivery, if a woman did "labor long," she usually squatted to speed the process. Generally the midwife would hold her hand, support her legs, and help her through what Mary insists were generally short and uncomplicated labors. "Back then, you start laboring and have it in a couple of hours . . . maybe three, because the midwives took care of them." After the delivery, she would stay for the first night, then return each morning to change and bathe the baby "until the navel dries out." She also wrapped infants in pieces of sheets cut to the width of ace bandages to keep them from moving around while sleeping.

The continuum of Mary's life was marked by her role as "helper" in many aspects of village life. It is so central to her self-image that she laughed when I asked when she "became" the health aide. "I don't know. I always was! My whole life, really, since I was young, I just wanted to help." She tried to foster the same sense of warmth that she created in the birth-setting in the clinic, in her other job as a kindergarten teacher, and in her home life. The last arena proved to be the most difficult. Her first marriage at fifteen, she reported, was arranged by her father in the hopes that he would have fewer mouths to feed. The pattern of choosing a man considerably older was common, Mary said, so that "he could take care of her." "Back then," she recalled, "as soon as a girl starts her menstruation, they marry her off."

Mary, in recalling how young women were treated during menarche, describes puberty seclusion as part of the "way things were." Documentation by early explorers describes the isolation of a young woman in a small, low hut for at least six months as the norm. After that time, she was welcomed back to her parent's home, fully initiated as a woman. During subsequent periods, a woman was sequestered for only the duration of the bleeding, after which she would wash herself and return to the village.[9]

Puberty seclusion practices on Kodiak were similar to those of other Native peoples and other cultural groups. There are varied interpretations of such practices a well as the attitudes towards women which surround them. On one hand, the seclusion of women is regarded as a negative reflection of their status as dangerous and potentially "polluting."[10] However, in some cultural settings, women identify puberty seclusion as a positive source of knowledge, power, sexual autonomy, or female solidarity. The "symbolic potency" associated with menstrual blood and accompanying practices has placed studies of menstruation at the center of many anthropological explorations of religion, taboo, and women's status.[11] On Kodiak today, women's stories affirm that these practices were continued until recent decades and that many of the attendant beliefs about women have been maintained. Mary recalls that:

> *They made a tent for us in the corner of the house.*
>   *We couldn't see anyone.*
> *And they don't let you see the light for five days.*
>   *If you do,*
>   *you might get blind.*
> *They don't want you around people.*
> *They didn't let you on a skiff*
>   *or around fish*
>   *especially summertime.*
> *Even older women,*
>   *after they have babies,*
>   *they won't let them on the skiff*
>   *or go to fishcamp*
>   *when they're having their period.*
> *They said that the odor of the blood is strong!*
> *In the spring,*
>   *why do you get a cold?*
>   *Why do you get sick?*
> *Cause the ground is thawing,*
> *and you see heat coming up.*
> *All that bacteria is coming up from the ground,*
>   *and we get sick.*
> *That's how they felt about a woman when she's having her period.*
> *And because of the odor,*
>   *and what we call bacteria.*
> *If I had TB now,*
>   *I couldn't even talk to you.*
>   *I'd have to wear a mask.*

That's how they felt about a woman with her period.
Especially the new ones,
* when they first start.*
For a whole year,
* they wouldn't go traveling in a boat.*
After a year,
* when they're not having their period,*
* they could go.*
Now, the real old people, they say,
* no wonder everything is disappearing...*
People get SICK *all the time*
* because the young girls are here and there...*
And the fish is disappearing.
* We don't have fish like we used to.*
They blame it on the girls traveling around
* when they're having their period.*
The old people get SO *mad.*

Mary's recollections about menarche reflect Kodiak women's ambivalence about cultural change. On one hand, "the way things were" is viewed with longing. However, traditional marriage patterns and Mary's father's plan to "marry her off" began a cycle of pain from which she only recently escaped. Initially, the plan backfired. Mary's first husband was not much of a provider, and she was soon back in her parents' house with her two young children. When her husband drowned a few years after their marriage, she remarried another man from the village.

Change: The Roots of Violence

Mary's other memories of village life are equally complex, full of bittersweet longing and painful recollection. On one hand, there are memories of the bountiful days of plenty from the land and the sea. These were times infused with ritual, when everyone helped one another and people were much healthier.

To me, it seemed like it was better then
* because everybody got along.*
It was hard to get food,
* but we never really ran out, you know,*
* because there was the* LAND
* where we could get food, and the ocean.*
The only other things would be sugar and flour and milk.
* And we hardly used them.*
Food was so CHEAP *then!*
My goodness, for fifty dollars, my dad would bring home a SKIFF *load of*
* groceries.*

My goodness! Everything in big sacks...
They all helped each other, too,
  and nobody was ever alone.
Everything that anyone ever did, they helped.

Mary's longing for the old days is sometimes overshadowed by more specific and often painful recollections of life in the villages. She grows distant when she recalls times of hardships and an undercurrent of neglect by her parents. When I asked what school was like, she remembered times when her parents simply "weren't there":

"American Christmas" was a sad day for me.
  when I was going to school,
My mom and dad never came to the school program.
All the other parents would be there but mine,
  but I tried to perform the best I could.
Sometimes my tears are coming down, you know.

Memories of violence in her own home emerge when Mary talks about changes in village life. She cannot fix a point in her own past when things began to be different, but she related the stories of things she has "always heard."

The old people,
  the way they talked about it,
    the Russians started it.
  they came and traded stuff.
One old man used to say
  that they had foxes all over the village.
They'd dry the furs, you know,
  and pile them as tall as a rifle or a shotgun.
For those, they'd get the gun.
They got gypped so much!
They brought diseases, all kinds.
  the White people brought them in,
  drinking and diseases.
We'd be better off without the White people.
They came and changed our way of life.
  "You'll be better off with this and that."
They try and make money out of us.
They didn't do so much drinking before,
  but I remember it already with my dad.
  I remember I was always scared.
My dad gets jealous
  even when he's not drunk
  and beats up on my mom.

But she never left him,
  and as he grew older,
    he got better.

The mark of violence on Mary's life, both as a child and as an adult, has become increasingly typical in Alaska for both Native and non-Native women, in villages and towns.[12] Statewide patterns are reflected on Kodiak, where social problems wrought by the extreme weather conditions, an erratic economy, and a transient fishing population have made violence endemic to life in town. Over half the reported cases are alcohol-related. Those problems were finally being addressed when I began working for the Kodiak Women's Resource Center in 1979. The center had been founded by a group of volunteers in 1976 as a grass-roots community project to address women's needs. They began with a crisis line and were eventually brought under the umbrella of a statewide network of women's organizations. Emergency aid to rape and domestic-violence victims was the funding priority, and most of the center's efforts were initially concentrated in town. Outreach to the villages, which began later, was an equally important but problematic arena. There was an understandable degree of mistrust of outside social service agencies, which had suppressed Native culture in the name of reform over a number of years. But through cooperation with KANA, the KWRC was eventually able to offer services to women in the villages.

At about the time that KWRC was beginning to reach the villages, Mary was working in the school until noon, then in the clinic until six in the evening. She would often be up all night with a patient, work all day, and return to a night of violence and fear. Of Mary's original eighteen children, the eleven who lived to adulthood were raised in the alcoholic household of her second marriage. She has nightmarish memories of never knowing what would happen, when and to where she would have to flee. Recounting nights of sleeping outside, hiding, running out in her nightgown without shoes, she says, "Oh, when I think about it, sometimes I wonder if it were true!"

When she married for the second time, Mary was unaware of the problems she would encounter. She had developed an "immunity," she said, "because I grew up in that kind of violent life." But her husband was also a radically different individual when he was sober. Mary tried to stay with him for the sake of the children and grandchildren and because, like so many abused women, she hoped he would change.

He was a DIFFERENT person altogether when he's sober.
  You wouldn't even know he's around!
  You wouldn't believe,
He could be good.
Some of my kids didn't really believe
  that he was that kind of man.

They never seen him in that violent way of his when he's drinking.
He made sure that the older boys didn't see him
because he knows what will happen to him.
They protected me.
He almost got killed by one of them,
the second from my first husband.
He's got scars on his face.
That's where I got this scar,
stopped that knife!
Just grabbed it,
just when it was hitting straight for his neck,
And they both weren't that drunk, either.
My older kids wonder
how I stayed alive,
and why I waited that long to leave him, you know. The older I was getting,
the more scared I was getting of him.
I couldn't stand it no more,
that constant drinking.

When Mary finally left that August night in 1980, she called the number on one of the small, yellow, crisis-line cards distributed by the Kodiak Women's Resource Center. A KANA employee who also served on the board of KWRC went down to the village to help, and she sought shelter first in Kodiak. "I didn't know anyone could help," she now says, "I lived in a village my whole life and I didn't know that people outside could be so nice." It was then that I initially heard pieces of her story, one that is both typical and unique. She came to Kodiak as one of an increasing number of village women who were beginning to discover that they could leave. Mary Petersen, however, was different in an essential way. Frequently, women from the villages seek temporary shelter and return home within a few days, often to the same violent situation. But Mary got on a plane to Anchorage, leaving her children and the village existence whose structure and rhythms had given her life meaning for so many years. I wondered then if she knew how much she would miss that life. The other feeling which assailed me that night when she first spoke of her past was one of tragic irony. I was amazed that women so powerful and central to village life had come to find themselves in such an extremely vulnerable position. As she took up the story when we met in 1985, unaware that I was the person she had met that summer night, an eerie sense of déjà-vu took hold.

They always ask me how did I do it.
How did I get the mind and strength to leave?
I was getting to where I was scared all the time.
I couldn't stand the drinking all the time.

I tried it,
  but I don't know how people could go
  for days and days and days...
I was getting sick and scared,
  and he kicked me out.
I knew I had to make a move sometime, I guess.
  I thought, "It's now or never."
  I decided.

Living in Exile

Mary Petersen is no longer afraid. "It feels so good not to be in fear now!" she says. "I do what I want to, and I'm not afraid and thinking, 'Oh, I shouldn't do that. He'll be mad.'" She has settled into her life in Anchorage now and recreated pieces of village life there. But it has taken time and painful years of readjustment. After the shock of leaving, the women from the shelter extended support, and her children in Anchorage helped as much as they could. But when the chaos settled, longing set in: longing for the fishing camp and the sweetness of salmon berries in summer, the Christmas traditions that she had lived for, and the satisfaction of her work as a midwife and health aide. She hated leaving behind her work and the familiar surroundings of village life, but those things, she says, she can recreate. "But me, I can't bring myself back."

Mary's escape from an abusive setting is also expressed in terms of "helping" others—in this case, protecting her children from trouble. She feared that in trying to protect her, they might instead have harmed themselves. Thus she views her departure not as cutting bonds, but rather of strengthening them.

My kids will feel hurt
  and blame their dad forever for it,
  and they might even hurt HIM.
They always told him not to touch mom on the face, you know.
So to save him
  and to save my sons from getting thrown in jail
  and save myself,
I HAVE to get out.
I HAVE to keep my sons from getting into trouble.

Fear of repercussions kept Mary from returning to Akhiok that first year. She met some new people among the city's large Native population and often saw her children who lived in Anchorage. The others flew the several hundred miles from Kodiak whenever they could, bringing fish and berries. She could not get the "tea" she missed so badly, the "medicine from the land," but she was managing. She got to church at St. Nicholas whenever she could find a ride. It was not the same—a big church, a big city—but she was getting by, until the holidays came. Then, she says, "Oh, when the holidays came, I just hurt! And I could just see it, just right there, picture it . . . right at twelve o'clock, the bell is ringing. . . . ." Mary grows very distant when she describes the yearning she experiences for the village. It is in the years of embedded memory, of knowing the landscape intimately—where the fish are, where to find the "medicine from the land," the steps followed from house to house behind the Russian "star." The pain is visceral, as raw as the violence that drove her away.

She now returns to the village at least twice a year, for Russian Orthodox holidays and in the summer to fish. She was afraid of seeing her ex-husband the first two years that she went back for the holidays, but now the fear has subsided. There is a sense of mission in Mary's return each year. Initially, she says, she went back because "they kept calling me to lead the 'starring' and I had to go because I want them to learn." She is firmly devoted to helping transmit the Native traditions which the village is so fearful of losing. She hopes that the Alutiiq language she once taught in a bilingual pilot program will start up again, but that is contingent upon government funds. She can teach the Alutiiq and Slavonic "starring" songs which have given her so much joy. In summer, she can climb the hills to look for herbs and medicines, maybe teaching her grandchildren how to spot the small, white flowers which promise good health. Fishing is again a central part of her year, as well as an economic necessity. When I asked if she would endanger her job by leaving Anchorage, she was indignant:

> If she don't let me go,
> I'll just pack up and leave ANYWAY!
> Because if I don't go fishing for the summer,
> I'll be miserable all the time.
> Next January and the holidays will be a LONG ways off yet, you know.
> I can't wait that long.
> I have to go home for the summer anyway
> to go fishing.
> I make more money there in three weeks than I do all year here.

Mary has changed, grown stronger in the time away. Living in Anchorage, she has also come to value her privacy after so many years of caring for others. Having raised eleven children and worked for years as a health aide and a village midwife, she had forgotten what it felt like to be alone. When I asked if she would consider going back for good or moving to Kodiak, she responded negatively. "If I do, you know what will happen to me. My house will be full all the time, and I will have no peace." She also cited the proximity to her ex-husband as a reason. He still bothers her when she is in the village if he has been drinking. "Here," she said, "at least I'm a little protected."

But Mary also realizes that village life has changed. Some of the changes, she hopes, will be positive, especially for women who are suffering from the effects of the kind of violence and alcoholism that ruled her life for so long. She also hopes that her example will help others to leave or take action in the face of violence. She does not want her daughters to live in the same cycle that she saw perpetuated from her earliest days in Karluk through her adult years in Akhiok. One daughter who is pregnant has chosen not to marry because of fear of violence. "She saw what life I went through," Mary says, "and now her sister's going through the same thing." She is philosophical with her daughters, telling them the thoughts which have served her well throughout seemingly unbearable years. "You have your ups and downs, but as long as you're still able, you know, but you have ups and downs." She added that life will be better for them because "the men are afraid now that the women are getting smarter. They know where to go, what to do. Sign a complaint on them, and they'll get thrown in jail." The Women's Resource Center has grown and built a permanent shelter since the days when Mary sought help in Kodiak. They have changed their name to the Kodiak Women's Resource and Crisis Center. They work in close contact with KANA on outreach to the villages, where violence is now on the decline. Perhaps the new health programs geared to cultural awareness have served to benefit women's safety by raising the level of self-esteem among men and women. Or perhaps, as Mary suggests, women are just "getting smarter." On another level, Mary knows that changes in the village have made it a place that she's not sure she could go back to. Life is not easy there for older people. "Helping" has been supplanted by cash exchange. "I can't roll a drum of oil," Mary says, "I'd have to hire someone. I have sons, but my mom, she has to holler and scream to get anything done. She has to cut her own wood. If I went back, I'd have the same problems. It's so HARD because they don't help each other like they used to." Other changes, in the realm of values, are less concrete. Mary believes that people think differently today, despite recent efforts to reinstitute Native traditions. Like other elders throughout Kodiak, she cites the unwillingness of the next generation to "listen" as the biggest problem. "They're getting so sassy now, you can't talk to them. If you try to tell them something, they say, 'Oh don't be so old-fashioned!' It's not old-fashioned. 'Old-fashioned people lived better than you do now,' I tell them."

Mary's account becomes part of the collective perspective of elders all over Kodiak: balancing the superiority of "old-fashioned" village life with the benefits of change. Like so many other women, she adamantly defends the "old ways," especially those surrounding midwifery, childbirth, and healing. But deeper in memory is lodged the recall of violence and unhappiness in her own home, even in the "old days." Change has intensified those problems, but also brought help in the form of outside agencies like KWRC. Life is better now, she tells herself, since she can live out her Native traditions at least part of the year in Akhiok and bring back the bits of village life that she selects. Her freezer in Anchorage is stocked with salmon and halibut, and there is a full supply of smoked and canned fish for winter. Perhaps she also knows that her exile is not simply from a place, but from a time—a mental landscape of the past where village life revolved around the dictum to "help" and to share, where healing worked because people believed, and the Church's role was, like its placement in the village, central.

> *The old people,*
>   *telling me stories,*
>   *telling me what not to do . . .*
> *Sometimes, now, when I'm by myself, you know,*
>   *and I go back,*
> *I wish,*
>   *Ooh, I wish them days were here now!*
>   *I WISH it was those days now!*
> *And summertime.*
> *Then I get to go by myself and pick berries*
>   *and I go fishing by myself,*
>   *no husband around.*
> *And then putting fish away.*
> *And Christmas.*
>   *They're the happiest.*
>   *They're the happiest.*

It was November, and gazing out the window at the traffic in the shopping mall, Mary was far away, thinking of the two short months until she could go back.

> *December will go by real fast!*
> *I'm getting worried . . .*
>   *will the weather be good?*
> *I get nervous . . .*
>   *I don't like to fly much.*
> *And I'm getting ready . . .*
> *In the old days, Russian Christmas is coming*
>   *and I'm getting ready,*
>   *preparing,*
>   *getting the house cleaned up.*
> *Everybody is trying to make their house look better than the other.*
> *Then everybody gets their home blessed,*
>   *all four corners with holy water.*
> *Then everybody drinks the water so you won't get sick.*
> *and I still believe.*

I always think,
  so many times I get sick,
  So many times I get sick,
    and somehow or another, I always get out of it.
I don't know . . .
I guess I believed.

Mary's belief constitutes an entire world of cultural values which have sustained her through a life of hardships, informing her ability to heal as a midwife and a health aide. Her greatest struggle now is to provide a critical link to the next generation by transmitting those values, a role she once filled as midwife and one from which she is now physically as well as emotionally displaced. Like many of the elders on Kodiak, she insists that the next generation just doesn't "listen." But as Native people throughout Alaska draw from the wellspring of tradition to find sources of strength to combat the social ills of alcoholism, violence, and cultural disruption, there is every reason to believe that this generation will turn once again to the ways of "helping" and "knowing" which informed the world of their grandmothers.

Epilogue: April 25, 1992

At 11:30 p.m. on a cool, clear spring night, I am preparing to attend the midnight service in celebration of Russian Orthodox Easter in the village of Akhiok. The small church on a bluff overlooking the water is already filling with people; preparations have begun for tomorrow's feast. In a small house in the center of the village where she now lives, Mary Petersen is making *kulich*, an elaborately decorated Russian Easter bread. For the first time in over a decade, she is spending Easter in her Native village, a place she never thought could be safe enough for her return. "It feels so good to be back," she says.

Earlier in the spring, Mary came back to a village transformed by sobriety. The Akhiok that she returned to is not the village of her youth, but far closer to a genuine community, one built on Native values and reciprocity rather than the alienated group of individuals that she left in 1980. The sobriety movement, which had taken hold in the 1980s, was temporarily disrupted by the Exxon Valdez oil spill and clean-up efforts, but now has gained momentum. Few villagers are drinking; most contribute to the collective story of how Akhiok is healing from the wounds of cultural destruction, fragmented family life, alcohol abuse, and violence.

Mary returned to a village equally transformed by a revitalization of Native life. Part of the recovery story is a renewed pride in what it means to be Alutiiq. As proclaimed on a t-shirt produced for a recent elders conference, Native people are "healing through our culture." In the past decade, villagers in Akhiok have stopped drinking, recreated a sense of their native identity, and relearned a number of traditional skills. Beyond the Orthodox church sits a "barabara," a traditional sod house constructed with grant funds from the Department of Health and Human Services. Masks and kayaks, replicas of artifacts used by their ancestors, are being built by students in the village school. The Kodiak Area Native Association has instituted an Alutiiq Studies Program that includes bilingual curriculum taught by village elders as well as via computer. All of these changes have strengthened Native identity and self-esteem and helped transform Akhiok into a village where Mary Petersen can again reside and participate in community life. This is the realization of many years of longing—to contribute once again to traditional life, to help ensure the maintenance of her Native language, to lead the Christmas "starring," to search for "medicine from the land."

In addition, Mary went back to Akhiok to work as the community health aide, a newer position in villages throughout Alaska that strongly resembles the role of the traditional midwife. Mary has come full cycle in her self perception as "helper" in realizing this continuity in women's roles as healers. As the health aide, she is once again a healer in a literal way. In a broader, metaphoric sense, she is contributing to the "healing through culture" that characterizes the contemporary movement among Alaska's Native people to reclaim their collective heritage. A central part of that process is the telling of stories, narratives of healing and renewal from which examples of how to live can be drawn. In searching for models, younger Natives are turning to the stories of elders like Mary Petersen, individuals who can provide an avenue for change as well as the knowledge of traditions. The Akhiok of 1992 to which Mary returned is, above all, a setting where her story can be heard, a place where she no longer needs to be silent and afraid.

Notes

1. Kodiak Natives employ "Aleut," "Alutiiq," and "Koniag" as terms of self-reference for their unique cultural identity. The elders in particular use "Aleut" to refer to their culture and language. There are differing explanations as to why "Aleut" was adopted in the nineteenth century for the language and culture of Kodiak's people. One version is that the word was mistakenly applied by the colonizing Russians to several groups of Native people they encountered in the early days of exploration. This has been a source of confusion, since Kodiak's Native people differentiate themselves from the Aleuts of the Aleutian Islands, with whom they share certain cultural and linguistic traits. Scholars have classified the Koniag as one group among a larger population of Pacific or Southern Eskimos, who, along with the Chugaches of Prince William Sound, speak the Alutiiq language. Today, one hears the term "Alutiiq" used more frequently by scholars and by Native people. For an overview of the Pacific Eskimo, see Nancy Yaw Davis, "Contemporary Pacific Eskimo," in *Handbook of North American Indians*, Vol. 5, ed. D. Dumas, (Washington, D. C.: Smithsonian Institution Press,

1984), pp. 185–97. For a further analysis of how the term "Aleut" evolved, see Father Michael Oleska, "What is the Proper Name for Kodiak Island Natives?", *Kodiak Times*, October 17, 1985, pp. 4, 6, and *Alaska Missionary Spirituality* (Mahwah, N. J.: Paulist Press, 1987). For a personal view of Alutiiq identity, see Gordon Pullar, 1992, "Ethnic Identity, Cultural Pride and Generations of Baggage: A Personal Experience." *Arctic Anthropology.* 29(2): 198–209.

2. Suicide among young Alaska Native men (approximately 20–24 years old) reached epidemic proportions in the 1980s, prompting a great deal of media attention, including a series of forty-four articles in a ten-day period in the *Anchorage Daily News* in January 1988. See also "Alaska's Suicide Epidemic," *Newsweek*, February 15, 1988, p. 61.

3. My conversations with Mary were infrequently interrupted, allowing her occasions to speak at length and display a level of verbal artistry not as evident in other interview settings. The linear arrangement of the text is intended to highlight the speaker's rhetorical skills, which would be obscured by presenting the text in prose blocks. Most of the texts show organization in pairs and three- and five-part elements, a pattern found in many Native American texts. For further details of the principles of ethnopoetics, see Dell Hymes, *"In Vain I Tried to Tell You"*(Philadelphia: University of Pennsylvania Press, 1981). For a perspective relying on auditory features, see Dennis Tedlock, *The Spoken Word and the Work of Interpretation* (Philadelphia: University of Pennsylvania Press, 1983).

4. For a history and overview of contemporary *Selaviq* practices in Western Alaska, see Ann Fienup-Riordan, "Following the Star: From the Ukraine to the Yukon," in *Russian America: The Forgotten Frontier*, eds. Barbara Sweetland Smith and Redmond J. Barnett (Tacoma, Wash.: Washington State Historical Society, 1990), 227–235. Folklorist Craig Mishler has documented similar traditions of starring as well as a folk drama known as "Nuta'aq" in English Bay and Port Graham on the Kenai Peninsula. These provide an interesting comparison with Kodiak's traditions. See Craig Mishler, "The Nuta'aq: Musical Folk Drama in English Bay." Paper presented at the Alaska Anthropological Association Meetings, March 25, 1988, Fairbanks, Alaska.

5. Women could also be shamans, although that position was more often held by men or by "berdaches" (often referred to in the ethnographic record as transvestites). Shamans were called upon to control weather conditions, to foresee the future, and to heal in cases which required a manipulation of the spirit forces underlying illness. Midwives, in contrast, attended to everyday needs, including surgical practices. Surgery was a well developed art among both the Aleuts and the Koniag, who used a variety of techniques—including lancing, bloodletting, piercing, and suturing—for both ornamental and medical purposes. For a more complete account of early health care practices, see Robert Fortuine, *Chills and Fever: Health and Disease in the Early History of Alaska* (Anchorage: University of Alaska Press, 1989). For an overview of the berdache tradition, see Walter Williams, *The Spirit and the Flesh* (Boston: Beacon Press, 1986).

6. For a cross-cultural view of birth, see Margarita Kay, *The Anthropology of Human Birth* (Philadelphia: F. S. Davis Co., 1982), and Brigette Jordan, *Birth in Four Cultures* (Montreal: Eden Press Women's Publications, 1980).

7. This plant is referred to in numerous accounts from people all over Kodiak. It is known to local people as "Labrador Tea" and "Mogulnik," technically as *ledum palustre de decumbens*. See Frances Kelso Graham, *Plant Lore of an Alaska Island* (Anchorage: Alaska Northwest Publishing Co., 1985), pp. 38–39.

8. Oleanna Ashouwak was a healer who lived on the southern end of Kodiak from 1909 until 1965. She was widely respected and sometimes feared by village residents, some of whom refer to her as a "witchdoctor." Her status was more akin to that of a traditional shaman than a midwife: although she rarely delivered children, she healed a wide variety of other ailments.

9. See Fortuine (1989).

10. Mary Douglas provides an analysis of women outside the social order as both dangerous and powerful, particularly in relation to menstrual blood and miscarriage. See *Purity and Danger: An Analysis of the Concepts of Pollution and Taboo* (London: Routledge and Kegan Paul, 1966). Also see Emily Martin's analysis of the metaphors of reproduction in *The Woman in the Body: A Cultural Analysis of Reproduction* (Boston: Beacon Press, 1987).

11. See the Introduction to *Blood Magic*, eds. Alma Gottlieb and Thomas Buckley (Berkeley: University of California Press, 1988) for an excellent overview of cross-cultural studies of menstruation. For an analysis of Native women's experiences which compares with that of women on Kodiak, see Julie Cruikshank's *Life Lived as a Story* (Lincoln: University of Nebraska Press, 1991). Cruikshank notes that for the three Yukon elders with whom she worked, puberty seclusion was a time for acquiring ritual and practical knowledge unavailable to men. She contrasts this view with the conventional assertions that women were perceived as "polluted" during these periods (p. 11). This analysis echoes a number of feminist studies which examine more carefully the meaning of symbols to women within different cultural settings.

12. The only statistical evidence prior to the late 1970s would exist in hospital and police records. One would have to do a fair amount of speculating in both cases, since domestic violence was frequently not reported as the cause of an accident. According to figures compiled by the Kodiak Area Native Association, incidents of domestic violence in the villages have been decreasing in the past few years. This may reflect new social programs intended to increase self-esteem and pride in Native culture while combatting alcohol and drug abuse.

Homesickness, Illness, and Death: Native-American Girls in Government Boarding Schools

BRENDA CHILD

Introduction

As part of the assimilationist impulse of the 1870s, federally funded boarding schools were created to help bring an end to tribalism and indoctrinate Indian children in the values, religion, and language of the ever-intruding American civilization. During the next fifty years, thousands of Native-American girls and boys were educated in government boarding schools. Early in the boarding school era, administrators and Indian agents were anxious to achieve high numbers. They persuaded Indian families, often by unscrupulous methods, to enroll their children.

Even after the schools declined in popularity among promoters of assimilation, boarding school attendance remained a common experience for Indians. Often the lack of adequate school facilities on the reservations, as well as the debilitating racial hostility Indian students encountered at off-reservation public schools, led parents to look for an educational alternative. Also, the poverty that characterized most Indian households forced parents to accept the idea of boarding schools as both temporary relief for their children and a possible means of escaping that poverty altogether. The fact that Indian families sometimes chose to send children away to boarding schools does not mean that the quality of education and life within the schools was high. Rather, it testifies to the bleak social and economic conditions that characterized so many Indian communities in the late nineteenth and early twentieth centuries.

169

Because assimilationists envisioned boarding school students as harbingers of civilization to their more unfortunate brothers and sisters back on the reservations, it was essential that girls as well as boys be educated in the institutions. Girls were expected to learn English, receive a rudimentary education, piously attend Christian church services, and embrace contemporary Western values concerning domesticity. Because traditional tribal work roles and other aspects of gender relations, including sexuality, incited so much negative controversy among reformers and policymakers, an education in the "correct" sexual division of labor and a strict monitoring of incipient adolescent yearnings were essential to boarding school life.

In an attempt to instill the desired values into Indian girls in a practical setting, they were sent out to work as domestic servants in local middle-class households. Indian girls who attended the Haskell Institute in Lawrence, Kansas, labored in the homes of white families in Lawrence and Kansas City in exchange for meager wages. Female students also baked and served as unpaid workers in the schools' kitchens. In another important lesson, girls toiled in the schools' laundries, washing and ironing the clothing for the male boarding school students.

Boarding school students and their parents hoped that education, and possibly the advantage of knowing a trade, would help alleviate the impoverishment of their families. Although parents sometimes saw the boarding schools as a way to help their children, they also learned that the schools offered their own brand of hardship. In fact, as parents and students alike would attest, boarding school life presented a myriad of problems for Indians, revealed in hundreds of letters sent between the schools and the tribal communities. The most serious of these problems were homesickness, illness, and death. Documentation herein of parental, student, and administration reaction to these health problems is drawn from the records of the Flandreau, Haskell, and Pipestone Indian schools, which are, or were, located in the states of South Dakota, Kansas, and Minnesota, respectively. Lakota and Chippewa students were in the majority at Pipestone and Flandreau. The student body at Haskell was even more inter-tribal, and many Indians came from areas farther west.

Health and the Boarding School Experience

Students often spent years in boarding school without being allowed to return to the home community. Prior to the 1930s, a period when home visits were strictly regulated by school officials, this loss of personal contact during the formative and vulnerable years of childhood and adolescence imposed tremendous emotional hardships on students and their families. Year after year parents pleaded with unyielding administrators to send their children home for a visit and promised to return them promptly at the beginning of the new term if only they could see them for a short time. In the following letter written in 1925 to Superintendent J. F. House of the Flandreau School in South Dakota, a Wisconsin mother begs for the return of her daughter, Margaret:

> So please be so kind Mr House and let her come home for this summer the poor girl has not been home for [a] long time and I know she will feel more like going to school next fall if she see her folks once more. I am willing to let her go as long as she wants I am proud of her to learn some thing. . . . Dear Sir if you please let her come home I am begging you Mr House so I will be looking for her I will thank you very much if you do this and also see that she go back to school. . . . Hopeing you will be kind. (National Archives, Record Group 75, Records of the Bureau of Indian Affairs, Flandreau Indian School, letters to Superintendent House from parent, Reserve, Wisconsin, July 1, 1925, and July 9, 1925)

In another letter to the school written the next month the same mother wrote: "This makes my third letter to you in regard of my daughter Margaret I dont see why you want to hold her . . . if you would only know how I feel longing to see her." She continued by saying, "Mr House please take my word send her home to me for a few weeks you know it wont be long school start just to see her before she goes to school again you know she will be gone good four years Mr House please do this for me I will be looking for [her] next week." After three such pleas to the school, the superintendent sent the forlorn mother a short reply saying that he could see no reason "that would justify me sending her home" (NA, RG 75, BIA Flandreau, letter from House to parent, July 11, 1925).

Mrs. Isabella Strong of Red Lake, Minnesota, a boarding school veteran herself, also tried to convince the superintendent of Flandreau that her "terribly homesick" daughter Claudia should be allowed to visit home. Mrs. Strong expressed the sentiments of many parents when she wrote: "It seems it would be much easier to get her out of prison than out of your school" (NA, RG 75, BIA, Flandreau, letter from parent, Redby, Minnesota, February 4, 1938).

Parents demonstrated a commitment to keep children who were away at boarding school actively involved in the life of the family and tribal community. In one very moving letter, the father of a deaf student named Mary pleaded with the Flandreau superintendent to allow his daughter to come home to Wisconsin, even at the risk of failing her school examinations. He was more concerned that his daughter spend time with her grandmothers in their old age, writing:

> Wont you please let me know if my poor girl is coming home this summer. I would very much like to have her come home. I know she is going to fail in examination. I know it. But for our poor sake please please let her come home this summer We have two old ladies here our mothers aged old

ladies. because if she dont come home this summer next year they might be gone. they old and sickly. Mary's grandmothers. and you know sir. Mary is a poor girl. a girl that can not hear. Mary didn't have to go to school But it was her own will to go she wanted to go and see the world. and our Doctor said as long as she wanted to go to let her go. Maybe she could learn something in domestic science. and that is why I let her go to school. I know she could not have special attention in school. . . . But won't you please be good & kind to let her come home vacation. my poor girl I feel bad about her. . . . please let me know if you are going to let her come home vacation. So I can get ready for her money We will send her some money. if she is coming home please let me know right away. I hope you will be kind to let my poor girl come home vacation. she is my oldest girl and I would like to have her come home vacation Because she will get lonesome when the other girls comes home. So please have pity on us and let her come home vacation. (NA, RG 75, BIA, Flandreau, letter from parent, Keshena, Wisconsin, May 6, 1924)

It is not known if Mary's father was successful at convincing the superintendent to allow his daughter a visit home. Usually when family members asked for the return of a child at boarding school, administrators were not inclined to grant their requests. In 1911, when Flossie, a young Chippewa girl at Flandreau, asked to be sent home to the White Earth Reservation in northern Minnesota to visit her relatives after a sister had generously offered to pay twenty-seven dollars, the cost of a round-trip fare, the administrator told the girl to "write your sister and explain to her the unwiseness of sending this amount of money for simply a visit" (NA, RG 75, BIA, Flandreau, Superindent correspondence to parent, Mahnomen, Minnesota, June 1911).

Homesickness was endemic at boarding school and was particularly hard on the very young students. Their plight sometimes aroused the pity of school personnel. In 1925 a Flandreau clerk wrote to the Wyoming reservation of a little girl named Grace to see if the forty dollars required for a round trip could be deposited. The clerk wrote:

[Grace] was at the office yesterday and complains that she is very homesick for her mother and father. . . . These children have not been home for two years and this is their second summer here, naturally they would get lonesome . . . the boys have more privileges and are well contented here but this little Grace she is small and at home for a short time with her mother will be fine. . . . Anything you can do for this little daughter will make her happy. (NA, RG 75, BIA, Flandreau, miscellaneous school correspondence, Parco, Wyoming, June 26, 1925)

Sometimes children grew so unhappy in boarding school that they became physically ill. This created problems for school administrators, who had to decide whether a student's illness warranted sending her home. When parents heard rumors that their children were unhappy or sick at school, they pressured administrators to return them. Such was the situation in the following letter, when a father wrote to the Flandreau school, concerned about his daughter Angeline's failing health. In 1924 he wrote:

> I understand you will let me know when Angeline is seriously sick but that might be a little to late then as she has been ailing for a long time. There must be something wrong with her as she spends most of her time in the hospital she might of caught cold or consumption is working on her. She should be examined by the Doctor very good. I dont want to take her out of school before the end of the year but if she's ailing all the time she might just as well be home. As she wrote to me herself she wasnt feeling any to good to go to school. We might wait a little to long and then it will be to late. (NA, RG 75, BIA, Flandreau, letter from parent, Fort Totten, North Dakota, April 5, 1924)

A few days later, the Flandreau superintendent responded: "Your daughter Angeline does not show any indications of serious illness. She is losing some in weight and does not seem to have much appetite, but the physician does not find any specific ailment and she does not run any temperature. I am inclined to think it is homesickness more than anything else. . . ." And despite the administrator's admission that "It is hardly permissible that I send pupils home on account of homesickness," he did make an exception in this case (NA, RG 75, BIA, Flandreau, Superintendent's correspondence, April 8, 1924).

Relatives frequently notified school administrators because their children were needed at home because of an illness, death, or other adversity in the family. In 1925 Joseph Big Bear of White Earth, Minnesota, wrote to Flandreau to say that his granddaughter Martha had a father at home who was "gravely ill." Mr. Big Bear spoke for his family when he said, "we all wish that you give [Martha] permission to come and see her father . . . just as soon as you can . . . while he is still alive." By return mail, Mr. Big Bear was coldly informed that "it is not the policy of the school to permit pupils to go home on account of sickness in the family . . ." (NA, RG 75, BIA, Flandreau, letter from relative, White Earth, Minnesota, March 1917; Superintendent's correspondence, March 17, 1925). That same year the father of another Flandreau student, Mattie, sent word to the school that the girl's mother had an advanced case of tuberculosis. Asking that their daughter be sent home as soon as possible, the father wrote:

> Her mother my wife is pretty sick and is nearly helpless now. I don't think she will ever get well. My wife would like to have her [daughter] home while she is alive you see Mattie has been away to school all her life and has never been home for any length of time. . . . Her mother wants her home very much right now. And I think in a case like this she ought to be

sent home right away don't you? (NA, RG 75, BIA, Flandreau, letter from
parent, St. Paul, Montana, January 10, 1925)

Apparently the school administrator did not agree that an immediate return
was warranted. Although the girl had a dying mother, Mattie's father was
told "it would be pretty bad for her school interests to leave now" (NA, RG
75, BIA, Flandreau, Superintendent House's correspondence, January 1925).

The homesickness of students and the lonesomeness of parents for
their children were dismissed as inconsequential by administrators. As one
man put it, "I have no authority to send pupils home for vacation unless there
is a necessity shown for their return to assist their parents or guardians in the
summer's work" (NA, RG 75, BIA, Superintendent's correspondence, 1911).
Parents realized the chance of having their children home for the summer was
greater if they had a reason judged worthy by the reservation bureaucrats or
school administrators. Those most successful at having their children home
for vacation were considered "industrious Indians," who required additional
labor to enhance the family's income. This was a policy that discriminated
against female students, whose parents generally asked for their return to care
for sick relatives or younger siblings. For many years officials expected the
majority of children to remain at school until their term of study had expired.
The routine of boarding school life presented problems for Indian families,
whose lives had long revolved around seasonal and natural rhythms. School
administrators grew frustrated because those students who did return home
for a vacation stayed away from school until tribal celebrations were over in
the summer. Because of this practice, one Haskell superintendent eventually
became convinced that it was useless to begin school until October. Most
parents opposed having their children at school during summer and lamented
the fact that they would not be home to partake in traditional seasonal
activities. This motivated a Chippewa father from Cass Lake, Minnesota,
to write to the school asking if his daughter, who had not been home for
three years, might return early because, "I am real anxious to have her here
while we make maple sugar." The man's request, however, was denied on
the grounds that it would be "disconcerting to the school" (NA, RG 75,
BIA, Flandreau, letter from parent, White Earth, Minnesota, November 1905;
Superintendent's correspondence, November 16, 1905).

Countless parents wrote to the schools pleading for the return of
their child because a brother had died, a mother was sick, a father injured,
or a grandparent aged. More than one parent encouraged the administrator
to "do the right thing because we never bother you about anything much"
and send their child home (NA, RG 75, BIA, Flandreau, letter from parent,
Couderay, Wisconsin, May 21, 1925). The lonesomeness of parents for their
children, who most often attended boarding schools at great distances from
their families and communities, sometimes even exceeded the homesickness

of their children. Still, many parents, persuaded of the importance of an education or learning a trade for their child's future, would have agreed with the Lakota father whose son and daughter attended Flandreau when he expressed his desire for their success in school and wish to keep them there, "as much as we can stand it" (NA, RG 75, BIA, Flandreau, letter from parent, Elbowoods, North Dakota, May 22, 1924).

With good reason, parents worried about the well-being of their children away at boarding school. Because of the presence of so many communicable diseases in the Indian boarding schools, many students contracted serious illness. Year after year, the superintendents chronicled epidemics of measles and influenza in the annual reports from their schools. In 1926, a year when a superintendent pronounced that there were "no serious outbreak of diseases at Haskell Institute," he still cited numerous cases of measles and mumps, several cases of tuberculosis requiring students to be sent away to sanatoriums, and two deaths due to meningitis. As late as 1935, the Haskell school reported eighty-two students with measles, nine positive cases of tuberculosis, and several active cases of trachoma, a highly contagious eye disease that could result in blindness. In one surprising letter sent from the Flandreau school to the Commissioner of Indian Affairs, the superintendent regretted to make known that one of the teachers had "a very pronounced case of small pox" and was "broken out" while he "met his classes." The superintendent expressed his hope that there would not be a "serious outbreak" as a result (NA, RG 75, BIA, Haskell, Superintendent's Annual Narrative Reports, 1910–1936, 1926, 1935; Commissioner of Indian Affairs Correspondence, 1929).

The boarding school setting was an atmosphere conducive to the spread of disease. Many of the Indian deaths during the great influenza pandemic of 1918–1919—which severely affected the Native American population—took place in boarding schools. At Haskell alone, over three hundred students grew critically ill, and many died. The administrators of the Haskell, Flandreau, and Pipestone schools often reported that their hospitals were "filled to overflowing" because their students were laid low with influenza.[1]

For many years trachoma, a contagious and painful eye disease, afflicted nearly half of the boarding school population. According to the Indian office rules, children stricken with contagious diseases were to be barred from attending government boarding schools, yet steps were never taken to discontinue the policy of enrolling trachomatous children. The disease spread easily in the communal environment of the boarding schools, where students shared not only pencils and books, but also soap, towels, washbasins, beds, and even bathwater. Girls who complained of sore and oozing eyes could be found working in the school's laundries, preparing food in kitchens, and milking the school's cows. In 1912, public health physicians argued that the trachoma epidemic on reservations was being spread by the government boarding schools. Trachoma was easily transmitted but difficult to cure. When afflicted Indians were treated for the disease, the method used was excruciatingly painful: it consisted of scraping or pinching the inflamed inner eyelid with small forceps, flushing the eye with a solution of boric acid, and a lengthy follow-up treatment where the eyelid was rubbed with a copper sulfate stick. Trachoma treatment was delicate for even the most skilled ophthalmologist, yet Indian students received follow-up care from unskilled school personnel, a situation that can only be considered cruel and irresponsible.[2]

The anxiety that parents felt regarding the health of their children in boarding school was exacerbated by the pervasiveness of serious diseases and by the fact that officials routinely concealed news of illness from family members. Not only did administrators fail to inform parents of their children's illness, they even resorted to confiscating letters written by sick children before they could be mailed. Many alienated parents wrote angry letters to school officials who neglected to inform them of their children's state of health. Distressed relatives frequently wrote to boarding school administrators expressing shock and anxiety because their children were sick or had been injured at school yet they were never notified. After a Wisconsin girl, Naomi, had been stricken with tuberculosis while at school, her mother wrote: "I did not know that she was not well and you cant tell what I feel. . . ." The mother had asked that her girl be sent home "for we want to take care of and watch over her while we can. that disease is no plaything" (NA, RG 75, BIA, Flandreau, letter from parent, West De Pere, Wisconsin, Octotber 28, 1926). In 1914, John Bonga, who worked at the Agency Trading Post in Onigum, Minnesota, also wrote to Flandreau, saying, "Somebody told me that my daughter [Sophia] is not feeling very good and . . . [I am] wondering how she is getting along." Mr. Bonga was informed that his daughter had developed tuberculosis and was being sent to a sanatorium. The father wrote back to the school expressing his despair. Mr. Bonga worried that his daughter might get lonesome at the sanatorium or would get lost en route because she was not used to traveling (NA, RG 75, BIA, Flandreau, letters from parent, Onigum, Minnesota, February 7, 1914, February 23, 1914).

Tuberculosis was commonplace in government boarding schools, where diseased and healthy students intermingled. Little effort was made to provide afflicted children with special care or enriched diets. School officials endangered the lives of healthy and sick pupils by ignoring the presence of tuberculosis among their students. In fact, H. B. Peairs, long-time Haskell superintendent and later chief supervisor of education, repeatedly ignored the advice of the school doctor, who recommended the quarantine of students obviously suffering from the disease. Haskell students who hemorrhaged on a regular basis were kept in the school hospital, although it was not an adequate facility for the tubercular.[3]

In 1924, Harriet, a young Chippewa girl from Ashland, Wisconsin, requested that she be sent to a sanatorium rather than attend school while suffering the effects of the disease. The girl, miserable because of painful lesions on her legs that refused to heal, complained about the constant drilling and marching that was so much a part of the boarding school regimen. Harriet tried to reason with the superintendent:

> . . . how do you expect me to learn and study when I suffer so[?] My parents are going to try and send me to a sanatorium . . . [so I] will get well quicker but they dont know how I am doing when I am here so I am going to ask you a question. . . . Would you rather have me go away to a sanatorium and get well and where I can learn and be happy or, Have me going to school and suffer? . . . its about time I was going to a sanatorium and get cured. (NA, RG 75, BIA, Flandreau, letter from student, Ashland, Wisconsin, February 1924)

For sound reasons, many parents became convinced that government boarding schools ravaged the health of their children. Mrs. Isabella Strong complained that her daughter and other Red Lake Chippewa children seemed always to return sick from school. Mrs. Strong contended that she did not want her daughter "to get all run down like my nephew Johnny Graves was when he reached home. He was so ill looking that he looked as if he had tuberculosis for years. He's picking up fast since he reached home" (NA, RG 75, BIA, Flandreau, letter from parent, Redby, Minnesota, February 9, 1938). Mrs. Strong and other parents criticized the schools because their children grew sick so often, lost weight, worked too hard, and did not have adequate food, clothing, or medical care. They complained about the outing programs, the long days, the work details, and the fact that boarding schools relied too heavily on unpaid student labor for their operation. Some parents believed their children were sickly because they were physically overworked. This prompted a Wisconsin Oneida mother to request that her daughter Ruth, who had lost thirty-four pounds since she first arrived at school, be relieved of some of her early morning work duties. The mother was well aware that weight loss was one of the warning signs of tuberculosis, and she cautioned the superintendent to go easy on her daughter, saying: "I with my husband can't spare her to run down in health. . . . we just buried a child a month ago and I can't see how we ever spared Ruth to go back [to school] for we love her so. . . . Watch her and be sure if she gets sick let me have her home. . . ." Ruth's mother closed with a necessary reminder to the superintendent: "health is as important as education" (NA, RG 75, BIA, Flandreau, letter from parent, Green Bay, Wisconsin, September 17, 1923).

Because disease was so prevalent in the Indian boarding schools, some students died. Imagine the feelings of the father addressed in the following letter, who received this belated news from Flandreau in the spring of 1906:

Dear Sir: It is with a feeling of sorrow that I write you telling of the death of your daughter Lizzie. She was not sick but a short time and we did not think her so near her end. On the evening of March 30th, I was at the girls building and the matron informed me that Lizzie had gone to bed not feeling well. I went up to her room with the matron and found her in bed with what seemed a bad cold. . . . She had quite a fever for several days and then seemed to improve, but did not rally as she ought to have done, and the doctor made a careful examination and said that she was without doubt going into quick consumption. . . . Last Wednesday I was called away to Minneapolis and. . . I was very much surprised upon my return Saturday evening to find she was dead, as the doctor had given us no information except she might live for a number of months. . . . Those that were with her say she did not suffer, but passed away as one asleep. Lizzie was one of our best girls, was always ready to do right, and will be missed by all who know her, and you will have the deep sympathy of all the employees of the institution in this your hour of affliction. . . . I am very sorry that you could not have seen your daughter alive, for she had grown quite a little and improved very much since you let her come here with me. Had we known that she was not going to live but so short a time, we would have made a great effort to have gotten you here before she died. (NA, RG 75, BIA, Flandreau, Superintendent's correspondence, April 16, 1906)

The letter was signed "Respectfully yours" by the superintendent of the Flandreau Indian School.

Conclusion

The boarding school experience posed many new dilemmas for Indian parents and their children. Homesickness was a persistent problem because children attended schools located at great distances from their own tribal communities. Home visits were far too infrequent, particularly for the very young pupils.

Parents had the additional burden of worrying about the health of their distant children. Although students with contagious diseases were theoretically excluded from attending government boarding schools, in practice tuberculosis, trachoma, and other serious diseases flourished in the overcrowded classrooms and dormitories. The diseases became a threat not only to the boarding school pupils, but also to the reservation population, as returning students carried sickness home. When school officials failed to inform parents of the health of their children, sometimes even after students contracted life-threatening illnesses, family members lost confidence in those who claimed that the interests of Indian children came first. And because the death of boarding school students was an all too common experience, family members often lived in a state of perpetual anxiety about the well-being of their children. Unfortunately, too many administrators flagrantly ruined the health of their pupils. In so doing, school officials alienated those Native-American families who most wanted their children to be educated.

Notes

1. Charles Roberts discusses the effects of this epidemic on the Cushman Indian School in Tacoma, Washington, where ten students died, in "The Cushman Indian Trades School and World War I," *American Indian Quarterly*, 11, no. 3 (Summer 1987): 221–41.
2. For a discussion of federal policy and the trachoma problem among the Indian population, see Diane Therese Putney, "Fighting the Scourge: American Indian Morbidity and Federal Policy, 1897–1928" (Ph.D. diss., Marquette University, 1980), 141–69.
3. See Putney, "Fighting the Scourge," pp. 78–109, for discussion of tuberculosis and federal policy.

Managing on Their Own: Ailing Black Women in Philadelphia and Charleston, 1870 to 1918

PRISCILLA FERGUSON CLEMENT

Introduction

At the end of the nineteenth century American cities were notoriously unhealthy places. The urban poor, often living in overcrowded and unsanitary housing, and working long hours for meager wages, were especially likely to experience serious medical problems and to require aid in times of illness. Both in the North and in the South, urban black mortality rates were high, much higher than those of whites. In 1900 the death rate for blacks in northern cities was twenty-seven per thousand, in southern cities, thirty-four per thousand. Yet the death rate for urban whites in both sections was less than twenty per thousand (U. S. Bureau of the Census 1918, 320; Hine, 1989, 8). Black women outnumbered black men in southern cities like Charleston and in northern cities like Philadelphia. Urban areas were particularly attractive to widowed and single black women seeking employment as domestics and laundresses. Such women worked hard but were paid little for their labor, and they were often unable to self-insure against illness and poverty (Jones 1985, 73–74).

The kinds of aid received by ailing urban black women in the North and the South in the postbellum years, 1870 to 1918, can be seen through a study of the records of medical charities in Philadelphia and Charleston. A close examination of one such charity in each city—the Philadelphia Protestant-Episcopal City Mission and the Associated Charities of Charleston—

reveals whether these northern and southern urban medical charities responded to black women differently. Both kept case records of their clients. Their records profile sick black women who sought aid in each city. These records reflect health care provided by whites to blacks through formal institutions, not assistance provided within the black community itself. Nonetheless, they demonstrate that impoverished black women were remarkably resourceful and determined to remain independent regardless of the physical infirmities they suffered.

Philadelphia and Charleston

Throughout the nineteenth century, partly because they were centers of medical education (Rosenberg 1987, 60–61, 210; Waring 1967, 87), both Philadelphia and Charleston had an array of hospitals and outpatient treatment programs. By century's end, Philadelphia had many more hospitals and medical dispensaries than did Charleston. This was largely due to Philadelphia's population, which was roughly twenty times greater than that of Charleston (Coclanis 1988, 116, table 4-6).

Philadelphia was never exempt from racism, although Philadelphia's Quakers were among the first white Americans to speak out against slavery (Nash 1988). As late as 1871, the city experienced a serious race riot. By the end of the century, even members of the Society of Friends had lost interest in aiding blacks (Lane 1979, 10, 24). In 1890, of the thirty-three public and private hospitals in the city, just eighteen (55 percent) were open to black women. In all of these, black and white patients were segregated (Wines 1895, 929–31; Civic Club 1896).

Segregation of patients was routine practice in hospitals throughout the country until well into the twentieth century (Rosenberg 1987, 301–03). It was certainly characteristic of Charleston, where by 1880 there were just two large public hospitals, only one of which admitted blacks to its segregated wards (Hill 1989, 321). This southern city's hospitals had not been open to blacks at all before the Civil War. After the war, through the prodding of the Freedmen's Bureau, Charleston's hospitals began to treat black patients (Williamson 1965, 320).

Statistics from twenty-three of the thirty-three hospitals in Philadelphia reveal that by 1890 the proportion of blacks in the total hospital population approximated their proportion in the city population: 4 percent (Wines 1895, 929–31; Civic Club 1896). Blacks did not have equivalent access to hospitals in Charleston. In 1880 only 51 percent of persons admitted to Charleston's City Hospital were black, although 70 percent of the city's population was black (*Charleston City Year Book* 1880, 203). Thus blacks were fairly represented in Philadelphia hospitals but not in Charleston medical facilities. Yet in both cities death rates among blacks in 1900 were much higher than among whites: in Charleston they were forty-four per thousand for blacks and twenty-three per thousand for whites, while in Philadelphia blacks died at a rate of thirty per thousand and whites at twenty per thousand. At any given time during this period, more blacks than whites were ill and in need of treatment (U. S. Bureau of the Census 1918, 320). Hence, considering numbers and medical need, black women and men were probably under-represented in hospitals in both cities.

Those few black women who were admitted to hospitals in either city were treated by white doctors and nurses. In the late nineteenth century black physicians and nurses were a rarity in both Philadelphia and Charleston (Gamble 1987, 19–21; Newby 1973, 117). Yet in both cities members of the black community were working to rectify this situation, and they succeeded. By 1896 Philadelphia's Douglass Hospital accommodated black patients and trained black nurses (Gamble 1987, 14), and in 1897 in Charleston's Hospital and Training School for Nurses on Cannon Street did the same (Newby 1973, 117; Hine 1989, 9, 15).

Whether administered by blacks or whites, hospitals in the late nine-teenth and early twentieth centuries were quite different institutions than they are today. In the past, medical therapies were fewer and less effective, and hospitals had a reputation among women and men of all races and classes as places where one went to die, not to get better (Rosenberg 1987, 298–99; Hine 1989, 21–22). Thus while racial prejudice kept blacks out of hospitals they as well as whites preferred treatment that allowed them to remain at home (Rosenberg, 1987, 4–5). Hospital outpatient departments and medical dispensaries provided such care fairly equitably to both black and white urban poor.

Dispensaries—neighborhood institutions where poor and working-class women and men could see doctors and receive medications—were either free or charged only minimal fees (Rosenberg 1987, 316–21). Dispensaries existed in both Philadelphia and Charleston. Records of two of the largest—one in each city—indicate that they treated disproportionately large numbers of black women. In 1870, 8.8 percent of the patients of the Philadelphia Dispensary were black (roughly double the proportion of blacks in the city population). Thus black women were well represented among the patient population (Philadelphia Dispensary 1870). In 1871 63 percent of the persons treated at Charleston's Shirras Dispensary were black women, at a time when such women constituted about one-third of the city's total population (Shirras Dispensary 1871). Dispensary records show that in the late nineteenth century, ailing black women in both Philadelphia and Charleston had good access to outpatient treatment—the preferred type of medical care in that period. Black women also could seek aid from other charities providing various types of assistance to ailing women, including food, fuel, and money.

Case records of the Philadelphia Protestant-Episcopal City Mission and the Associated Charities of Charleston provide what demographics of hospital and dispensary patients cannot: insight into how equitably black women were treated by white-operated medical charities and information on the circumstances and coping strategies of indigent, sick, black women.[1]

Philadelphia's Protestant-Episcopal City Mission was founded in 1870 to assist the poor who had no church affiliation. Within a year it established mission churches throughout the city and dispatched male, and later female and male, missionaries to canvas the poor door-to-door. By 1890 most of its staff in direct contact with the poor were women (Philadelphia Protestant-Episcopal City Mission 1871, 1872, 1879, 1890). In contrast, Charleston's Associated Charities, begun in 1888, was part of a national movement to organize urban charities and prevent duplication of services to the poor. It was a central clearinghouse for Charleston charities. Poor persons would apply there first and, after proper investigation by a female general secretary, be referred to appropriate charities for assistance (Jordan 1987). Within a few years of their founding, both agencies came to care principally for the sick and aged poor. In 1875 Philadelphia's City Missionaries discovered widespread illness, especially consumption, among the city's poor. They opened the first of several neighborhood-based Sick-Diet Kitchens, providing free food to the ailing poor on a daily basis. The next year the mission opened its first sanitarium for consumptives. Its second opened in 1886, and its third in 1896 (Philadelphia Protestant-Episcopal City Mission 1879, 1885, 1900).

As for Charleston's Associated Charities, initially a large proportion of its applicants were ill. Its general secretary either aided the sick poor herself or referred them to the Ladies Benevolent Society. The latter had provided medical aid to the city's poor since 1813 (Charleston Associated Charities). Ailing women were willingly assisted by the Associated Charities of Charleston. There is no evidence that blacks were turned away, yet the agency's clientele was overwhelmingly white. Although the Associated Char-ities never pronounced itself "whites only," clearly it was more interested in aiding the white population than in aiding blacks. In a sample of two hundred women assisted by the agency between 1888 and 1909, just sixteen (or 8 percent) were black women, even though in 1910 black women made up 34 percent of the city's population. Moreover, while the incidence of tuberculosis was very high among blacks in South Carolina (in 1884 it was two times that of whites [Waring 1967, 177]), of the sixteen black women in the sample, only one suffered from consumption. This medical charity was minimally concerned with helping black victims of (arguably) the most common and debilitating disease among the urban poor (Trattner 1984, 142).

Speaking before the National Conference of Charities and Corrections in 1894, Associated Charities General Secretary Mrs. M. A. Rhett remarked: "Of the negroes, who compose more than one-half of our population, few apply for aid . . ." (National Conference 1894, 35). This may have been because the application process was especially difficult and demeaning to blacks. A black woman had to be acquainted with a white person respected by the Associated Charities, confess her poverty to that person, and request a recommendation. In the South an unwritten code governed this "personalism." Black women had to be deferential and prove their "respectability" by displaying "decorum, piety, and sobriety" (Johnson and Roark 1984, 10–11). Their deference is confirmed by the dearth of black women recorded in the Associated Charities' application books described as other than "respectable and polite." If a black woman had no established connection with well-known white Charlestonians, she was given minimal aid by the Associated Charities. For example, Julia Roland, a black newcomer to Charleston, became ill, lost her job, and was denied the wages owed her as a house servant. Roland had no references except for "an old colored woman" who had "nursed her when sick." The agency's only assistance was in the form of information about two advertisements for house servant jobs (SCHS, AC, case 533, book 4). Other black female clients of the Associated Charities in the sample, all of whom had proper white references and behaved submissively to agency officials, received such concrete aid as food, fuel, rent money, or admission to an asylum.

Overt prejudice against black women was much less evident in Philadelphia's Protestant-Episcopal City Mission. Black women were over-represented among its clients. They were likely to receive aid whether favorably described by agency officials or not. The number of black women in a sample of two hundred aided by Philadelphia's Protestant-Episcopal Mission, from 1902–18, was eighteen (or 9 percent). Yet in 1910 black women constituted just 3 percent of Philadelphia's population, compared with 34 percent in Charleston. Thus black women were over-represented among the northern charity's clients. In Philadelphia, as in Charleston, black women had to have references from established whites in order to obtain aid. But in Philadelphia it was easier for black women to secure referrals than it was for black women in Charleston. Apparently, there were more white persons—doctors, churchmen, employers, charitable officials—willing to recommend black women in the northern city. No evidence exists that this difference was due to more poor or sick black women in Philadelphia. In fact, the much higher death rate of blacks in Charleston indicates that the opposite was probably true.

Black women found it easier to apply to the Philadelphia charity. They were also accorded aid even if they did not behave exactly as City Missionaries wished. One-third of the ailing black women who applied to the Philadelphia agency were described negatively by its officials. Yet all of the women (as well as all of those more positively described) were recommended for aid. For example, City Mission officials repeatedly objected to Mollie Avery's "begging letters" to all sorts of charities. Yet Avery herself received several grants of food and money from the City Mission (UAC, PECM, case 192, book 68). Not that mission visitors treated all black women alike, regardless of behavior. Particularly difficult women were denied aid in their own homes. They were referred to the city's public hospital—a facility many poor Philadelphians feared. There they were stigmatized as paupers and experimented upon by doctors (Rosenberg 1987, 298–99, 325). Thus, chronically ill Eliza Whitman insisted to a Mission worker that "the city has a right to keep her as she wished to be kept" in her own home. The Mission official labeled her "impertinent" and insisted that she enter the Philadelphia Hospital (UAC, PECM, no case number, box 71, admittted May 17, 1905).

Mission officials were also not entirely exempt from racism. They assisted more black women suffering from consumption (three of the fifteen ailing blacks in the sample) than did officials of Charleston's Associated Charities. Yet these women were treated in only one of the mission's two sanitariums for consumptive women; the other was reserved exclusively for young white women (Philadelphia Protestant-Episcopal City Mission 1900). Black women were treated in a prejudicial fashion by both the Philadelphia City Mission and by Charleston's Associated Charities. Not surprisingly, they faced more discrimination from the southern than from the northern agency.

Nonetheless, cross-race and cross-class sympathy existed in both agencies. The white, economicallly well-to-do women who interviewed black applicants for both charities initially doubted their worthiness but ultimately recognized their need. When Mrs. M. A. Rhett, member of a prominent white Charleston family, heard from another white female social worker that Amelia Farr, a poor black woman, was ill with pneumonia, the Associated Charities General Secretary wondered why Farr's church or her family did not aid her. After visiting Farr, Rhett reported, "A most deplorable case. Applicants are living in a miserable hut. The woman critically ill with pneumonia and her son with rheumatism. Their sickness the result of exposure in the bitter cold weather. . . . They have had to take the money given them by the church for wood and medicine." Rhett paid Farr's rent and arranged for her and her son to get their medicines free (SCHS, AC, case 1308, book 7).

Similarly, a white female social worker for Philadelphia's Protestant-Episcopal City Mission doubted whether black applicant Mary Flemming was truly without resources. The worker found Flemming "in bed with pneumonia." Her husband had died three years before, her brother was "not to be depended upon for help, drinks. . . . Her eldest child stays home from school with her mother." Although "visited daily" by a member of her church, she had "no money coming in." Convinced that even with the help of her daughter and church this ill black woman could not get by, the City Mission supplied her with food (UAC, PECM, case 3190, box 72). Initially wary of black female applicants, white female charity workers ultimately came to sympathize with them. White racial distrust and patronization never disappeared entirely, but they were mitigated when prosperous white women met and became caregivers to indigent, ailing black women within medical charities.

The stories of Amelia Farr in Charleston and Mary Flemming in Philadelphia reflect a pattern: in both cities the circumstances of ill black women applying for aid were remarkably similar. So were the ways in which these women coped with their illnesses. In both cities, black female applicants were not entirely helpless and without resources. They probably would have been patients in a hospital had they been so. Few black women were in either the Charleston or the Philadelphia hospitals. This means most ailing black women in these cities resembled those in the care of Philadelphia's City Mission and Charleston's Associated Charities. These women did everything in their power to avoid hospitalization.

Family was the first recourse of black women when they became ill. In Charleston approximately one-third, and in Philadelphia half, of the women reported that relatives helped them. Such relatives were themselves poor and not able to provide adequately for the applicants. For example, Tenah Gilbert, a fifty-year-old black suffering from rheumatism, had three daughters, two of whom helped her financially. One, who was married, gave her money occasionally. The youngest paid her mother's rent. Gilbert applied to the Associated Charities of Charleston for food. She lived independently with the help of her daughters and charitable aid (SCHS, AC, case 504, book 4). The Philadelphian Helen Astor was in similar circumstances. She was in "poor" physicial condition. She had a sixteen-year-old daughter who worked as a waitress. With her help and a little coal and food from the Philadelphia City Mission, Astor got by (UAC, PECM, case 284, box 68).

Black women without relatives to aid them worked even though physically incapacitated. Thus, according to the records of the Protestant-Episcopal City Mission in Philadelphia, Mollie Avery, paralyzed from the waist down and confined to her bed, still sewed, told fortunes, and kept boarders in order to support herself. She managed with occasional grants of food and money from charities (UAC, PECM, case 192, book 68).

No black women in the Charleston sample reported themselves employed. Two-thirds of them did not mention any relatives providing them assistance. Conceivably, these black women were much worse off than those in Philadelphia. They were likely living a very precarious existence. Possibly many of the Charleston women were working, at least occasionally. More may have received assistance from relatives, but it is difficult to determine, since the general secretary of the Associated Charities of Charleston did not record as much information about black clients as did her northern counterparts. In South Carolina two-thirds of black women were employed in 1910, usually as maids or laundresses (Newby 1973, 141). It may have been presumed that adult black women not in an institution were employed, and thus their jobs not recorded. Further, black women, fearful that aid might be denied unless they were entirely dependent, may have failed to report assistance from relatives.

In addition to relying on their families and on their own earnings, some black women took action to insure themselves against need if they became ill. Membership in black churches or beneficial societies self-insured urban black women in the nineteenth and twentieth centuries (Jones 1985, 75). When they became ill, women appealed to their churches for aid. They also claimed weekly sick payments from beneficial societies to which they had contributed.

The first black church in the United States was founded in Philadelphia in 1786. Charleston had two all-black churches before the Civil War and many more thereafter (Williamson 1965, 188–201). As early as 1837, Philadelphia black women had organized sixty-two mutual benevolent societies (Nash 1988, 252–53). Black women in Charleston and in other cities did the same after the Civil War. Almost three-fifths of the black women who applied to the Philadelphia Protestant-Episcopal City Mission were members of black churches. Another one-fifth belonged to beneficial societies. Only one-quarter of the black women on the rolls of Charleston's Associated Charities belonged to black churches. None belonged to beneficial societies. It is possible that this information was simply not recorded or not reported by the applicants.

Other evidence suggests black women willingly took the initiative to provide for themselves when sick. Virtually all charities in both cities were administered by whites. In order to receive aid from many, including the Associated Charities and the Protestant-Episcopal City Mission, black women requested recommendations from white persons. Nearly all black applicants to both agencies had managed to get such recommendations—no mean feat. Several black Charlestonians applied to white female members of the Associated Charities for aid. Thus Annette Rowley, "ill and in need," and Lula Call, a "respectable negro woman quite sick and in need of wood," obtained referrals to the agency. They were granted aid (SCHS, AC, case 1842, book 8 and case 1553, book 9). In both cities, ailing black women often asked white doctors for a charitable referral. Bertha Ramey, whom her doctor reported as too "old and feeble to care for herself," came to the attention of the Associated Charities (SCHS, AC case 192, book 2). And Emily Brook, whose doctor reported her as suffering from consumption (but whose case was "hopeful"), obtained admission to the Protestant-Episcopal City Mission's sanitarium at Chestnut Hill (UAC, PECM, case 650, box 68). Moreover, black Philadelphian applicants also sought aid from other charities. Mollie Avery, totally bedridden, wrote requests to at least four charities, including the City Mission; all of these aided her (UAC, PECM, case 192, book 68). Eliza Cooper used various pseudonyms when applying to Philadelphia charities, and most of them assisted her (UAC, PECM, case 1443, box 72).

Far from helpless, these black women were determined to receive aid on their own terms. Although impoverished and dependent on the good will of white-administered charities, they still managed to assert their rights. There is greater evidence of this assertiveness in Philadelphia's records. Because Charleston's Associated Charities aided so few black women, those who managed to secure aid from this agency were fearful of losing it. Nonetheless, evidence suggests that ill black women in Charleston were not docile. On several occasions, black women required to report back to the general secretary of the Associated Charities did not. One case involved Tenah Gilbert, who, in a "respectful and polite" manner, asked for provisions from the Associated Charities. She was recommended for a food allowance from the city. She was also advised to go to Ashley, the city's home for aged blacks. Gilbert agreed, "if she cannot be cured." The general secretary expected to hear how Gilbert "was getting on." She never reported back (SCHS, AC, case 504, book 4). She apparently had secured what she wanted from the agency and abhored the secretary's recommendation that she enter an asylum.

There are several examples of Philadelphia's black women showing an equally determined attitude. They accepted aid in time of illness exclusively on their own terms. Harriet Irwin, who had suffered "for several years with intestinal trouble," insisted she go to a "first class hospital" for treatment (UAC, PECM, no case numberr, box 69, admitted June 19, 1902). Mollie Avery, though virtually bedridden, refused suggestions that she go to the Philadelphia Hospital for treatment. She remained persistent in her demands for money and food, and the City Mission and several other charities relieved her (UAC, PECM, case 192, box 68). Eliza Whitman, not as fortunate in securing aid, was just as determined. She suffered from both Bright's Disease (characterized by high blood pressure and albumin in the urine) and "heart trouble." Whitman, like Avery, refused suggestions to enter a hospital. An agent from the City Mission came to her home on several occasions. The agent spent "an hour trying to persuade Eliza to go to a hospital—but she absolutely refused to go." When the agent denied Whitman any other assistance, she "said as she had been helped before she was determined she would be helped now." On another occasion Whitman insisted "that she will not go to a hospital and says that the ladies of Phila [*sic*] have a right to support her at home." She did not enter a hospital, but neither did she receive aid from the City Mission (UAC, PECM, no case number, box 71, admitted May 17, 1905).

Conclusion

Between 1870 and 1918, black women in the North found hospitals somewhat more accessible than did those in the South, if Philadelphia and Charleston can be taken as representative cities. In both regions, black patients' accommodations were on segregated wards, and they were remanded to the care of white doctors and nurses. In both regions, urban black women preferred to avoid hospitalization at a time when hospitals were more likely to be asylums for the dying than facilities for the recuperating patient. Medical dispensaries, whether in the North or in the South, treated them equitably with whites. Other charities, however, providing food, fuel, and money to indigent sick women, were more discriminatory. Southern charities, in particular, were likely to demand extreme deference from sick black women. They assisted them only if they had proper references from respected white residents. With recommendations, both southern and northern black women usually received aid, because the white women who dispensed it sympathized with their plight. When black women took the initiative and applied for aid, white female caregivers often recognized the seriousness of their need and gave relief. Applying for charity was only one of the variety of strategies urban black women used to get by, according to the records of the Associated Charities of Charleston and the Philadelphia Protestant-Episcopal Mission. Many remained employed, even when physically disabled. Others relied on assistance from family members, churches, and beneficial societies, along with occasional aid from various charities. Despite discrimination and physical infirmity, most black women managed to persevere by utilizing a variety of resources, both within their own communities and within the larger, white-dominated society.

Note

1. All of the information on black women in the care of these two charities is drawn from random samples of case histories of 200 women in the care of the Philadelphia Protestant-Episcopal City Mission, 1902–18 and 200 women in the care of the Associated Charities of Charleston, 1888–1909. When individual women's records are cited, I have changed the last, but not the first names of women to preserve their anonymity. The case records of the City Mission are in Philadelphia at the Urban Archives Center, Temple University Libraries, Episcopal Community Services, Protestant-Episcopal City Mission (referred to in citations as UAC, PECM), Boxes 68–72. The case records of the Associated Charities are in Charleston at the South Carolina Historical Society, Associated Charities (referred to in citations as SCHS, AC), Applications Books, numbers 1 through 9.

Works Cited

Charleston Associated Charities. 1888 to 1902. Minutes. In South Carolina Historical Society. Record 11/612.
Charleston City Year Book for 1880. 1880. Charleston, South Carolina.
Civic Club of Philadelphia. 1896. *Civic Club Digest of Educational and Charitable Institutions and Societies in Philadelphia.* Philadelphia: George Buchanan and Co.

190 | Priscilla Ferguson Clement

Coclanis, Peter A. 1988. *The Shadow of a Dream: Economic Life and Death in the South Carolina Low Country, 1670–1920*. New York: Oxford University Press.

Gamble, Vanessa N. 1987. "The Negro Hospital Renaissance: The Black Hospital Movement, 1920–1940." Ph.D. diss., University of Pennsylvania.

Hill, Walter Byron. 1989. "Family, Life, and Work Culture: Black Charleston, South Carolina, 1880 to 1910." Ph.D. diss., University of Maryland, College Park.

Hine, Darlene Clark. 1989. *Black Women in White: Racial Conflict and Cooperation in the Nursing Profession, 1890–1950*. Bloomington: Indiana University Press.

Johnson, Michael P., and James L. Roark. 1984. *No Chariot Let Down: Charleston's Free People of Color on the Eve of the Civil War*. Chapel Hill: University of North Carolina Press.

Jones, Jacqueline. 1985. *Labor of Love, Labor of Sorrow: Black Women, Work, and the Family from Slavery to the Present*. New York: Basic Books.

Jordan, Laylon Wayne. 1987. "'The Method of Modern Charity': The Associated Charities Society of Charleston, 1888–1920." *South Carolina Historical Magazine* 88:34–47.

Lane, Roger. 1979. *Violent Death in the City: Suicide, Accident, and Murder in Nineteenth-Century Philadelphia*. Cambridge: Harvard University Press.

Nash, Gary B. 1988. *Forging Freedom: The Formation of Philadelphia's Black Community, 1720–1840*. Cambridge: Harvard University Press.

National Conference of Charities and Corrections. 1894. *Proceedings*.

Newby, I. A. 1973. *Black Carolinians: A History of Blacks in South Carolina from 1895 to 1968*. Columbia: University of South Carolina Press.

Philadelphia Dispensary. 1870. *Annual Report*.

Philadelphia Protestant-Episcopal City Mission. 1871, 1872, 1879, 1885, 1900. *Annual Reports*.

Rosenberg, Charles. 1987. *The Care of Strangers: The Rise of America's Hospital System*. New York: Basic Books.

Shirras Dispensary. 1871. Quarterly Report of Sick and Wounded Destitute Poor, Eastern Division and Western Division. In City of Charleston, Division of Archives and Records, Record Group 31.

Trattner, Walter I. 1984. *From Poor Law to Welfare State: A History of Social Welfare in America, 3rd ed.* New York: Free Press.

United States Bureau of the Census. 1918. *Negro Population, 1790–1915*. Washington, D. C.: Government Printing Office.

Waring, Joseph Ioor. 1967. *A History of Medicine in South Carolina, 1825–1900*. Columbia: South Carolina Medical Association.

Williamson, Joel. 1965. *After Slavery: The Negro in South Carolina During Reconstruction 1861–1877*. New York: W. W. Norton.

Wines, Frederick H. 1895. *Report on Crime, Pauperism, and Benevolence in the United States at the Eleventh Census, 1890*. Washington, D. C.: Government Printing Office.

Empowered Caretakers: A Historical Perspective on the Roles of Granny Midwives in Rural Alabama

SHEILA P. DAVIS AND CORA A. INGRAM

"That baby won't live through the night." These words of the doctor resounded in the mother's ears like the reverberating sound of an old church bell after the bellringer has left the belfry. The death sentence was pronounced by the doctor after he had arrived and examined the tiny infant. His pronouncement was in direct conflict with the assertion of the midwife who had "caught the baby" and assured the mother that the baby would be fine. A rush of thoughts filled the mother's head, and her mind began to replay the events that surrounded the birth of her tiny baby. When the labor pains began she had been stunned; she was only in her seventh month and feared that something was amiss. She awakened her husband and asked him to summon her mother and the neighbor woman who attended to "women's business." Since cars and telephones were virtually unheard of in Alabama's rural African-American communities in the 1940s, her husband set out on foot to summon the women. Once the women attendants were in place, her husband, responding to her request, began the three-mile walk to the doctor's house. But babies, when they're ready to be birthed, do not adhere to people's imposed schedules. So the baby was delivered by Miss Janie, a granny midwife, just minutes before the doctor arrived.

Following examination of the infant, the doctor had recommended hospitalization for the child's prematurity and low birth weight. However, the mother and her husband, with the support of the gathered women, adamantly opposed hospitalization. The racism and segregation that characterized the

191

South also extended to its health care system. The hospital in Lauderdale County, Alabama, adhered to the prevailing practices of the day and had a "ward" in its basement for "colored patients." At that time, the "colored ward" was being used to isolate polio patients. So African Americans, be they adult or infant, were hospitalized in the "colored ward" of a hospital in a neighboring county. The mother was sure the baby would die if torn from the love, caring, and knowledge of the women caretakers who had gathered in her home. She believed the women possessed knowledge grounded in a collective unconscious born out of the necessity for cultural, physical, and spiritual survival. The women's store of information had been handed down from mother to daughter, from generation to generation. Their wisdom was rooted in their African heritage and had supported them through the horrors of the middle passage, slavery, and second-class existence. Surely they held the keys to her baby's survival! Nonetheless, her baby's premature entrance into life at a weight of 2 lbs. 2 oz. stirred fears of death. Large tears welled in her eyes as she looked upon her tiny infant daughter. Miss Janie, the granny midwife, sensing the mother's need for comforting, softly patted the mother's arm and said: "Now chile don't you worry none. This baby gon be fine; she too fisty to die. Ma Jane done seen um live way littler than this. I brought her here and with the help of the good lawd, I'll keep her here. You don't pay no 'ttention to no Doctor, he human just like us. The only Doctor I trust is in Dr. Jesus cause he ain't never failed me yet." The other women who had gathered echoed Miss Janie's proclamation and recounted tales of their deliveries and others they had attended.

The childbirths of these women, as with thousands of other African-American women in rural Alabama in the 1940s, had three common characteristics. Childbirth was natural, requiring no surgical intervention; it occurred at home; and granny midwives performed the deliveries. According to Laura Blackburn, a practicing public health nurse in South Carolina in the 1940s, midwives attended more than 60 percent of childbirths by black women in Alabama, Arkansas, Florida, Georgia, Mississippi, and South Carolina (Blackburn 1942). These lay granny midwives lived in rural communities and had no formal education. However, they were held in high esteem and were believed to be endowed with special ability and wisdom related to birthing babies. Several midwives were in their church's most recognized position of spiritual wisdom, Mother of the Church (Holmes 1986), a designation determined by consensus of the church membership. This revered position was reserved for an elderly person who demonstrated a high degree of compassion, caring, and wisdom and who led an exemplary Christian life. Some midwives participated in brief courses sponsored by the local health departments, but the practice of midwifery in African-American communities was perceived as a traditional art and calling that one generation of women had handed down to another from the eighteenth century to the 1940s. "Catching babies" was "women's business" and was perhaps the only arena in which males willingly deferred to the authority and knowledge of women. During childbearing and for a short time thereafter, African-American women experienced a temporary emancipation from a life typified by white oppression and male domination. These women-centered patterns had their precedents in African heritage and culture. In Africa, one of women's primary roles was that of motherhood. Much value was placed upon bearing and raising children, and those roles were retained as much as possible during and after the practice of slavery (White 1985).

Thus the process of pregnancy and childbirth empowered both the granny midwives and the women they tended. Midwives believed that they were called to this noble work and ordained by God. This enabled them to transcend the limitations placed on "ordinary people" and access a higher power, their own power being a special gift from God. When asked about the source of her ability and skill in delivering babies, an eighty-four-year-old retired midwife in rural Alabama in 1990 gave the following reply: "Well, I think that was a gift God gave me. Cause, I tell you, when I do go. . . it must have been something from God. . . . I always was pushing him in front to do things for me and he did. Wherever I go, I always put him in front and he would help me. And I always did it. I had a little trouble, but with the Lord, I went through it" (Davis and Ingram 1990). These women functioned as autonomous independent practitioners. They engaged in complex decision making coupled with empathetic, compassionate caring. The power of granny's empathetic caring is best described by a middle-aged woman who was attended by a midwife during the birth of her children in the 1940s. Sharing her ideas on the differences in the care provided to her by a physician and by a granny midwife, she stated:

> Granny midwives did more caring . . . there was more hands on, they touched you and made you feel [safe]. Yes, she would be sitting right there by your side, you wouldn't have a hard time like we do in the hospital, you hurting and nobody there to touch you. The midwife would probably be there, your grandmama [would be] there. It wouldn't be like she was out to lunch or out of the house. (Davis and Ingram 1990)

In addition to being skilled, compassionate birth attendants, granny midwives also provided prenatal and postpartum care. They would visit the pregnant mother, telling her how to take care of herself during pregnancy and advising her about what was needed in preparation for the new baby. Typically, the midwife stayed with the mother during labor, helped her through the delivery, and monitored and cared for her through the early post-delivery period. She would go home for a day or so, only to be back on the third day. On that visit, she would "take the mother up," which meant getting her out of bed for the first time, giving her advice on her care and that of the baby, and "do up the wash." She advised new mothers to stay inside for two to three weeks before getting out to do anything. As one midwife put it "getting out is a strain and you ain't doing nothing but catching cold. Your veins are open" (Davis and Ingram 1990). She cared and nurtured not only the mother and the new baby, but the whole family. From all accounts the granny was in charge. During the postpartum period she placed a number of restrictions on the mother's functioning. Another woman who was cared for by a granny in the 1940s recalls that the granny attending the delivery of her children recommended postpartum restrictions related to diet and physical activity. These included staying in bed for three to nine days following delivery and not lifting anything heavier than a skillet. The dietary restrictions focused on the elimination of fish, cabbage, "anything like inside a hog," and alcohol (Davis and Ingram 1990).

Midwives also functioned as fertility specialists. Recounting her care by a granny midwife, one woman recalled:

> I had went to several doctors and they said that I would never get pregnant. But I went to a midwife in a place called Pineapple, Alabama, and she said they say you can't have a baby but I'll show you that you can have babies. She said what you do is take nine eggs, raw eggs, fresh laid eggs, not refrigerated. And she said the only eggs that is going to make you sick is the ninth egg. I did what she said. Morning, noon, and night. And that ninth egg, I just got sick. And I got pregnant. Now, I don't know whether I believe that or it was true, but it happened. And I had kids like '57, '59, and '62. (Davis and Ingram 1990)

Information received from interviewees demonstrated that midwives were empowered through their specialized knowledge and by the local folks who believed that they had special skills and powers. The efficacy of the midwife-recipient relationship is revealed again in the testimony of another infertile woman. Asked about the midwife's knowledge of fertility, she answered: "I think they were strong. Just wise. They were strong women. They were wise. But I believed her. I believed every word she said. And it happened" (Davis and Ingram 1990).

Granny midwives handled not only normal deliveries, but everything with which they were called to assist. This meant they attended breech deliveries and other abnormal presentations; premature and excessively large babies; and, on occasion, babies with such abnormalities as hydrocephalus, an abnormally large head resulting from an accumulation of cerebro-spinal fluid because of a blockage in the brain. For many, the success rate in such situations was very high—midwives who were interviewed reported no instances of infant deaths among those they attended. Premature babies and babies with other problems would often be sent to the hospital for care after delivery, but not always. Sometimes the midwife would supervise care of the premature infant in the home. In addition to dealing with the physiological problems directly associated with the delivery, midwives oftentimes worked in environmental and material surroundings that were less than ideal. As one midwife said: "Oh, Lord, I had a white uniform and when I come home, I look like I been up the chimney and slid down. Nowhere to sit but on a keg or something like that. And the goat be in the house, and the chicken be in the house" (Davis and Ingram 1990). There are ample historical precedents for instances such as these.

Historical Development of African-American Granny Midwives

Historically, African-American granny midwives were women who had endured against formidable odds. The safety and sanctity they offered came from a spiritual calling to service. African-American women had to learn quickly to be self-forgiving, for often exterior events conflicted with their internal beliefs and sense of integrity. Still, they managed to survive (Angelou 1989). On antebellum plantations, African-American females performed the same labor as African-American men and were subjected to the same kinds of physical abuses. In addition, slave women endured sexual violence (Davis 1971). The historian and theorist Bell Hooks has written that it was common on a plantation to see female slaves stripped naked, tied to a stake, and whipped with a hard saw or club. White slavers often freely exercised their absolute power in relationship to female slaves, who were their legal property. They brutalized and exploited them economically and sexually without fear of retaliation; the women were legal property (Hooks 1981; see also Giddings 1984).

Yet African-American women survived verbal, psychological, physiological, and sexual abuse. Granny midwives, we contend, represented the high point of authority and control—and provided a pivotal empowering element—in plantation communities. They bestowed healing among women. Midwives whose hands linked generations through the miracle of birth were seen in their communities as models of strength, wisdom, and power. At a time when blacks were relegated to a legal status equalling three-fifths of a person, African-American midwives experienced high cultural autonomy and prestige. They also earned stature in the eyes of white owners as they attended a significant number of white births. How could these women "care" for those who separated their families, sold their children, and abused them sexually and physically? They stoically believed they were called by God into the profession. This gave them a special status that enabled them to transcend racial, cultural, environmental, and oppressive forces to do the Lord's work: deliver babies.

Up until the eighteenth century, for women of European descent of all social classes, midwifery had been the undisputed province of women. With the invention of forceps by the Chamberlains of Britain, a new era of obstetrics was begun. Hence, in the early nineteenth century, male physicians successfully usurped the midwives' role among middle- and upper-class white urban women, both in Europe and America (Aveling 1977; Cutter and Viels 1964; Robinson 1984). As one might expect, granny midwives remained the dominant birth attendants in rural areas and among ethnic, immigrant, and working-class communities. There is little significant evidence of midwifery among the "elite" from the nineteenth century onward (Wertz and Wertz 1977).

As men entered the lying-in chamber, critics of male midwives accused these physicians of turning to "ergot, chloroform, crushing forceps, and the perforators" in order to bring about more prompt deliveries. Other proponents of female lay midwives argued that the presence of a male in the lying-in chamber offended the modesty and delicacy of parturient women. The strongest argument against women pursuing the newly "scientificized" profession was the claim that women's uteri and central nervous systems rendered them incapable. The medical community hypothesized that shock to the nervous system, incurred from intense academic study (now a requirement for birth attendants), prohibited a woman student's reproductive organs from growing to full maturity. Thus women were excluded from the new science of obstetrics (Litoff 1978).

With the introduction of males into the birthing chambers, childbirth was transformed from a group domain of women conducting women's business to an individualized medical crisis requiring the services of a male medical practitioner. With the incorporation of forceps, anesthetic agents, and surgical procedures by the medical profession, the grannies' practices were increasingly viewed as mystical, rudimentary, and obsolete. Yet among common folk the popularity of midwives continued. As among African Americans, a large number of immigrant midwives attended the childbirths of fellow immigrant women. They fulfilled needs unique to their own group, such as commonalities of language, religious practices, and cultural rituals.

The suppression of African-American and ethnic midwives extended beyond concerns of inadequate academic preparation to questions of prejudice. Also at play were complex issues of medical professionalization. To further the exclusivity and profitability of the new science of obstetrics, another argument used against midwives was that there was an excess of practitioners. Garrigues, a medical doctor writing in 1890, argued that there was a superabundance of medical men in the United States who were in great need of obstetrical cases. He reported that there was one physician for every 150 women of childbearing age (Litoff 1986). The question that arises is, who was Garrigues counting? As late as 1930, there was approximately one black physician for every 3,300 blacks (Robinson 1984). Surely, Garrigues' statistics did not consider African Americans or the effect of the elimination of granny midwives in their communities. Disproportionately few white physicians served rural and African-American communities. Thus the burgeoning medical profession recognized midwives who practiced in these communities as "necessary evils."

The stop-gap solution proferred by physicians was to provide midwives with limited education to facilitate their effectiveness. Physicians were in the forefront of those blaming midwives for maternal-infant mortality figures in the United States. In 1918, twenty-three thousand women in the United States died from conditions related to childbirth; and in 1921, the maternal death rate in America was higher than that of almost every foreign country for which statistics were available (Litoff 1986). Ironically, many foreign countries utilized midwives, yet their mortality rates were lower than those in the United States. The American Medical Association (AMA), recognizing that lower infant mortality rates during the early part of the twentieth century in European countries were attributable to midwife education, sought to abolish the midwife problem by placing midwives under control of state educational requirements. Hence only the "intelligent" (i.e., those privileged enough to have access to formal training) could continue to practice, until even they were eventually phased out in favor of physicians (Litoff 1986). Debate over the licensing of midwives led to the passage of the Sheppard-Towner Act of 1921, and as a result, Congress provided training grants to states. At monthly meetings, public health nurses gave instruction to granny midwives on asepsis and basic maternity care and informed health officials of problems encountered in practice. Identifiable problems consisted mainly of children failing to achieve appropriate weight for age (used as an index of the nutritional status) (Robinson 1984). A granny midwife from rural Alabama interviewed in 1990 recalled her experience at one such meeting: "I went to the county health department and they had a nurse coming from Montgomery. They taught us how to make bed paddings with newspapers that you put under the mother when she was delivering" (Davis and Ingram 1990). At this meeting public health nurses praised granny midwives for identifying women and children who were at risk in their communities or who had health problems that needed the attention of medical personnel. Once clients at risk were referred to health care officials, they were not attended by midwives. Ironically, by complying with regulations, grannies contributed to their own demise. Midwives were credited with identifying and relocating eleven thousand patients into prenatal clinics in the state of South Carolina in 1941–42. According to the state health office, ethnic and African-American patients did not wish to come to the clinics, and they used every device in their power to outwit the midwife who was to bring them there. But the midwives stood firm in refusing to take any case in which the expectant mother did not get approval for midwifery services from a physician (Blackburn 1942). These regulations continued. A granny midwife from rural Alabama stated that during her practice as a midwife in the 1960s: "I could not deliver any babies without the approval of the physician. He had to say that she was okay to deliver at home" (Davis and Ingram 1990). Granny midwives who were interviewed asserted that they could not deliver a baby unless the mother had a card from the health department approving her delivery by a midwife. In short, the control of midwives by the medical profession was very pronounced, placing the granny in an awkward middle role and limiting her autonomy. Rather than inhibiting obstetrical prenatal care, granny midwives complied and served as facilitators.

In the midst of the early-twentieth-century debate over the role of midwives, the creation of trained nurse-midwives (with formal academic education in nursing and midwifery) was suggested by a few physicians and public health officials. The first concrete effort to establish a nurse-midwife service in the United States occurred in 1925, with Mary Breckinridge's service in Kentucky. Despite the excellent records of trained nurse-midwives, over the next several decades nurse-midwifery failed to make significant headway as a recognized profession and did little to quell the midwife debate (Litoff 1986). The more powerful and articulate professional medical associations continued to blame high infant mortality rates on midwives, as they had done in the mid- and late-nineteenth century (Litoff 1978). By 1936 most states had closed their midwife training programs, claiming they were too costly for the numbers of recipients involved. Alabama offers an exception to this trend. There, the Tuskegee Institute established a midwifery training program for African-American public health nurses in 1941. During its five-year period of operation, a total of twenty-five African-American midwives were graduated (Robinson 1984). At this time, approximately half of all births in the United States still occurred in women's homes (Leavitt 1986).

In 1976 Alabama's Lay Midwifery Practice Act was repealed and replaced by the Nurse Midwifery Authorization Act, which aimed to replace folk midwives with professionally trained nurse midwives. Under the new law, no new permits were issued to lay midwives. However, existing lay midwives were "grandmothered" (they could continue to practice) until their permits expired or were revoked by a county board of health. Under the 1976 law, a nurse midwife was defined as a registered nurse (RN) whose practice was regulated by a joint task force of the Board of Nursing and the Board of Medical Examiners. Regulations required: a) graduation from an approved Alabama Certified Nurse-Midwifery program; b) American College of Nurse-Midwife certification (ACNM)—granted if the midwife graduates from an accredited midwifery program, is recommended for certification by the program director, and passes an examination administered by the ACNM; c) a current Alabama RN license; d) compliance with ACNM continuing education and recertification requirements; and e) submission of the name of a licensed physician-sponsor actively engaged in the practice of obstetrics and gynecology to whom the nurse-midwife is accountable (*Journal of Nurse-Midwifery* 1984). This law signaled the official end of the granny midwife in Alabama. However, her legacy lives on.

Contrary to what advocates of contemporary nurse-midwifery argue, we do not see drastic improvements in maternal-infant mortality rates. According to Claude Fox, an Alabama State Health Official speaking in 1990, prenatal care—not the birth attendant—is the closest determinant of mortality statistics. His findings reveal that Alabama ranks fifth in the country in infant mortality. The major contributor to infant mortality is low birth weight. For African Americans in Alabama, infant mortality rates and incidences of low birth weight are twice that of whites. However, for African-American mothers who had prenatal care (of at least eleven to thirteen visits), infant mortality rates were vastly improved over those who recieved no prenatal care (Fox 1990).

When she was interviewed in her home in 1990, an eighty-five-year-old granny midwife from rural Alabama who had successfully delivered over three thousand babies shared her thoughts on the causes of the alarmingly high infant mortality rate among blacks. Recalling her own days at the bedside, she said:

> I would tell them what they supposed to do and you know cut down their habits if they had one for nine months for goodness sake. A lot of the time, people get pregnant, they not healthy themselves. And quite naturally their baby not going to be what you think he ought to be. He going to be defective some way. I wouldn't go back for nothing now, cause I see so much happening to people who is pregnant and they ain't stop none of their ways. Some of the babies come wrong or be deformed or they don't be right. (Davis and Ingram 1990)

Among the types of care she advocated were improved diet, exercise, rest, and temperance. Today, the voices of granny midwives are largely silenced within their own communities. They have been labeled as ignorant and superstitious, as a problem or unhygienic. Yet when they were allowed to practice, they diligently carried out their duties and achieved excellent results. Their people listened to them and respected their directions because they thought midwives were filled with the Holy Spirit. Without the aid of sophisticated modern equipment, the midwives who were interviewed for this study successfully delivered over four thousand babies. They were empowered and provided care that was both medically safe and heartfelt. This compels us to ask: what have we gained compared to what we have lost?

Notes

This essay is dedicated to the memory of Carrie M. Ingram, one who was empowered by a "Granny." The authors wish to extend special thanks to Dr. Ann Clark, director of the Center for Nursing Research, University of Alabama at Birmingham, School of Nursing.

It is based upon secondary historical material and primary data from a qualitative research study conducted by the authors in 1990. The respondents in the study were drawn from four southwestern Alabama counties. Granny midwives and recipients of care by granny midwives were interviewed using open-ended, semi-structured questionnaires. The respondents were identified from information provided by state and local health employees. Conversations with lay community residents were also helpful in identifying and locating respondents. Respondents were contacted by telephone, and the interviews were conducted in a health care agency and in the homes of the respondents. The individuals interviewed remain anonymous in order to protect their privacy. Transcripts of the interviews are housed at the University of Alabama at Birmingham Nursing Research Center, Birmingham, Alabama.

Works Cited

Angelou, M. 1989. Interview in B. Lanker, ed. *I Dream a World*. New York: Stewart, Tobari and Chang, 162.

Aveling, J. 1977. *The Chamberlains and the Midwifery Forces*. London: Churchill.

Blackburn, L. 1942. "The Midwife as an Ally." *American Journal of Nursing* 42:57.

Cutter, I., and H. Viels. 1964. *A Short History of Midwifery*. Philadelphia: W. B. Saunders.

Davis, A. 1971. "Reflections on the Black Women's Role in the Community of Slaves." *Black Scholar* 3 (4).

Davis, S., and C. Ingram. 1990. Unpublished research interviews in Central and Southwest Alabama. University of Alabama–Birmingham School Of Nursing, Birmingham, Ala.

Fox, C. "The State of Black Health in Alabama." Paper read before the State of Black Health Conference at the University of Alabama–Birmingham, Birmingham, Ala., March 2, 1990.

Giddings, P. 1984. *When and Where I Enter: The Impact of Black Women on Race and Sex in America*. New York: Bantam.

Holmes, L. 1984. "Alabama Granny Midwives." *Journal of the Medical Society of New Jersey* 81:389–91.

———. 1986. "Traditional Afro-American Midwives." In Pamela S. Eakins, ed. *The American Way of Birth*. Philadelphia: Temple University Press.

Hooks, B. 1981. *Ain't I a Woman: Black Women and Feminism*. Boston: South End Press.

Editorial. 1984. *Journal of Nurse-Midwifery* 29:63.

Leavitt, J. 1986. *Brought to Bed: Childbearing in America 1750 to 1950*. New York: Oxford University Press.

Litoff, J. 1978. *American Midwives: 1860 to the Present*. Westport, Conn.: Greenwood Press.

————. 1986. *The American Midwife Debate.* New York: Greenwood Press.

Robinson, S. 1984. "A Historical Development of Midwifery in the Black Community: 1600-1940." *Journal of Nurse-Midwifery* 29:247–50.

Wertz, R., and D. Wertz, 1977. *Lying-in: A History of Childbirth in America.* New York: Macmillan.

White, D. 1985. *A'rn't I a Woman? Female Slaves in the Plantation South.* New York: W. W. Norton Co.

Childbirth, Lay Institution Building, and Health Policy: The Traditional Childbearing Group, Inc., of Boston in a Historical Context

GLORIA WAITE

Introduction

A non-profit, black midwifery group, the Traditional Childbearing Group, Inc. (TCB), was founded on Mother's Day, 1978, in Boston, Massachusetts. The uniqueness of the TCB stems from the fact that, in its origins and objectives, it draws on two distinct traditions, namely, modern lay midwifery and traditional African-American midwifery. It has an organizational structure appropriate for carrying out its projects in an urban environment and is attuned to the needs of the African-American community. Thus, while specializing in home birthing, the TCB is also actively involved in the African-American community in Boston, promoting and providing information on breastfeeding, prenatal and postpartum care, child care, nutrition, adolescent parenting, and non-maternal health care.

TCB and Modern Lay Midwifery

Modern lay midwifery emerged in America in the late 1960s and early 1970s, a period of great cultural and social transformation for both blacks and whites that was spawned by the civil rights movement of the early 1960s. In this period, black and white health care reformers in the civil rights and feminist movements began to raise questions about the quality of health care and, in particular, about male physician and technological dominance of obstetrics and gynecology (Ruzek 1978, 62–64). Women opened alternative clinics, founded self-help health groups, and began utilizing "natural" and home birthing services (Ruzek 1978, 9, 47–49, 58–62). Some modern African-American midwives were not motivated as much by medicine's technological dominance as by the inadequate service their people were receiving. For instance, Shafia Monroe co-founded the Traditional Childbearing Group, Inc., out of a concern for the "high rate of adverse reproductive outcomes within the black community and the medical care system's difficulty in providing community-oriented care" (Sakala and Ekstein 1987, 4). Betty Watts Carrington, an African-American nurse-midwife in New York City, said she was "motivated by the desire to improve the quality of health care rendered to the mothers and babies with whom I worked" (Carrington 1978, 34).

Monroe and other contemporary lay midwives who do home birthing differ from their predecessors—such as the "granny midwives" of the South, the partera of the Mexican-American communities, and the midwives of the Amish and Mormons—since they began practicing at younger ages, have college educations, and are raising children of their own (Reid 1989, 223–24). For example, Monroe is in her early thirties. She assisted her first home delivery when she was nineteen-years old. Over the next five years, Monroe trained and worked as a nurse's aid, earned a bachelor's degree in arts, and began raising children of her own (personal interview, Shafia Monroe, 1 March 1990).

Like their predecessors, however, modern lay midwives acquire their skills through apprenticeship with another midwife and express the feeling of being "called" to their profession (Reid 1989, 223). As a child in Boston, and in Alabama where she spent her summers, Monroe brought home sick animals and homeless people. She wanted to be a veterinarian when she grew up. At the age of fifteen, however, she converted to Islam within two months of her mother's sudden death. A Muslim who did not know of her interest in healing nevertheless intuitively detected something of this and gave her the name "Shafia," which means "the healer" in Arabic. Monroe lived with a Muslim family, learning some aspects of childbearing and child care from a woman in the home. This woman had many children of her own but was not a practicing midwife, although she had a great deal of interest in the subject. Monroe received her inspiration from this woman and decided that she "wanted to help black women give birth to healthy babies" and would become an obstetrician. She entered college as a pre-med student. While taking courses related to reproductive medicine, she began training in Boston with midwives from Zaire, Pakistan, Ghana, and Alabama (Gaskin 1990, 7; personal interview, Shafia Monroe, 1 March 1990). Subsequent to her apprenticeship, Monroe, like many other lay midwives (Lee and Glasser 1974, 539), attended local midwifery classes, acquiring in the process more legitimacy than she otherwise might have had with physicians and others who value credentials (personal interview, Shafia Monroe, 1 March 1990). Monroe points out, however, that a midwife "doesn't need training as such"; she adds: "There's a role for training; it can help, but it's not essential. There's a spiritual aspect [to the work] and there's not a lot to having a baby, anyway" (personal interview, Shafia Monroe, 1 March 1990). (The belief in guiding spiritual forces is widespread among lay midwives, but at a secular level they also know that childbirth is a natural experience. Their use of natural techniques to assist the process, such as teas to stimulate labor and oil and massages to help the baby pass through the birth canal, is nothing more than the application of what one midwife called "motherwit" [DeVries 1985, 93; Logan 1989, 89,135–57].) Unlicensed modern midwives such as Monroe are also like their predecessors in having considerable autonomy over their work. Their independence distinguishes them from licensed midwives and nurse-midwives, both of whom are under state control and are trained and supervised by doctors (DeVries 1985, 90–117; Reid 1989, 237).

In the 1970s, the number and percentage of out-of-hospital births increased nationwide (DeVries 1985, 49–50). Women began turning to planned home birthing for several reasons, among which the desire to have a natural birthing experience that they could control may be the most significant (DeVries 1985, 110; Lee and Glasser 1974, 541; Logan 1989, 127–29). Many women were uncomfortable with the services provided by hospitals and clinics, which they regarded as too fragmented, impersonal, often insulting, and unnecessarily medicalized (Lee and Glasser 1974, 542; Macintyre 1977, 479). Others preferred home birth because they had no one to care for their children, while some women wanted to be certain that they were attended by another woman (Lee and Glasser 1974, 542). For women without health insurance, home birthing was a low-cost option they could afford (Hart 1990, 1; Lee and Glasser 1974, 542). Studies show that fully 80 percent of the women who have given birth at home and in the hospital prefer home birthing (Devitt, 1977, 49).

Increased demand for midwifery services increased the expenses of the midwives. They spent more time on bookkeeping and needed to maintain small libraries for themselves and their clientele. They also needed beeper services, answering machines, or second phone lines. Many clients lived beyond walking distance of their midwives, who thus incurred the additional costs of gasoline and car maintenance. Furthermore, having young children of their own, many midwives must arrange for child care while attending to their clients (Reid 1989, 230). As a result of these added expenses, therefore, modern midwives became increasingly business-oriented, a process that distinguishes them from earlier midwives.

In these circumstances, the midwives began charging fees for attending home births. Generally, the fees range from $400 to $600, which is still considerably less than the $2000 to $3000 charged for obstetrician-attended hospital births (DeVries 1985, 52). The Traditional Childbearing Group charges $5 and $10 for individual prenatal care visits, $45 to $60 for a series of seven childbirth classes, and $600 for comprehensive maternity services (Hart 1990, 21; Sakala 1989, 898). Clients who cannot afford these fees pay what they can or are not charged at all, with the hope that they will spread the word about maternal health or do volunteer work for the TCB (Hart 1990, 21; Sakala 1989, 898). Fees collected by the TCB are shared with assistants, including apprentices and lactation experts (personal interview, Shafia Monroe, 1 March 1990).

Yet despite the rising demand for home birthing service, most lay midwives are not financially independent and must rely on the incomes of their spouses to sustain themselves and their children (Reid 1989, 229). Since their method of practice is labor intensive, the midwives are able to serve only a limited number of clients at any given time. For instance, Monroe presently has only twenty to thirty clients a year (Hart 1990, 21; personal interview, Shafia Monroe, 1 March 1990), and, as noted, not all of her clients can afford to pay. Between 1977 and 1987, however, she delivered 350 babies (Adams 1987, 26), or an average of thirty-five babies a year.

Like other lay midwives, Monroe provides personalized service, which makes her relationship with her clients different from that of an obstetrician (DeVries 1985, 106). In this regard, Monroe says, "there's a relationship there that will continue, I believe, until death do us part. And obstetricians cannot say that. They assist the mother . . . and then they don't have that connection again." She adds, "Catching the baby is the quick, easy, technical part of assisting childbearing families. Building relationships of trust and influence is the hard part that requires sustained effort" (Sakala and Ekstein 1987, 5). Monroe has contact with her clients long after delivery (personal interview, Tijuana Tillery, 6 March 1990; telephone interview, Rhonita Harris, 6 March 1990) and does not charge them for services such as counseling and referrals that she provides before and after delivery (personal interview, Shafia Monroe, 1 March 1990). The fact that people respect her advice and continue to call her years after childbirth demonstrates the trust families place in her.

The business orientation of modern lay midwives is not limited to their home birthing service. Some of them have opened offices in order to promote their work and present it in a professional manner (DeVries 1985, 106–7; Reid 1989, 235). For instance, the TCB was founded in order to advocate home birthing. It is a cooperative organization with a small staff of trained midwives and lactation experts. The group writes proposals for private grants, for which it must hire part-time consultants and bookkeepers. When it has sufficient funding, it hires a secretary and rents office space, which it uses as a reading room, for centralization of services, and for holding meetings (Hart 1990, 21; personal interview, Shafia Monroe, 1 March 1990).

Yet, though similar to other modern lay midwifery groups in terms of structure, business orientation, and the backgrounds of its personnel, the Traditional Childbearing Group is different from them in the relationship it has with the community it serves. This orientation derives from the older practice of traditional black midwifery in America, with its focus on the community. Nor is this orientation restricted to the TCB. Another midwifery group, the Houston-based Childbirth Providers of African Descent, is also reported to have a community focus (Sakala 1989).

Traditional African-American Midwifery and Community Service

From the colonial period to the twentieth century, traditional African-American midwives, commonly known as "granny midwives," were an enduring feature of southern society. Each plantation had a midwife who served it and the surrounding neighborhood. Midwives attended the births of 90 percent of the blacks and at least 50 percent of the whites (Savitt 1978, 182–84). These traditional midwives were generally the older, more intelligent women in their communities (Campbell [1946] 1984, 7). It has been said of them that they were "the repository of folk wisdom concerning the inscrutable ways of nature, and the guardian of the younger generation" (Frazier [1939] 1948, 119–20). Traditional midwives were particularly proficient in attending breech births, treating hemorrhage with herbal therapies, and accelerating the pace of labor (Sakala and Ekstein 1987, 4; Logan 1989, 84, 90–91, 141). They learned their craft through apprenticeship to other midwives and through self-education (Campbell [1946] 1984, 7). After slavery, in some southern counties traditional midwives were informally organized, with a well-established apprenticeship system, clear lines of command and succession, and sanctions to maintain the integrity of their profession (Mongeau et al. 1961).

A common feature in traditional and modern African-American lay midwifery is the role of religion in the work. Traditional midwives and their clients were Christians (Dougherty 1978; Logan 1989). Some women spoke of praying with the midwife, which helped distract them from the labor and gave them great comfort (Carrington 1978, 45). Modern lay midwifery, on the other hand, emerged at a time when an increasing number of African Americans were converting to Islam. Thus, as noted, Monroe is a practicing Muslim. There are no apparent Islamic features in the program or structure of the TCB, however, and its members and clients belong to different faiths. Yet the fact that Monroe, like many traditional midwives, attributes the success of her work to a higher source and regards her profession as a "calling" clearly indicates a persistent religious influence in African-American midwifery.

Traditional African-American midwives, like their modern successors, provided services other than assisting childbirth. They gave massages to expectant mothers and supplied patent medicines and home remedies made from Native-American roots and herbs (Logan 1989, 53). This practice continues today among modern black and white lay midwives (DeVries 1985, 93; personal interview with Joyce Lawrence, 7 March 1990; personal interview with Shafia Monroe, 1 March 1990). Traditional midwives did not give prenatal care (Logan 1989, 55, 65), but they provided postnatal care and helped mothers with various domestic chores, including cooking, washing, and taking care of small children within the home.

Onnie Lee Logan, an Alabama traditional midwife who was born about 1910, told her story in 1984. In practice in Mobile for close to four decades, Logan provided a vivid description of the extreme poverty of most of the black (and many white) residents from the 1940s through the 1960s, and of the tasks she performed for "her families," as she referred to her clients. One of the most daunting problems Logan faced in home birthing was having a clean setting for delivering babies. Many homes lacked soap, clean clothing, and clean bedding. Logan described her help as follows:

> When I went home after delivery I would carry whatever they needed back. Food, soap, sheets, clothin that I could make. I would sit down alot a days and just make not only the lil baby somethin to put on, the other babies too as well somethin to put on. Alot of em was hungry. Alot a times they didn't really have hardly bread for the lil ones in the family that was there in those times. (Logan 1989, 96)

Logan worked as a maid in the home of a wealthy white doctor and received about a dollar-and-a-half a week for unlimited hours of service (Logan 1989, 86, 104–6). She recalled not having "hardly anything myself. . . .but I shared whatever" little she had (Logan 1989, 96).

When she was a child, Logan aspired to be a nurse; she first tended her wooden dolls, then helped bathe her nephews and nieces, and cared for the sick people her mother nursed (Logan 1989, 66–71). Unable to go to high school, Logan could not fulfill her dream of becoming a nurse. When she was about twenty-one-years old, she assisted a doctor who came to deliver a baby in a family she was working for in Magnolia, Alabama. Impressed by her skills, the doctor told her, "You would make a good midwife. Not only make a good midwife. I think you'll make a good doctor" (Logan 1989, 80). She was determined from that day to become a midwife. While encouraged by the doctor's comment, however, Logan's inspiration to pursue her goal came from the pride she felt for her mother and grandmother, both of whom were midwives. Her grandmother, about whose work Logan grew up hearing stories, was particularly inspiring (Logan 1989, 48–50). Her memories of her own mother sacrificing to help people encouraged her to help families (Logan 1989, 96).

Logan took her sense of social responsibility to new levels in the 1950s. If a man was working but not taking proper care of his family, Logan reported those families to the county welfare department, which then took the father to court and garnished his wages. When it was simply a case of a family having no money because of unemployment, she reported the matter to the field nurse of the board of health (Logan 1989, 97). In all cases, even before turning to state services, Logan brought her own relief to these families (Logan 1989, 97–98). She did not limit her work to maternity cases. As a counselor in her church, she advised young women to delay pregnancy, since she was concerned about unwed teen mothers (Logan, 1989, 112–13). She gave massages and applied a grease and turpentine-based remedy to women who complained of "female troubles." From her own description, this was probably prolapsed uterus (Logan 1989, 117–19), a protrusion of the uterus through the vagina in women who have borne children and who do strenuous work.

Onnie Lee Logan's story is especially valuable, not only for its details of the services she and other traditional midwives rendered, but also because there are very few, if any, traditional midwives still practicing in the South. Their days were numbered when, in the early decades of this century, American midwifery came under attack from public health advocates and obstetricians. At the time, many public health issues were being raised, and public health reformers alleged that lay midwifery was an unhygienic practice. Additionally, a general medicalization of life in the early twentieth century led obstetricians to convince the public that childbirth was a pathological condition requiring technological intervention. In an age when specialist and monopoly medicine were becoming the norm (Brown 1979, 80–97), obstetricians attacked midwifery in order to build up their own clienteles (DeVries 1985, 39–42).

State boards of health, with funds provided under the federal Sheppard-Towner Maternity and Infancy Protection Act of 1921, began to institute programs for midwife education and registration (DeVries 1985, 38). Midwives in northern cities were primarily European immigrants serving members of their own ethnic groups. Their numbers rapidly declined after World War I through a combination of factors, including restrictions on European immigration and an increase in the number of hospital beds (DeVries 1985, 38). Midwives had attended 40 percent of all births in 1915, but only 11 percent by 1935 (Devitt 1977, 48). The rest went unattended or were attended by doctors at home or in hospitals. Increasingly, however, births took place in hospitals, and from 1930 to 1960 the proportion of hospital births rose from 37 to 96 percent (Devitt 1977, 47). In 1935, by contrast, 54 percent of all black babies were still being delivered by midwives (Devitt 1977, 48). This practice, however, was restricted to the South, since African Americans who were migrating to northern cities in the interwar period generally delivered their babies in municipal hospitals (Carrington 1978, 40). Because of its segregationist policies and its endemic poverty, the south had both a dearth of hospital beds and a shortage of doctors, especially for black people.

At the beginning of the regulatory period, public health nurse-midwives nationwide were trained for work with the poor (Campbell [1946] 1984, 9–10; DeVries 1985, 39), but in the South there were too few of them. Thus, due to economic and social reasons, southern doctors could not eliminate African-American midwives altogether, despite their desire to do so. Instead they sought instead to regulate and control them and to teach them hygienic practices (Kobrin 1966, 353–54). Midwives were blamed for the high incidence of infant and maternal mortality among their clients, without any reference to the underlying socioeconomic causes (Logan 1989, 65–66). As Logan points out, however, it was not the fault of the midwives that as a result of inadequate diets black people were deficient in vitamins and minerals. Nor were the midwives responsible for the filthy conditions in which many people lived (Logan 1989, 56).

Following federal initiatives, however, in the 1920s the regulation and control of "granny midwives" began with state licensure. In the early 1940s, their supervision, training, and evaluation were placed under public health nurse-midwives (Campbell [1946] 1984, 10–11; Hine 1989, 71–73, 154–55). Traditional midwives were required to attend monthly meetings with the nurses, who drilled them in sanitary and safe maternity care and in state regulations, or what the midwives called "The New Law" (Campbell [1946] 1984, 8–43). The nurses inspected their bags, making sure that they contained only the supplies furnished by the health department and no "contraband" substances, such as roots, herbs, patent medicines, and homemade salves, all of which were forbidden (Campbell [1946] 1984, 27–28; Logan 1989, 53, 137–40). The regulatory measures resulted in a serious decimation in the ranks of traditional midwives. Annual licenses were not renewed for any number of reasons, including missing the monthly mandatory classes or simply because the state boards decided that some midwives were too old to practice (Campbell [1946] 1984, 18–20, 137–38; Logan 1989, 172–73; Mongeau et al. 1961, 500).[1] After the 1940s, the number of practicing midwives was further reduced when federal funds were made available for new maternity clinics. These gave southern women, both black and white, more childbirth options. Additionally, practicing midwives found it difficult to recruit from the next generation, whose members were able to find jobs with more regular hours and steady pay (Campbell [1946] 1984, 7).

Today, women in the South who employ traditional African-American midwives for home birthing do so because they want a natural delivery without medical intervention or, occasionally, because they are unwilling to pay the few thousand dollars for delivery in the hospital that their income would require of them (Logan 1989, 127–29). In some cases, midwives practice surreptitiously (Logan 1989, 174–75). In Alabama, for example, lay midwifery was outlawed in 1976, although Logan was allowed to practice legally until 1984, when her license was not renewed. The last "granny midwife" in Mobile, she was determined to continue practicing, even without a license (Logan 1989, xiii).[2]

The Health of the Contemporary African-American Community

In order to appreciate the context for the resurgence of African-American midwifery in contemporary urban settings, it is necessary to consider the health status of current African Americans, as well as the centuries-old institutional development within the black community that helps it confront its oppressive reality. The African-American community took root over two hundred years ago in two places, namely, in the slave quarters of the South, where over 95 percent of African Americans lived (Blassingame [1972] 1979; Rawick 1972), and in early American cities like Boston, where there were relatively large concentrations of free blacks (Curry 1981; Horton and Horton 1979). This community, slave and free, was distinct from the larger society in which it existed by virtue of its condition of servitude, poverty, discrimination, and, significantly, its resistance to these injustices. As a result of their exclusion from the dominant white society, blacks built separate institutions, such as churches, schools, small businesses, and self-help organizations. Thus, the emergence of the Traditional Childbearing Group and similar groups cannot be seen in isolation. They are an integral part of a long-standing process of institution building within a community continually finding ways to survive against formidable odds.

African Americans are not excluded from white society because they are "deviant" or "different." There are no profound cultural differences between white and black Americans. Rather, it is the American practice of white supremacy that keeps blacks from full participation in American society. What is not commonly realized is that long before the twentieth century black and white Americans began to share the same culture, including religious affiliation, family structure, and basic values. African Americans became Christians in very large numbers in antebellum America and in even larger numbers after the Civil War (Woodson 1921). Practically their entire social life and organization revolved around their church—whether this was the institutional church of free blacks or the "invisible" church of the slaves. Philosophically, they share in the "American messianic culture," which fuels a sense of destiny and the quest for upward mobility on the part of both blacks and whites (Moses 1982). Just as white Americans, blacks of all classes aspire to financial independence and social mobility. Their middle class, small as it was before the 1960s, has always lived according to the ideals of the white middle class (Bruce 1989). And for over a hundred years, until the 1960s, three-quarters of African-American families were headed by males.

The subject of the family needs further elaboration, since it is central to a discussion of maternal and child welfare. In the past twenty years there has been considerable debate regarding the extent to which the black family is comparable to or different from the white family. The sociologist E. Franklin Frazier ([1939] 1948) established the view that continued to be held up to and beyond the publication of the controversial study by Daniel P. Moynihan (1965): that blacks had a pathological family pattern, because they had more female-headed households than did whites. Frazier called the pattern "matriarchial." It was Frazier's emphasis on this model that [mis]informed the literature after him. Yet both his (Frazier [1939] 1948, 103–4) and Moynihan's (1965, 9) findings concurred with the revisionist studies in the 1970s, which show, irrefutably, that until the mid-1900s 70 to 80 percent of black families lived in male-headed, generally nuclear, households (Farley and Allen [1987] 1989, 163–65). Even during slavery, when blacks were separated at the whim of slave masters, the two-parent household was the ideal, if not always the reality (Gutman 1976). The great majority of the unmarried female heads of households were widowed women caring for their grandchildren or middle-age women who, in most cases, had men in the home while their children were growing up. To their credit, Frazier and others discussed the impact of poverty on the black family. One way in which African Americans coped with the poverty in their community, and with the high incidence of premature adult deaths, was by sharing the care of children. Black people attached great status to adopting motherless children. Older, widowed women, in particular, looked upon adoption as a privilege rather than a burden, and women of all ages willingly cared for the children of mothers who worked elsewhere (Johnson [1934] 1979, 71).

In the last two decades there has been a rapid expansion of poverty in , the African-American community (Wilson 1987). By 1984 the incomes of 34 percent of blacks, in contrast to 12 percent of whites, were below the poverty line (Farley and Allen [1987] 1989, 55). In the inner cities, where the majority of blacks live, there is widespread street crime, frequent violence against women and children, high infant mortality, child neglect, drug and alcohol addiction, teenage pregnancy, welfare dependency, increased school dropout and illiteracy rates, and high proportions of female-headed households due to high rates of divorce, separation, and non-marital childbirths (Farley and Allen [1987] 1989; Helmore and Laing 1986a–d; Wilson 1987).

The poverty of African Americans is concentrated mainly in female-headed households, since women, whether black or white, have historically earned less than men and their families are more financially disadvantaged than are poor, male-headed, black or white families (Wilson 1987, 27). By 1982, 71 percent of all poor black families were headed by single women, an enormous increase from less than 30 percent in 1959 (Wilson 1987, 71). Of the poor, black, female heads of families in the 1980s, 86 percent were under the age of twenty-five (Helmore and Laing 1986b, 29). The sharpest decline in employment, from 1960 to 1984, was of black males aged sixteen to twenty-four (Wilson 1987, 43). In 1948 pregnant teens married the fathers of their children in 35 percent of the cases, while in 1985 this rate was only 5 percent (Helmore and Laing 1986b, 29). In 1970 only 5 percent of all black children lived with a never-married parent, but by 1984 the proportion had increased to 24 percent, although at this later date only 2 percent of all white children were living with a never-married parent (Hilmore and Laing 1986b, 26).

At the same time that enormous structural changes were taking place in the American economy, as heavy manufacturing industries began closing, cutting back, or relocating abroad, the civil rights movement of the 1960s raised the hopes of African Americans for fuller participation in American society. The rising tensions and resulting riots in the urban ghettos prompted a federal response in the form of social programs which partly filled the social gap created by de-industrialization. Neighborhood health clinics (multiservice centers) were built; free milk and other supplementary foods were distributed through the Women, Infants, and Children program (WIC); free meals were provided in some elementary schools; and, thanks to Head Start, many children from low or zero income families received an early childhood education. Participation in these programs was based on income, but from the mid- to late 1970s, and especially in the 1980s, these and other "Great Society" programs were cut back or eliminated. Conservative federal administrations, taking their cue from the dominant white working- and middle-class majority that refused to pay for human services which were of no benefit to them, justified the cuts by arguing that poverty was increasing because of the very programs that had been created to alleviate it. The programs benefitted families living below the poverty line due to low wages or unemployment, yet cuts were made at the very time when poverty was on the rise in America and female-headed families were increasing to unprecedented levels.

The health status of African Americans has been seriously compromised by the cuts, compelling even a conservative periodical, which in the early 1980s helped lead the intellectual charge against social programs, to comment on the tragedy of "healthy babies fall[ing] low on the scale of priorities in today's White House" (*New Republic* 1985, 5). For instance, by 1983 almost half-a-million fewer children were receiving Medicaid, yet between 1981 and 1985 three million children joined the ranks of the poor (*New Republic* 1985, 5). Instead of placing the responsibility on budget cuts, however, the Reagan administration sought to blame poor women themselves for the resulting increase in infant mortality. Thus in 1985 Dr. James Mason, the acting U. S. assistant secretary of health, expressed the belief that prenatal care was widely available but pregnant women were not using it, ascribing this to "an apathy factor" (*New Republic* 1985, 6).

Because of the cuts in human services, increased social dislocation, and the continuing rise of poverty, the life chances of African Americans took a dramatic turn for the worse. A recent study by the state of Massachusetts of its Head Start population revealed some of the consequences of cuts in government-funded nutrition programs, namely, WIC and food stamps. Of 3,500 children aged two to six, in selected Head Start programs across the state, 90 percent live in families whose incomes are at or below the poverty line. Due to nutritional deficiencies in their diets, 10 percent are at risk for overweight, 9 percent have shorter than normal height, and another 8 percent are anemic because of iron deficiency (Reid 1990, 23). The problem was anticipated to grow worse, since more unemployment was expected in the state and the 1990 state budget resulted in substantial cuts in social and human services.

The most disturbing trend in this worsening health situation is the rising infant mortality rate. For instance, the city of Boston, which boasts one of the highest concentration of medical facilities in the nation—and some of its most renowned—had a black infant mortality rate of 26 deaths per one thousand births in 1985, an increase of 32 percent over the previous year (Knox 1987a). For white babies, by contrast, the rate in 1985 was 10.1 per thousand. By 1988, the black infant mortality rate in Boston had dropped to 24.4 deaths per thousand births, but the rate for whites declined even more, to 7.1 (Hart 1990, 21). The infant mortality rates for blacks in Boston are duplicated in every city and are twice as high in the rural South.[3] Thus black babies are dying in their first year at a rate over three times that of white babies.

The racial difference is thought to be caused by several factors. African-American women have a greater risk of infant loss because of compounding health and stress factors, and they have a high rate of low-birth weight babies due to a legacy of malnutrition (Kiple and King 1981). As a result of prematernal conditions, African-American women may need prenatal care more than other groups in the United States. A smaller percentage of them, however (62 percent, compared to 79 percent of white women in 1983), are receiving prenatal care within the first three months of conception or continuing to receive care throughout their pregnancy (Farley and Allen [1987] 1989, 50–52). Women generally fail to get prenatal care because of lack of available care, personal indifference, and lack of money.

Many women on Medicaid, for whom prenatal and obstetric care are free, are finding that an increasing number of doctors are unwilling to serve them, since the government reimburses them at a lower rate than do private insurance companies. In one New York county, for example, several hundred maternal Medicaid recipients received little or no prenatal care in

1984 because no obstetricians would treat them (*New Republic* 1985, 6). For women who can obtain free or low-cost prenatal care, there is often a two- to four-month waiting period (*New Republic* 1985, 6; Wilkerson 1987, 1), which delays the beginning of this care. Some women do not make their pregnancies a priority because they are living from crisis to crisis. They have reason enough to worry about finding rent money and food to eat. Other women are discouraged by poor public transportation systems, while some lack babysitters for their children while they spend several hours monthly making trips to clinics or hospitals. Some cities are making efforts to eliminate the transportation and child care problems, but the waiting lists grow longer, and more time is spent waiting to be seen (Wilkerson 1987, 1). Some women regard the trip to the doctor's office as a waste of time, especially if previously they had trouble getting care and then gave birth to healthy children. As one woman put it, "you wait four hours to see the doctor for five minutes. He just pokes at your stomach and tells you everything's O.K." (Wilkerson 1987, 1). Monroe describes her own experience getting prenatal care at a clinic, which she undertook in order to understand the experience of other women. She was not seen until two hours after her scheduled appointment, after which she was referred to several different locations for services. The only food to which she had access during this time was junk food in vending machines. Additionally, Monroe found the interview process demeaning in both tone and scope (Sakala and Ekstein 1987, 4–5).

Many low-income African-American women have no health insurance and do not qualify for Medicaid. As a result, they have difficulty receiving prenatal care. One of Monroe's clients, a secretary with no health insurance, told of how she could not afford to pay for prenatal care at a hospital, but could afford to pay Monroe for biweekly visits (Hart 1990, 21). A study of insurance coverage in Boston found that in 1987, 15 percent of the city's residents had no health insurance. Of this proportion, 64 percent had jobs and 45 percent earned more than twice the federal poverty level. Furthermore, blacks in Boston are one-and-a-half times as likely as whites to be uninsured. As a whole, the uninsured are fifteen times as likely as the insured to postpone needed medical care (Tye 1987, 1).

While poor teenage mothers have a higher proportion of low birth weight babies—probably attributable to their inadequate diets (Helmore and Laing 1986b, 29)—Monroe notes that many mature black women have nutritionally deficient diets. Birth outcomes are affected by poor diets that cause anemia, obesity, high blood pressure, and depression. Monroe also observes that many black women are preoccupied with the excessive crime and drugs in their neighborhoods and with the problem of getting a decent education for their children. She concludes that these stresses, together with the hostile and discriminatory attitudes of the dominant society, impact negatively on pregnancy (Sakala and Ekstein 1987, 4). Indeed, scientists are beginning to quantify the links between the excessive mortality of African Americans, the psychological impact of oppression (Kong 1990, 1), and the concomitant development of low self-esteem (Lee 1989, 1).

The Traditional Childbearing Group, Inc., and Community Service

Monroe and her colleagues organized the TCB out of an acute awareness that African-American women are not receiving quality prenatal health care. They chose the word "traditional" for the name of the group in order to emphasize "the tradition of women being supported and nurtured through the childbearing period by the family-centered care of midwives" (Sakala and Ekstein 1987, 4). Monroe regards herself, and midwives like her, as "community midwives." Their role is special, she says, because as members of the same community they can inspire respect and trust and are more influential than people who do not live and work in the community. Monroe explains:

> Community midwives provide comprehensive services—from nutritional guidelines to information on signs of labor to parenting advice—through one person and in one location. They have an advantage over clinical personnel because they see the environment in which their clients live and thus can develop a more accurate understanding of the kind of help they need. . . . People are able to be warmer and more open in the home setting. (Sakala and Ekstein 1987, 5)

Monroe maintains her most important functions are simply taking time to explain the importance of prenatal care and helping to alleviate the stress of her clients' poverty. Many of these women, she notes, "are just struggling to survive." In contrast to clinics and health centers, where pregnant women are generally scheduled for fifteen-minute prenatal visits, Monroe spends an hour with her clients. In this hour, she explains, "fifteen minutes is prenatal care. The rest is hugs, talking, learning to cook and learning to eat well" (Hart 1990, 21).

Midwives, whether traditional or modern, are familiar with and attentive to the home settings of their clients (DeVries 1985, 106). They have what Monroe describes as "a holistic approach to the care of women and families." Since they share, or at any rate are familiar with, the cultural assumptions of their clients, midwives are in a much better position to discourage behavioral patterns that have negative consequences for mother and child. When necessary, the midwife links women to doctors, health clinics, detoxification centers, social workers, food vouchers, heating fuel, and even housing, and in the process teaches them how to use the system (Hart 1990, 21). Since the TCB is independent and community-oriented, it can help its clients become informed and assertive consumers. They can be advised to avoid unnecessary medical procedures, gain access to their records, and give priority to preventive health practices (Sakala 1989, 897).

Monroe regards midwifery as the first line of defense in a community riddled with a multitude of illnesses. "My midwifery is not just catching babies," she says. "You can't isolate it. We have to deal with all the illnesses at once. Midwifery is bringing people back together . . ." (Gaskin 1990, 12). In order to attain this goal, the TCB educates the community, local doctors, and other professional health care providers about the important contributions made by midwives. It formulates its programs and services to serve the particular needs of the African-American community. Members of the TCB go to laundromats, grocery stores, community centers, and the streets to hand out pamphlets it produces on the importance of breastfeeding, the need for prenatal care, and the benefits of home birthing (Sakala 1989, 897). The TCB provides sexuality education for teens at state juvenile detention centers and in a summer work program (Gaskin 1990, 8–10; Sakala 1989, 898). It holds prenatal and breastfeeding workshops on a regular basis at the women's state prison, in ghetto high schools, and at the Boston City Hospital (Prescott 1990; Sakala 1989, 898). Some services, such as its teen childbirth and parental education classes and the breastfeeding support services, are provided free of charge (Sakala 1989, 898). The TCB places particular emphasis on breastfeeding, in part because the medical system has de-emphasized it (Sakala and Ekstein 1987, 5), despite its well-documented positive value. The TCB's childbirth education classes reach over 1,000 adults and teens per year. An estimated 1,800 callers per year receive information, advice, and referrals on its twenty-four-hour phone line. Up to three hundred clients are helped annually through its breastfeeding workshops, which are held separately from the classes it conducts at public institutions. About forty-five teenage girls come to TCB parenting classes each year (Sakala 1989, 897–98).

The TCB is active at other levels as well. When the eight nurse-midwives at Boston City Hospital resigned in 1988 due to limits placed on their practice by the chief of obstetrics (Knox 1988, 17), TCB developed videotapes on childbirth issues for television and organized community support for the nurse-midwifery services at the hospital (Sakala 1989, 898; personal communication with Shafia Monroe, June 1988). Monroe also trains other women to become community midwives, under the slogan: "If you want to save an unborn's life, become a midwife" (Sakala and Ekstein 1987, 5). Her dream is that "In Roxbury [the center of Boston's black community], there would be a midwife every five blocks in the next five years" (Gaskin 1990, 12).

Non-maternal care is also addressed by the TCB. It annually measures the blood pressure of about 150 people at various sites and serves about forty families a year in its family counseling service (Sakala 1989, 898). Since 1988 it has annually held all-women's symposiums, which are announced through various means, including distributing leaflets in public places in Roxbury and north Dorchester—the two Boston black neighborhoods in the immediate vicinity of the TCB's office. At these annual symposiums an increasing number of African-American women of diverse backgrounds share an evening of food and music. They are presented with lectures and demonstrations by African-American women healers and others on such topics as massage, chiropractic, nutrition, sisterhood, herbal medicines, the technique of wrapping babies on the back, and the history of African-American women healers. In addition to empowering its clients, the TCB empowers women working within the group (Sakala 1989, 898), helping them to build skills, become more aware of policy issues in their city, and get involved in working on some of the social problems in their community. In the past decade, through its work on behalf of this constituency, TCB has established itself as a major grass-roots organization within Boston's black community.

Community Midwifery and Public Health Policy

The extent to which the TCB or any other community midwifery group can be effective depends upon the support it receives from the community and health care professionals. Unlike Onnie Lee Logan, who came from a long line of midwives whose services were respected and needed by the people they served, (Logan 1989, 60, 65), Shafia Monroe began practicing at a time when over 95 percent of all births were taking place in hospitals. Home birthing in the last two decades has been sought mainly by middle-class white women. Monroe's earliest clients were African-American women who chose home birthing for political reasons.

> These were women who were close to the Sixties, who were talking about cultural genocide, didn't trust the system, and who were going back to our roots of self-determination. They didn't want to have their babies delivered into a kind of system that never did us justice. They were alternative-type people, and they were well-educated. (Gaskin 1990, 8)

It is more difficult to convince young or less well-educated women about the values of home birthing and breastfeeding. The contemporary African-American community, taking its cues from the dominant white middle-class culture (which idealizes hospital delivery), has become estranged from its midwifery tradition (Sakala and Ekstein 1987, 5). Yet it is interesting to note that although studies find that most African-American women think hospital delivery is safer, many of them are ambivalent about technical interference in labor. A study of childbearing beliefs in a group of lower-class black women in the late 1960s found that "quite a few preferred staying home until the last possible moment in order to avoid 'them doctors messing you around' during labor" (Frankel 1977, 68). These women showed a strong interest in controlling their labor. The legacy of women-centered childbearing and of traditional African-American midwifery has not entirely vanished, since modern midwives permit the mother to remain in control of her experience (Frankel 1977, 66–67; Logan 1989, 152). Monroe's advice to women—"You can take charge and have a healthy baby"—applies to prenatal care as well as childbirth options (Sakala 1989, 897). Monroe also struggles against the indifferent and even contemptuous attitude that public health officials, obstetricians, and politicians have toward African Americans and independent health care services. With reference to the problems afflicting the black community today, she notes that "Few people really care about women of color and their babies, that is obvious. Drugs, the housing shortage, crime, violence, AIDS—none of it is a coincidence for black people. We are being hit from all sides" (Hart 1990, 21).

The TCB is one response, and an early one, to the crisis affecting the contemporary African-American community. More recently there has been a greater amount of internal rethinking and renewed institution building in the community. Many activists and intellectuals are seeking solutions to the problems, especially of the working poor and the underclass. Beginning in the early 1980s and accelerating at the end of the decade, older black institutions—ranging from religious groups such as the Methodist, Baptist, and Pentecostal churches and the Nation of Islam, to civil rights groups such as the National Association for the Advancement of Colored People, the National Urban League, and the National Council of Negro Women—began making the plight of the black family a priority at their conferences and in sponsored activities. Numerous grassroots organizations have been emerging in cities throughout the U. S., fighting drugs and crime and helping young people with job-training, literacy training, tutoring, counseling, and support groups (Helmore and Laing 1986b, 27; 1986c, 21–23, 25; 1986d, 35; *New York Times*, 1988, A10).

The work being undertaken by the TCB and others fills a gap created in part by the failure of black elected officials to affect the quality of life in the inner cities. Since the civil rights movement of the 1960s, hundreds of black public officials, many of whom represent predominantly African-American constituencies, have been elected to various offices. Like other elected officials, they can provide two kinds of benefits, namely, public and private or class benefits (Kilson 1989, 530). Unfortunately the class benefits which profit their middle-class constituencies, such as businessmen, lawyers, developers, and the like, have thus far received most of their attention. There are numerous instances of capital formation for these emerging black capitalists, but few cases of better service for the public, such as crime protection and improved schools (Kilson 1989, 530–32). This fact is not lost on the working-class public, however, as interviews with residents in Boston's black neighborhoods indicate (Graham 1990,1). City residents are beginning to ask why their elected officials, as well as activists and clergy, have failed to put forward a social and political agenda that will deal with the chronic ills of the community. This question is also being asked in other cities (Helmore and Laing 1986d, 33).

African-American city councillors and state representatives in Massachusetts are vocal in their support for renewed funding of hospital-based prenatal services (Martins 1987, 1). They came out in support of the nurse-midwifery program at Boston City Hospital when the eight nurses in this program resigned in 1988. The councillors complained that poor and minority women would no longer have the option of being treated by midwives (Knox 1988, 17)—as though these eight were the only available midwives. In contrast, Monroe received no support from local politicians (personal interview, Shafia Monroe, 1 March 1990) after it was reported in early 1990 that the $35,000 grant that TCB received from the Boston Foundation in 1988 was running out and there were no prospects of new funding (Hart 1990, 21). Despite extensive coverage of the TCB in the Boston newspapers since 1985, elected officials act as if it does not exist. Perhaps this is because TCB is independent of the medical establishment. Yet the comprehensive, family-centered service Monroe gives her clients cannot be duplicated by nurse-midwives or public health nurses.

Political elites, like doctors, generally regard hospital and clinical care as more appropriate than the home for birthing. With respect to the TCB, they engage in what could aptly be called "benign neglect." Their support for conventional health care has deep roots, even among radical politicians like Mel King—a 1972–82 Massachusetts state representative from Boston and Boston mayoral candidate in 1983—who originated the concept of the Rainbow Coalition, that Jesse Jackson used in his two presidential bids in 1984 and 1988 (Marable 1985, 274). At a 1969 conference on health care in the ghettos, (which was dominated by white medical planners and providers) King, then director of the Boston chapter of the National Urban League, raised the issue of services. He made no mention at all of programs that could emanate from within the black community, even though this was the era of "black power" (King 1969). At the same conference, Nathan Hare, at the time a sociologist at San Francisco State College, called for the creation of independent "Black Mothers Clubs" to encourage and provide prenatal care (Hare 1969).[4] But to my knowledge no politician has ever seriously considered the creation of "Black Mothers Clubs" or any other service that would be independent of the medical establishment. Instead, black elected officials have concentrated on establishing and expanding conventional health facilities and maternal and child care programs controlled or supervised by doctors.

It would be ludicrous and irresponsible to suggest that such facilities and programs are insignificant. The use of hospital facilities for childbearing is now a well-established practice in the United States and is not likely to change any time soon. Additionally, midwives do not serve, or else refer for doctors' care, women whose pregnancies threaten their lives or those of their infants (Devitt 1977, 51; DeVries 1985, 98; Hart 1990, 21; Lee and Glasser 1974, 541). On the other hand, most pregnancies are normal and do not require medical intervention. Indeed, some pregnancies might not become abnormal if the mothers received adequate prenatal care.

Studies undertaken since the large-scale movement toward hospital birthing began in the 1930s show unequivocally that healthy women with normal pregnancies have nothing to gain by having hospital deliveries (Devitt 1977, 57). In fact, there is a greater incidence of birth injuries and mortality in hospitals than in planned home birthing, since obstetrics interferes with a normal process (Devitt 1977, 57). Members of the Massachusetts Midwives Alliance, of which Monroe is a member, attended 853 planned home births between 1984 and 1986, and had not a single maternal death. They had complications in 26 percent of the cases, were able to manage 14.4 percent of them in the home, and transferred the rest to the hospital prior to or immediately after delivery (Massachusetts Midwives Alliance 1987). In contrast, a study by the Massachusetts Medical Society found that half of the seventy-nine maternal deaths in the state between 1976 and 1985 were among women who received little or no prenatal care and the other half were caused by physician error, including "inadequate monitoring" in anesthetics, "surgical mishaps," and "someone who wasn't attentive to the patient's symptoms" (Knox 1987b, 1). The report also faulted doctors for failing to recognize signs of postpartum depression—a condition which may lead to suicide, a significant factor in maternal mortality (Knox 1987b, 1). It noted that black women died, in childbirth or within the first three months of giving birth, at a rate three and a half times that of whites. Furthermore, obstetricians do not monitor a mother's progress once she leaves the hospital to the extent that midwives do. Monroe gives the mothers a supportive environment in the first twenty-eight days after birth, when many maternal deaths occur (Sakala and Ekstein 1987, 4). She follows up a birth with three consecutive days of home visits, another visit a week later, and telephone calls thereafter (Adams 1987, 26).

Health officials and doctors are generally hostile to groups like the TCB that advocate home birthing and freedom of choice in birthing. For instance, for the past five years the Massachusetts Midwives Alliance has been lobbying for a bill that would recognize midwifery through certification and by giving consumers the right to choose home birth—including letting them pay for it with insurance. Doctors argue against this bill, saying that home births are unsafe. Opponents of home birth, however, refuse to distinguish planned home births from unattended home births and premature deliveries (Phillips 1985, 8). The Alliance's own outcome data for the period 1984–86 give fetal (stillborn) and neonatal death rates of 2.3 and 3.5 per thousand births, respectively. That is, of 853 home deliveries in that period, two were stillborn and three died in the first twenty-eight days (Massachusetts Midwives Alliance 1987). This record compares to similar findings from other states which the Alliance also submitted to the state legislature in support of the bill. It is far superior to the national rates of 10 percent infant mortality and the almost 25 percent black infant mortality. Yet Monroe says that doctors regularly tell her that her clients are "at risk" and, therefore, should give birth in hospitals. She notes:

> Someone once told me that it's okay for white women to have their babies at home because they have oil [heat] in their houses, while Black women may not. I replied, "What if a woman leaves a cold house to go to the hospital and have a baby? Three days later she'll be coming back to the same cold house with a newborn baby. What are you going to do—give her oil or move her to the hospital forever?" (Sakala and Ekstein 1987, 4)

Monroe believes that behind the doctors' resistance is a concern about economic competition and a resentment that blacks want to take charge of their lives (Sakala and Ekstein 1987, 5).

The failure of city officials and doctors to formulate a program that takes into consideration the needs of the community and its resources can also be seen in the work of the Boston Perinatal Capacity Task Force, a joint city-state venture in 1989–90 which, after a decade of rising African-American infant mortality rates, was charged with determining the reasons for the racial differences (Boston Perinatal Capacity Task Force 1990). It proposed establishing a paramedical class of low-wage workers to provide prenatal care. However, it expressed no interest whatsoever in utilizing community midwives. This is unfortunate, since a very strong case can be made for supporting and expanding the work of community African-American midwives and encouraging more women to use their services. African-American health care providers and recipients will necessarily have to play a leading role in resolving the infant and maternal health crisis in their community, and the TCB offers an excellent model of what can be done through a community-based and socially-conscious organization.

Notes

1. From approximately 9,000 midwives practicing in the state of Georgia in 1925—the year the state board of health began to license them—the numbers had decreased to 2,200 by 1944. They attended 26 percent of all births in Georgia in the early 1940s, down from 42 percent the previous decade (Campbell [1946] 1984, 7–8). The percentage of black births attended by midwives in Georgia during this period is unknown, but in Alabama, where African-American midwives were still attending 20 percent of all births in the late 1940s, they attended 50 percent of the black ones (Logan 1989, xii). In the more poverty-stricken state of Mississippi,

by comparison, midwives were still attending 80 percent of black births in the early 1940s (Frazier [1939] 1948, 120).

2. By the late 1980s, Alabama's infant and maternal mortality rates were once again among the highest in the nation, in part because of the nationwide tendency of obstetricians to relinquish practices because of the rising costs of malpractice insurance (Logan 1989, xiv).

3. For instance, in Alabama's Greene County, historically the state's second poorest county, 40 of every 1,000 black babies died in 1985, twice the number of black babies dying in cities and over four times the national average (Wilkerson 1987, 1).

4. Perhaps these were to be modelled on the mothers clubs that African American women established in the South at the turn of the twentieth century, during a period of intensive institution building and social welfare work (Neverdon-Morton 1989).

Works Cited

Adams, Jane Meredith. 1987. "A Baby Is Born at Home, with the Help of Friends." *Boston Globe*, 12 October 1987, 26.

Blassingame, John W. 1979. *The Slave Community: Plantation Life in the Antebellum South*. Rev. ed. First published 1972. New York and Oxford: Oxford University Press.

Boston Perinatal Capacity Task Force. 1990. Minutes of Meeting 2 April 1990. Boston, Mass., 31 May 1990.

Brown, E. Richard. 1979. *Rockefeller Medicine Men: Medicine and Capitalism in America*. Berkeley: University of California Press.

Bruce, Dickson D., Jr. 1989. *Black American Writing from the Nadir: The Evolution of a Literary Tradition, 1877–1915*. Baton Rouge and London: Louisiana State University Press.

Campbell, Marie. 1984. *Folks Do Get Born*. First published 1946. Reprint. New York and London: Garland Publishing.

Carrington, Betty Watts. 1978. "The Afro-American." In *Culture, Childbearing, Health Professionals*, edited by Ann L. Clark, 35–52. Philadelphia: F. A. Davis Co.

Curry, Leonard P. 1981. *The Free Black in Urban America, 1800–1850—The Shadow of the Dream*. Chicago and London: University of Chicago Press.

Devitt, Neal. 1977. "The Transition from Home to Hospital Birth in the United States, 1930–1960." *Birth and the Family Journal* 4:47–58.

DeVries, Raymond G. 1985. *Regulating Birth: Midwives, Medicine, and the Law*. Philadelphia: Temple University Press.

Dougherty, Molly C. 1978. "Southern Lay Midwives as Ritual Specialists." In *Women in Ritual and Symbolic Roles*, edited by Judith Hoch-Smith and Anita Springs, 151–64. New York and London: Plenum Press.

Farley, Reynolds, and Walter R. Allen for the National Committee for Research on the 1980 Census. 1989. *The Color Line and the Quality of Life in America*. First published 1987. Reprint. New York and Oxford: Oxford University Press.

Frankel, Barbara. 1977. *Childbirth in the Ghetto: Folk Beliefs of Negro Women in a North Philadelphia Hospital Ward*. San Francisco: R. & E. Associates.

Frazier, E. Franklin. 1948. *The Negro Family in the United States.* Rev. ed. First published 1939. Chicago and London: University of Chicago Press.

Gaskin, Ina May. 1990. Interview with Shafia Mawshi Monroe. *Birth Gazette* 6:7–12.

Graham, Renee. 1990. "City's Black Leadership Must Unite to Address Violence, Say Activists." *Boston Globe*, 10 April 1990, 1.

Gutman, Herbert G. 1976. *The Black Family in Slavery and Freedom, 1750–1925.* New York: Random House.

Hare, Nathan. 1969. "Does Separatism in Medical Care Offer Advantages for the Ghetto?" In *Medicine in the Ghetto*, edited by John C. Norman, 43–49. New York: Appleton-Century-Crofts.

Harris, Rhonita. 1990. Client, Traditional Childbearing Group, Inc. Interview with author. Boston, Mass., 6 March 1990.

Hart, Jordana. 1990. "She Fights for Healthy Black Babies." *Boston Globe*, 4 January 1990, 21.

Helmore, Kristin, and Karen Laing. 1986a. "Exiles among Us: Part 1: A World Apart." *Christian Science Monitor*, 13 November 1986, 20–24.

———. 1986b. "Exiles among Us: Part 2: The Fragile Family." *Christian Science Monitor*, 18 November 1986, 25–32.

———. 1986c. "Exiles among Us: Parts 3 and 4: Superfluous People?; Crime and the Underclass." *Christian Science Monitor*, 19 November 1986, 19–26.

———. 1986d. "Exiles among Us: Parts 5 and 6: The Need for Education; Building Bridges." *Christian Science Monitor*, 20 November 1986, 28–35.

Hine, Darlene Clark. 1989. *Black Women in White: Racial Conflict and Cooperation in the Nursing Profession, 1890-1950.* Bloomington and Indianapolis: Indiana University Press.

Horton, James Oliver, and Lois E. Horton. 1979. *Black Bostonians: Family Life and Community Struggle in the Antebellum North.* New York and London: Holmes & Meier.

Johnson, Charles S. 1979. *Shadow of the Plantation.* First published 1934. Reprint. Chicago and London: University of Chicago Press.

Kilson, Martin. 1989. "Problems of Black Politics: Some Progress, Many Difficulties." *Dissent*, Fall 1989, 526–34.

King, Melvin H. 1969. "Can the Medical Profession Share Power with the Community?" In *Medicine in the Ghetto*, edited by John C. Norman, 51–57. New York: Appleton-Century-Crofts.

Kiple, Kenneth, and Virginia King. 1981. *Another Dimension to the Black Diaspora: Diet, Disease, and Racism.* Cambridge: Cambridge University Press.

Knox, Richard A. 1987a. "Hub Infant Deaths up 32%: Blacks Bear the Brunt of 1985 Mortality Hike." *Boston Globe*, 9 February 1987, 1.

———. 1987b. "Two Causes Cited in Maternal Deaths." *Boston Globe*, 12 March 1987, 1.

———. 1988. "Maternity Services Struggling at BCH." *Boston Globe*, 27 July 1988, 17.

Kobrin, Frances E. 1966. "The American Midwife Controversy: A Crisis of Professionalization." *Bulletin of the History of Medicine* 40:350–63.

Kong, Dolores. 1990. "Social Factors Linked to Black Death Rates." *Boston Globe*, 4 February 1990, 1.

Lawrence, Joyce. 1990. Midwife, Traditional Childbearing Group, Inc. Interview with author. Boston, Mass., 7 March 1990.

Lee, Felicia R. 1989. "Doctors See Gap in Blacks' Health Having a Link to Low Self-Esteem." *New York Times*, 17 July 1989, 1.

Lee, Florence Ellen, and Jay H. Glasser. 1974. "Role of Lay Midwifery in Maternity Care in a Large Metropolitan Area." *Public Health Reports* 89: 537–44.

Lewin, Tamar. 1990. "Rise in Single-Parent Families Found Continuing." *New York Times*, 15 July 1990, 17.

Logan, Onnie Lee. 1989. *Motherwit, an Alabama Midwife's Story: Onnie Lee Logan as Told to Katherine Clark*. New York: E. P. Dutton.

Macintyre, Sally. 1977. "The Management of Childbirth: A Review of Sociological Research Issues." *Social Science and Medicine* 11:477–84.

Marable, Manning. 1985. *Black American Politics: From the Washington Marches to Jesse Jackson*. London: Verso.

Martins, Gus. 1987. "Poverty Is Blamed for Infant Deaths." *Bay State Banner*, 19 February 1987, 1.

Massachusetts Midwives Alliance. 1987. Outcome Data for Midwife-Attended Home Births in Massachusetts 1984-1986. Boston: Massachusetts Midwives Alliance.

Mongeau, Beatrice, Harvey L. Smith, and Ann C. Maney. 1961. "The 'Granny' Midwife: Changing Roles and Functions of a Folk Practitioner." *American Journal of Sociology* 66:497–505.

Monroe, Shafia. 1990. Executive Director and Midwife, Traditional Childbearing Group, Inc. Interview with author. Boston, Mass., 1 March 1990.

Moses, Wilson. 1982. *Black Messiahs and Uncle Toms: Social and Literary Manipulations of a Religious Myth*. University Park and London: Pennsylvania State University Press.

Moynihan, Daniel Patrick. 1965. *The Negro Family: The Case for National Action*. Washington, D. C.: United States Department of Labor: Office of Policy Planning and Research.

Neverdon-Morton, Cynthia. 1989. *Afro-American Women of the South and the Advancement of the Race, 1895–1925*. Knoxville: University of Tennessee Press.

The New York Times. 1988. "Black Family Unit Promoted in Drive." 12 September 1988, A10.

The New Republic. 1985. "Milk for Babies." 2 September 1985, 5–6.

Phillips, Vicki. 1985. "Local Midwives Rally to Ensure Home Births." *Bay State Banner*, 16 May 1985, 8.

Prescott, Jennifer, M.D. 1990. Member, Board of Directors, Traditional Childbearing Group, Inc. Speech, Traditional Childbearing Group, Inc.'s, Third Annual All-Women's Symposium. Boston, Mass., 7 April 1990.

Rawick, George P. 1972. *The American Slave: A Composite Autobiography*, v. 1: *From Sundown to Sunup—The Making of the Black Community*. Westport, Conn.: Greenwood Publishing Company.

Reid, Alexander. 1990. "Study Targets Low-Income Diets in Children." *Boston Globe*, 1 August 1990, 23.

Reid, Margaret. 1989. "Sisterhood and Professionalization: A Case Study of the American Lay Midwife." In *Women as Healers*, edited by Carol Shepherd McClain, 219–38. New Brunswick and London: Rutgers University Press.

Ruzek, Sheryl Burt. 1978. *The Women's Health Movement: Feminist Alternatives to Medical Control.* New York: Praeger Publishers.

Sakala, Carol. 1989. "Community-Based, Community-Oriented Maternity Care." *American Journal of Public Health* 79:897–98.

———, and Marlena Ekstein. 1987. "Shafia Monroe's Keynote Address." *Midwife Advocate* 4:4–5.

Savitt, Todd L. 1978. *Medicine and Slavery: The Disease and Health Care of Blacks in Antebellum Virginia.* Urbana, Chicago, and London: University of Illinois Press.

Tillery, Tijuana. 1990. Client, Traditional Childbearing Group, Inc. Interview with author. Boston, Mass., 6 March 1990.

Tye, Larry. 1987. "Hub Study: 15 Percent Have no Health Plan." *Boston Globe,* 30 June 1987, 1.

Wilkerson, Isabel. 1987. "Infant Mortality: Frightful Odds in Inner City." *New York Times,* 26 June 1987, 1.

Wilson, William Julius. 1987. *The Truly Disadvantaged: The Inner City, the Underclass, and Public Policy.* Chicago and London: University of Chicago Press.

Woodson, Carter G. 1921. *The History of the Negro Church.* Washington, D. C.: Associated Publishers.

Nutrition, Breastfeeding, and Ethnicity: Understanding Maternal and Child Health Beliefs among New-Wave Immigrants

CAROLINE WESTBROOK ARNOLD

Introduction

While African Americans remain the largest of the "old" minority groups in the United States, in recent years there has been a marked increase in the growth of Hispanic and Asian populations, largely because of immigration. Given the declining birth rate of the native-born American population, immigrants now comprise a greater percentage of the nation's total population growth than they have since the first two decades of the twentieth century: approximately 25 percent of the population increase (U. S. Bureau of the Census 1984). Even conservative estimates indicate that Hispanic and Asian populations are likely to double, to thirty and ten million, respectively, by the end of this century (U. S. Bureau of the Census 1984). Unlike the older immigration from Canada and Europe, new-wave immigrants come increasingly from the Third World. Of all immigrants who have entered this country after 1970, for example, 78 percent came from Latin America and Asia. At present, the predominant sources of immigration to the United States are Asia, the Caribbean, and Central and South America. A decade ago, the leading countries of origin for immigrants were Mexico, the West Indies, Vietnam, the Philippines, Cuba, Korea, the Dominican Republic, China, and India, in that order (U. S. Bureau of the Census 1980).

Historically, immigrant populations have been highly susceptible to adverse health and social consequences and attendant problems of displacement. Yet despite inordinate need, these highly vulnerable groups receive less efficacious health care than native-born majority groups. Although considerable progress has been made in recent years to lessen disparities, children who are born to mothers who are poor, non-English-speaking, minority immigrants or refugees are at the greatest risk for health deficits (Gortmaker 1979; Egbuonu 1982; Binkin et al. 1985). Immigrant minority mothers are more likely than non-immigrants to suffer from poor nutritional status; greater maternal morbidity, infection, and mortality; a lack of prenatal and overall medical care; and greater exposure to occupational diseases and health hazards due to lack of protection in employment, poor environmental and living conditions, and substandard housing. They are also more likely to experience the adverse social consequences of low educational attainment, low income, and underemployment (Aykroyd 1971; Gortmaker 1979; Egbuonu 1982). Children born to immigrant minority mothers are more likely to be underweight, premature, or suffer from birth abnormalities than children in the population at large (Gortmaker 1979; Malina and Zavaleta 1980; Egbuonu 1982; Binkin et al. 1985).

Because maternal and infant risk factors are sensitive indicators of individual, family, and community health status, the imperative to respond to these issues among immigrant populations is clear. Moreover, the health care system and other institutions of society must be called upon to reflect the pluralism and diversity of the nation and move to elevate the health status and well-being of all its peoples.

The Significance of Nutrition and Breastfeeding in Elevating the Health Status of New-Wave Immigrant Groups

Nutrition is one important way to address concerns about maternal and infant health deficits among immigrant groups, specifically the problems of high infant mortality rates and low birth weights. Improving nutritional status before, during, and after pregnancy greatly improves the viability of the fetus during gestation, the health of the newborn during the critical first year of life, and the well-being of the child during its formative years. Another key way of promoting greater health and survival rates is to encourage the practice of breastfeeding among immigrant mothers.

There is much evidence that the fetus is sensitive to the pre-pregnancy and gestational nutrition of the mother (Wittenberg 1983). There is also considerable proof that maternal under-nutrition and malnutrition in pre-pregnancy and during pregnancy significantly affect the birth weight of the newborn and the health of the infant up to six to nine months of age, as well as the nutritional health of the child during the critical transition to preschool, up to three years of aged (Jelliffe and Jelliffe 1981; Wittenberg 1983). A nutritional diet in pregnancy is beneficial to both mother and fetus. It lowers the risk of small-size infants resulting from fetal malnutrition by increasing the levels of fetal stores of nutrients such as vitamin A, ensuring optimal nutrient stores in both the fetus and the mother, and laying down adequate lactation reserves during pregnancy in the form of fat needed as a major source of calories, fatty acids, and subsequent breast milk production (Jelliffe and Jelliffe 1981).

Breastfeeding can best be understood as nutritional, psychological, biological interaction and communication between mother and offspring, with each affecting the other. While the dyadic link, both transplacentally and in breast milk, between mother and fetus would appear to be biologically obvious, much of the practical significance and mutually beneficial nature of the breastfeeding process is still under-appreciated. The newborn can be thought of as an external fetus, with the breast taking the place of the placenta as the primary source for meeting nutrition needs. Indeed, the complex, species-specific nature of the nutritional and immunological components of breast milk are uniquely suited to meet the changing needs of the infant and are impossible to duplicate (Newton and Newton 1967; Jelliffe and Jelliffe 1981, 1984).

There is no way to replicate the ever-changing physiological, psychological, and developmental interaction which occurs between the nursing mother and her offspring (Jelliffe and Jelliffe 1981). The superiority of human milk and breastfeeding over formula and bottle-feeding applies to rich and poor families alike and persists whether the family lives in a wealthy community or a poor inner-city neighborhood (Mohrer 1979). Until recently the relative consequences of the two methods of feeding were considered to be of no real importance in urban societies. We now know, however, that recognition of the public health significance of breastfeeding and of human milk can make a particularly positive difference in poor urban communities (Mohrer 1979; Bryant 1982; Rassin et al. 1984). In 1981, 57.6 percent of American newborns were reported to be breastfed when discharged from the nursery (Martinez 1981). More mothers are continuing to breastfeed for as long as six months. However, this increase is not particularly evident in lower socioeconomic groups and among women of color. One study shows wide differentials in breastfeeding practices between ethnic groups—43.5 percent for whites; 9.2 percent for blacks; 22.6 percent for Hispanics; and 42.1 percent for others (Rassin et al. 1984). Another study shows a smaller variance, concluding that "blacks were less likely to breastfeed than whites by 21 percent and 26.8 percent respectively" (Kowlessar 1986).

Research on patterns of breastfeeding among immigrant women indicates striking urban-rural differences in the number of women who breastfeed, the duration of breastfeeding, and the child's age at weaning (Graitcer et al. 1984). It appears that the abandonment of breastfeeding is principally an urban phenomenon, often not so much because urban mothers work as because bottle-feeding is one of the sophistications of city life adopted by immigrants. This phenomenon is evident both within the United States and in areas where large numbers of immigrants to the United States originate. The case of Haitian migrants is illustrative of this point (Graitcer et al. 1984). In rural areas of Haiti almost all mothers breastfeed their children up to twelve months, but in Port-au-Prince, nearly 23 percent have stopped breastfeeding before the child is a year old. In both urban and rural areas younger women wean their children earlier than do older women. Women in urban areas are more likely to wean children before one year, or to never begin breastfeeding at all, in comparison with rural women. Likewise, data on Southeast-Asian women show that their infants tend to be weaned early from breast to formula. This practice is partly related to the mother's need to work outside the home and partly because of the perceived association of higher status and formula (Groppo et al. 1981; Wadd 1983).

This trend is especially disturbing given the decided benefits of breastfeeding for both mother and infant. For example, there is convincing evidence that in contrast to formula, breastfeeding establishes a bond between mother and child, helps ward off or minimize postpartum depression, helps the uterus resume normal size, and delays ovulation, thus contributing to the spacing of children and aiding in the restoration of the physique. Breast milk provides antibodies and friendly bacteria that help babies resist infection and fortifies the immune system through the transfer of antibodies, hormones, enzymes, and other biologic substances, a process crucial to early physical and mental development. Breastfed babies have fewer illnesses and are particularly less likely to have allergies and diarrhea, the leading cause of hospitalization of infants. They are also less likely to be overweight in infancy and later as well. Breast milk is easily digested and contains the nutrients that babies need in the correct proportions. Importantly, it is a steady and ready supply of sterile fluid of exactly the right composition and ideal temperature. Thus it helps mothers avoid having their infants contract diseases associated with non-sterilized bottles or watered down formula tainted by unsafe or contaminated water supplies. In communities where food supplies are inadequate, or where there is little money for the purchase of food, breastfeeding costs nothing and aids in the mobility of mothers and infants (Jelliffe and Jelliffe 1981, 1984). While breastfeeding has these positive consequences, the use of powdered milk and formula in bottles can have disastrous results for infant health, including problems associated with nursing-bottle syndrome—severe dental caries, oral malocclusions, and nutrient deficiencies.

Health Education, Outreach, and Cultural Awareness Regarding Breastfeeding and New-Wave Immigrant Patients

The promotion of breastfeeding is, of course, a multifaceted process. It includes the need for programmatic services and activities designed to inform, educate, and advocate breastfeeding among health workers, health care institutions, and public policy makers. Providers and facilities must modify their attitudes, approaches, and policies to recognize and respond to the high-risk need of immigrant populations. They must make the promotion of breastfeeding an integral component of their maternal and infant health ideology.

Results of current surveys demonstrate that this is not presently the case. For example, a 1986 survey conducted in Boston-area hospitals showed that ". . . 15 of 28 area hospitals routinely distribute formula milk gift packets to all new mothers, including those mothers who intend to breastfeed" (Frank et al. 1986). The results of another study conducted at Boston City Hospital and reported in the April 1986 edition of the *American Journal of Disease of Children* were equally disturbing. This study showed that women who were given commercial packets of formula were less likely to breastfeed, regardless of their intent when they first entered the hospital, than women who were given non-commercial packets containing breast pads and health education pamphlets which advocated breastfeeding. The study also found that when bedside lactation counseling supplemented the non-commercial packets and there was follow-up telephone counseling after discharge—accompanied by encouragement and support of the decision to breastfeed—the likelihood that mothers would begin and continue to breastfeed is even greater.

According to A. Naylor (1984), the promotion of breastfeeding is a multifaceted process; health care providers who understand the complexities of lactation and suckling, are trained to convey this understanding to women, possess supportive attitudes, and are staunch proponents of the practice are essential to the socialization of mothers. Unfortunately, such training is uncommon, and any clinical exposure to the subject is coincidental. While other areas of medical or nursing education have undergone numerous revisions in response to the many advances made during the past three decades, attention to lactation and breastfeeding declined to near-extinction. Obstetrics instruction taught students how to inhibit lactation and speed the postpartum involution of the breast, while pediatrics training concentrated on the fine points of providing infants with artificial formula. The breast became a topic discussed primarily in pathology classes and surgical clerkships, where the details of how to temporarily or permanently eliminate its basic function were the focus. Nothing was taught about how to encourage and enhance its normal processes, nor how to prevent, diagnose, or treat deviations from normal functions. As a result, most physicians remain uneducated, untrained, indifferent, or ambivalent about breastfeeding. They embark upon their practice unprepared to assist the nursing mother, and they often give advice and carry out procedures that lead directly to breastfeeding problems and failures (Naylor 1984; Ettner 1988).

Social support from key influential people, family members, and friends can be important in a woman's decision to begin and continue breastfeeding, and this has implications for outreach programs and policies. A study which examined the influence of social support systems and the decision to breastfeed found that among Anglo-American mothers, the male partner is clearly the single most important source of support in promoting breastfeeding. In this group, support from a best friend was influential, but not as great as from the male partner. In contrast, among African Americans the most influential person was the best friend. The male partner had little influence among Mexican-American families, where the mother of the birthing mother was the primary source of social support for breastfeeding (Baranowski et al. 1983). Reaching the people who are most influential in the birth mother's support system can have implications for the ways in which programs and services to promote and encourage breastfeeding are devised among various ethnic groups. For example, programs targeted to Anglo-American families should include male partners, whereas educational programs targeted to blacks should involve female peers, including school, social, or church groups. Among Mexican Americans groups which involve prospective grandmothers are good places to promote breastfeeding.

Many myths, misconceptions, and superstitions have been perpetuated about breastfeeding, both within and without the medical establishment. Understanding the cultural implications of illness and health care is crucial when dealing with new minority groups coming from cultures alien to traditional American health ideology. Health care providers need to know about the health problems of immigrants that might differ from those they ordinarily encounter. They also need to be aware of the traditional health practices and cultural and religious beliefs of the immigrants, and how these might affect their ability to receive and maintain care.

It is well, for example, to consider the cultural mystique surrounding breastfeeding and breasts within American culture among American women. Despite the fact that a growing number of American women breastfeed, breasts are still more closely associated with eroticism than with reproduction and infant feeding. A widely held belief is that large breasts are a measure of sexuality and denote greater sexual responsiveness. For many women, the size and shape of the breasts are a defining component of their self-concept, self-image, and self-worth as sexual beings. Because of such cultural interpretations, many women have feelings of inadequacy and self-consciousness about their bodies, even if nursing, and experience discomfort and shame if their breasts are exposed in public to nurse their children (Strong and DeVault 1988).

When patients come from a different country, culture, or social milieu, health workers must know something about how they conceive and conceptualize their condition in order to communicate with them effectively about a treatment regimen. Practitioners must familiarize themselves with patients' views of etiology and therapeutics and develop a special understanding of the cultural constructs and context of traditional and folk beliefs and practices.

Traditional Health Belief Systems and Ideas of Well Being and Illness

For many newcomers traditional and folk health belief systems and Western medicine are not mutually exclusive. For example, central to the folk systems of Latin America, Haiti, and Southeast Asia is the concept of humoral medicine, which has its roots in Hippocratic, Western medicine. In this belief system, illnesses are classified as either hot or cold. Food and medicine, also classified this way, are used to restore the body's natural balance (Logan 1975). Embodied in the concept of humoral medicine is the notion of health as a state of opposing forces: balance/imbalance, positive/negative, male/female, hot/cold, Yin/Yang. For example, H. G. C. Wiese (1976) describes traditional Chinese beliefs about humoral medicine as follows:

> Although the particulars of humoral theory vary widely among various cultural groups, the underlying premise remains the same. The concept rests on the assumption that the elements exist naturally in a state of binary opposition and the effects of one element upon the other equalizes the balance of each. One common manifestation of humoral medicine is a hot/cold classification of foods. This classification does not depend on any physical property of heat or cold, but rather on an innate quality of that food to generate heat or cold on or within the body. The classification of foods is just one aspect of humoral medicine; the classification of body states and illnesses is another. Like that of foods, this system varies considerably among cultures. The premise upon which it is based, however, is the same: the equilibrium between hot and cold. Maintenance of health in such cultures is believed to depend upon meticulous care of this balance in everyday activities. Where these humoral classification systems intersect, they greatly affect behavior.

In many Latin-American cultures, the hot/cold (*caliente/frio*) dimension of the humoral concept dominates traditional medicine. Diseases are grouped into hot/cold classes, while medications and foods are trichotomized as hot, cold, or an intermediate category, "cool" (*fresco*) (Harwood 1971). Cold-classified illnesses are treated with hot medicines and foods, while hot illnesses are treated with cold or cool substances thought to neutralize them.

Although the terminology of the hot/cold system suggests that it is based on temperature, the thermal state in which food or herbal medicines are taken is not relevant to the classification scheme (Logan 1973; Logan 1975). When new foods are introduced into the diet or medications are prescribed, they are incorporated into the hot/cold system according to the effect they have on the body (Logan 1975).

The hot/cold classification has implications for maternal and infant health care. For example, during pregnancy a Latin-American woman is careful to avoid hot foods or medications to prevent her baby from being born with an "irritation" (a rash or red skin). An important consequence of the avoidance of hot substances during pregnancy is that many women will not take "hot" iron supplements or vitamins. However, to "cool" or neutralize these "hot" medicines women can be encouraged to take them with fruit juices or herbal teas (Harwood 1971; Logan 1975). Another example of food avoidance concerns post-partum practices. A. Harwood (1971) reports that, "Many women avoid eating cool foods after delivery on the grounds that they impede the flow of blood and therefore prevent complete emptying of the uterus and birth canal." As discussed previously, like most other minority mothers, Hispanic mothers tend not to breastfeed. Therefore, perhaps the most important implication of the hot/cold system concerns the feeding of infants and the use of commercial formula. Evaporated milk, the formula base usually recommended to mothers upon leaving the hospital, is considered a hot food, whereas whole milk is considered cool. Because "hot" evaporated milk is thought to cause rashes in the infant, mothers prefer to feed their infants "cool" whole milk and almost immediately begin the transition from evaporated milk to whole milk. This transition can be abrupt or gradual, using cool substances such as barley water, magnesium carbonate, and marnitol to supplement the formula and neutralize the effects of evaporated milk. Health workers should be alert to this practice, because these neutralizing foods have a cathartic and diuretic effect when taken in sufficient quantity and may cause dehydration, diarrhea, and other side effects in infants (Harwood 1971).

Similarly, the hot (cho)/ cold (fret) system is a salient feature of traditional medicine in Haitian culture (Wiese 1976; Laguerre 1979). In addition to being a classification system for illness, medications, and cures, the system ascribes qualities of "light" and "heavy" to foods, and the method of preparation affects food groupings (Wiese 1976). According to Haitian tradition, there is a belief that not all foods are good at all times for the human body; the use of food must be in harmony with the individual life cycle. There are foods for babies, foods for adults, foods for menstruating women, foods for the sick, and foods for the elderly. Some foods are forbidden to people at different stages of the life cycle. Pregnant women are particularly subject to food taboos or special food practices (Laguerre 1979). They are permitted to "eat for two" (*manger pour deux*) and therefore gain considerable weight during pregnancy. They are also cautioned to avoid spices, but red fruits and vegetables (for example, beets or pomegranates) are thought to build up the baby's blood. Another example of Haitian food taboos relative to maternal and infant nutrition is eating "cool" tomatoes or white beans after childbirth, because they are believed to induce hemorrhage. The body of a woman is believed to be "hot" during the weeks after childbirth. Lactating women are thought to be particularly susceptible to illness, and any illness, it is believed, affects their milk in various ways. The milk of a lactating mother is believed to be stored in her breast, and the mother must eat very well to be able to produce healthy milk for her child. Although breast milk is believed to be a nutrient for both mother and baby, it can also be detrimental to the health of both if it is too "thin" or too "thick." If milk is too thick, it is said to cause impetigo (*bouton*) in the child. It is believed that breast milk can become thick when a mother is frightened, which causes the milk to move to her head, inducing acute headaches or postpartum depression in the mother and imparting diarrhea to the baby (Laguerre 1979). Breast milk itself is classified as neutral, neither hot nor cold, and is thought to have a balanced effect on infants. If, however, an infant develops a condition—such as a rash—which is considered hot, mothers supplement breastfeeding with "cool" liquids—such as herbal teas or fruit juices—to restore humoral balance.

Among Southeast-Asian cultures the humoral notion is evidenced in the concept of Yin-Yang, which postulates that the universe, and consequently each human being, is composed of two opposing forces: male, positive energy, or Yang, that produces light, warmth, dryness, and fullness; and Yin, or female, negative energy that produces darkness, cold, wetness, and emptiness (Manderson and Matthews 1981). An illness or imbalance is attributed to metaphysical forces. Therapeutic adjustment of the diet requires consideration of the hot/cold qualities of food, cooking methods, and the nature of the illness. Although among Oriental cultures notions of hot-cold are similar to those in the Hispanic and Haitian cultures discussed above, Asian systems are more difficult to decipher and translate with precision. However, in general, most fruits and vegetables, along with fish, duck, and other things that grow in water, are considered "cold"; most meats, sweets, coffee, and spicy condiments, such as garlic, ginger, and onion, are "hot." "Hot" foods and beverages are believed to replace and strengthen one's blood; therefore, after surgery or childbirth, "hot" drinks are preferred and cold drinks, jello, and juices are avoided (Muecke 1983). Pregnant women are encouraged to eat special herbs and food to insure the babies' health as well as their own. Various "health" foods are carefully prepared and provided for the mother. One such health food is ginseng herb, which is believed to be a general-strength tonic for both the expectant mother and the postpartum mother (Chung 1977).

Religious Belief and Health Practices

Traditional and religious beliefs and practices are intertwined with health belief systems. Often there is not a clear distinction between orthodox religion, folk religion, folk healing, and Western medicine. For example, although Catholicism is the predominant, official religion of Haiti, many Catholic Haitians strongly hold and combine the beliefs and practices of Vodum (voodoo)—a complex system of beliefs and rituals derived from African traditions—with Catholicism. They experience no contradiction in the simultaneous practice of both systems. Moreover, the distinction between physical and spiritual healing is not fully drawn. Disease and illness are frequently attributed to supernatural causes and possession by spirits (*mystere*). Therapeutics and cures may be sought singularly or in combination from parish priests, voduum priests (*Houngon*) and priestesses (*Mambo*), spiritual doctors, healers, readers, or diviners, as well as Western medical doctors (Laguerre 1981).

Catholicism in Latin American cultures combines with traditional healing systems. Depending upon the nationality and ethnic group, the folk-healing system includes the practice of *Espiritismo* (a religious cult of European origin based on an ethical code which is concerned with communication with spirits and the purification of the soul through moral behavior) or *Santeria* (a blend of African beliefs and Catholic practices which, unlike *Espiritismo*, takes no moral position). The leader, or *santero*, works solely on behalf of the practitioner of the faith, and his activity can be beneficial, of no import, or harmful to others (Scott 1974).

Less familiar to Anglo-Americans are the non-Christian, non-Western religions prevalent in Asian cultures where conversion to Christianity has been minimal. The majority of Southeast Asians identify with the orthodox religions indigenous to Oriental cultures. According to Hoang (1984), *Buddhism*, the main religion of Southeast Asia, is much less a matter of organized and institutional orthodoxy than a state of mind. Buddhism teaches that suffering is a reality of life and can be seen as a divine punishment for wrongdoing, and therefore it is not universally accepted as a symptom of disease. Adherence to this belief system can lead to undue delay in seeking medical care. Further, *Confucianism* is described as a code of ethics emphasizing hierarchy in society and stressing the worship of ancestors. The opinion of the elders of the family is sought in making decisions about medical care. Taoism or *Naturalism* advocates taking no unnatural action to achieve conformity with the "Tao," or creative principle, that orders the physical universe. When things are allowed to take their natural course, they move toward perfection and harmony. This belief reinforces passivity and procrastination in seeking medical care. And finally, Hoang describes *Animism* or Animistic belief as the philosophical system most commonly practiced by the hill tribes of Laos. The Laotians believe in gods, demons, and evil spirits as a way of life, and they feel they must communicate with the spirits of deceased ancestors to obtain their beneficial protection. When illness occurs, cures are sought through the rituals of shannan or by wearing symbolic objects on the body to ward off harmful spirits.

It should be noted that within each of these major religions, there is much variation and diversity. Additionally, variations occur in different forms among various nationalities and ethnic groups, as well as within each ethnic group of Southeast Asia (Groppo et al. 1981; Manderson and Matthews 1981; Wadd 1983).

Religious, dietary and health beliefs are inextricably related, and the food habits of any group of people must be seen systematically as an integral part of their social matrix. It is important to recognize that in almost every society there are close associations between food and religious symbolism, food and the body as it relates to states of health, and food as it is interpreted through the disciplines of medicine and nutrition. And while people bring their food habits with them when they move from one country to another, their eating patterns are inevitably disturbed. This is especially true when the countries are as different as the United States and the countries of Southeast Asia, the Caribbean, and South and Central America in terms of culture, climate, and the availability of foodstuffs, in ways of preparing, purchasing, and storing food, and so forth. In addition, factors such as taste, smell, and appearance strongly influence the acceptability of new foods. These elements must be taken into account by health care practitioners who hope to encourage the introduction of new foods among people with traditional eating habits (Logan 1973; Carlson et al. 1982; Hargreaves 1982).

There is substantial evidence that immigrants and refugees are in general more likely to suffer from deficits in nutrition status and that the adverse effects of inadequate nutrition are intergenerational (Aykroyd 1971; Greener and Latham 1981; Carlson et al. 1982; Harwood 1971). Similarly, since food preferences—and, often, the poverty that limits food choices and availability—are continued through generations, nutrition status becomes a part of family history. In the same way, social class, and the economic and political factors that condition it, are also integral to family history. Inadequate diet is not only a question of personal volition, but, rather more likely, a factor of social status. Because food, diet, and eating habits are a learned way of life and are passed on from generation to generation, conditions fostered by six or eight generations of inadequate diet cannot be completely remedied by the current generation of mothers breastfeeding their infants and revising their own and their families' diets. Nutrition status can be improved, however, and good nutrition does make a difference in overall health and well-being (Aykroyd 1971).

At the same time, there is substantial support and precedence for the view that American health care workers should be obligated to become aware and knowledgeable about, but not necessarily to alter, the food ideologies of other cultures. To do otherwise, either by design or default, severely compromises the ultimate effectiveness and diminishes the quality of the health enterprise. Moreover, it is imperative that the American health care system take culture and ethnicity (including the social and economic character of newly-arrived consumers' lives and the environmental conditions that influence them) into account and make an effort to translate cultural considerations into clinical practices, treatment protocols, and institutional policies. Indeed, to encourage heightened cultural literacy in the health care system poses no contradiction. It is both desirable and appropriate that the system reflect the diversity and differences of all the people whom it serves.

Works Cited

Aykroyd, W. R. 1971. "Nutrition and Mortality in Infancy and Early Childhood: Past and Present Relationships." *American Journal of Clinical Nutrition* 24:480–87.

Baranoswki, T., et al. 1983. "Social Support, Social Influence, Ethnicity and the Breastfeeding Decision." *Social Science and Medicine* 17:1599–1611.

Binkin, N. J. et al. 1985. "Reducing Black Neonatal Mortality: Will Improvements in Birthweight Be Enough?" *Journal of the American Medical Association* 253: 372–75.

Bryant, C. A. 1982. "The Impact of Kin, Friend, and Neighbor Networks on Infant Feeding Practices." *Social Science and Medicine* 16:1757–65.

Carlson, E. et al. 1982. "Feeding the Vietnamese in the U. K. and the Rationale Behind Their Food Habits." *Practice of Nutrition and Society* 41:229–37.

Chung, Hyo Jin. 1977. "Understanding the Oriental Maternity Patient." *Nursing Clinics of North America* 12:67–75.

Donley, J. 1990. "Lactation Consultant and La Leche League Contact Person for Lakewood, California." Interview, July 1990.

Egbuono, L. 1982. "Child Health and Social Status." *Pediatrics* 69:550–57.

Ettner, F. 1988. "Do Health Professionals Encourage Breastfeeding?" *New Beginnings* July–August: 99–103.

Frank, D., et al. 1986. "Duration of Breastfeeding among Low-Income Women: A Randomized Trail of the Effects of Commercial Hospital Discharge Packs and Hospital-Based Telephone Counseling." *American Journal of the Diseases of Children* 140:311.

Gortmaker, S. L. 1979. "Poverty and Infant Mortality in the United States." *American Sociological Review* 44:280–97.

Graitcer, P., et al. 1984. "Breastfeeding and Weaning Practices in Haiti. *Journal of Tropical Pediatrics* 1:10–16.

Greener, T., and M. C. Latham. 1981. "Factors Associated with Nutritional Status among Young Children in St. Vincent." *Ecology of Food and Nutrition* 10:135–41.

Groppo. C., et al. 1981. "Bridging Cultures: The Vietnamese American Family–and Grandma Makes Three." *Maternal Child Nursing* 6:177–80.

Hargreaves, A. 1982. "Ann Hargreaves Returns from Fact-Finding in El Salvador." *Massachusetts Nurse* 52:6.

Harwood, A. 1971. "The Hot-Cold Theory of Disease: Implications for Treatment of Puerto Rican Patients." *Journal of the American Medical Association* 216:1153–58.

Hoang, G .N. 1984. "Bridging the Cultural Gap: Issues in Health and Mental Health Care for Southeast Asian Refugees." Technical Assistance Paper prepared for the National Institute for Planned Change, Washington, D. C.

Jelliffe, D. B. and E. F. P. Jelliffe. 1981. *Advances in International Maternal and Child Health*. Oxford: Oxford University Press.

———. 1984. *Advances in Maternal and Child Health*. Clarendon Press.

Kowlessar, M. et al. 1986. "Breastfeeding and Ethnicity." *American Journal of Diseases in Children*. 140:311.

Laguerre, M. S. 1979. "The Haitian Niche in New York City." *Migration Today* 7:12–18.

———. 1981. "Haitan Americans." *Ethnicity and Medical Care*. Cambridge: Harvard University Press.

Logan, M. H. 1973. "Humoral Medicine in Guatemala and Peasant Acceptance of Modern Medicine." *Human Organization* 32:385–95.

———. 1975. "Selected References on the Hot-Cold Theory of Disease." *Medical Anthropology Newsletter* 6:8–11.

Malina, R. M. and A. N. Zavaleta. 1980. "Secular Trend in the Stature and Weight of Mexican-American Children in Texas Between 1930 and 1970." *American Journal of Physical Anthropology* 52:453–61.

Manderson, L., and M. Matthews. 1981. "Vietnamese Attitudes Towards Maternal and Infant Health." *Medical Journal of Australia* 1:69–72.

Martinez, A. 1981. "Minority Response to Disease Concepts in the Barrio Today." *Community Nursing Research* 6:197–200.

Mohrer, J. 1979. "Breast and Bottle Feeding in an Inner-City Community: An Assessment of Perceptions and Practices." *Medical Anthropology* 3:125–45.

Muecke, Marjorie A. 1983. "Caring for Southeast Asian Refugee Patients in the USA." *American Journal of Public Health* 73:431–38.

Naylor, A. 1984. "Learning the Management of Lactation and Breastfeeding: Experience at San Diego Lactation Clinic." *Advances in International Maternal and Child Health* New York: Clarendon Press.

Newton, N., and M. Newton. 1967. "Psychological Aspects of Lactation." *New England Journal of Medicine* 277:1179–80.

Rassin, D. K. et al. 1984. "Incidence of Breastfeeding in Low Socioeconomic Group of Mothers in the United States: Ethnic Patterns." *Pediatrics* 73:132–37.

Scott, C. S. 1974. "Health and Healing Practices among Five Ethnic Groups in Miami, Florida." *Public Health Reports* 98:356–59.

Strong, B., and C. DeVault 1988. *Understanding Our Sexuality*. New York: West Publishing.

U. S. Bureau of the Census. 1980. *Current Population Reports*.

———. 1980, 1981, 1984. *U. S. Population Series and Supplementary Reports*.

Wadd, L. 1983. "Vietnamese Postpartum Practices: Implications for Nursing in the Hospital Setting." *Journal of Gynecological Nursing* 12:252–58.

Wiese, H. G. C. 1976. "Maternal Nutrition and Traditional Food Behavior." *Human Organization* 35:193–200.

Wittenberg, C. K. 1983. "Summary of Credit Research for 'Healthy Mothers, Healthy Babies' Campaign." *Public Health Reports* 98:356–59.

PART 4

BREAST CANCER:
IMAGES OF SELF

Introduction

Part Four focuses on a particular illness of special concern to women of color, breast cancer, together with the importance of early detection and possibilities of self-help, attitudes of women toward it, and the experience of treatment. The detection of breast cancer and its treatment through mastectomy, lumpectomy, diet, and/or chemotherapy and radiation, raise issues not only of attitudes toward cancer of all types and toward death, but of a woman's sense of her own identity, her womanliness, her role as a mother, her concept of her body, and her sexual relationships with significant others who will have their own reactions to the changes her body has undergone.

Breast cancer is the leading cause of cancer mortality among African-American women. Poorer prognosis and higher mortality rates among African-American and Hispanic women who develop breast cancer are directly attributable to lack of awareness about the disease and to poor-quality health care. Both can result in late diagnosis of the condition and delay in treatment. For women of all ages, breast examination, which can lead to early treatment, is critical for survival.

Health professionals Teresa C. Jacob, Leslie E. Spieth, and Nolan E. Penn detail the special health risks of African-American women with regard to breast cancer and explain that there are three levels of breast examination: mammography, clinical breast examination by a health professional, and breast self-examinations. Early detection through examination makes it possible for a cancerous lump to be removed before the malignancy has spread to other parts of the body. Mammography, an imaging technique, can reveal the existence of lumps that are so small they cannot yet be felt through touch. Mammography is a relatively expensive procedure, however, especially for those without health insurance and/or those with a low income. Clinically based, the procedure is also not readily available to many women outside major urban areas. Additionally, it is not as effective for younger women. Breast examination by a health professional also depends on access to, and ability to pay for, medical care. Breast self-examination thus remains an extremely important factor in maintaining the health of women of color. Jacob, Spieth, and Penn recommend greater emphasis on health education to enhance women's awareness of the importance of self-exams and their proficiency in performing them. They call for health professionals to show greater concern in taking the time to instruct women in the method when they have the opportunity to do so. They also encourage the growth of self-help-style groups, in which women proficient in self-examination teach other women the technique. They end their essay with seven practical steps to empowerment through breast self-examination.

Jacob, Spieth, and Penn's arguments are supported by researchers Michelle Saint-Germain and Alice Longman's study of older Hispanic women's attitudes and responses to breast cancer. Saint-Germain and Longman used bilingual methods to survey over four hundred older Hispanic women living in Tucson, Arizona. They point out that for many Hispanics, health care is a luxury. Like the women who Gregoria Rodriguez spoke with and described in her essay in Part Two, the Latina respondents in Saint-Germain and Longman's research noted the priority of obtaining basic necessities—food, clothing, shelter—over paying for health care. Availability of care and transportation to it are issues related to the ability to pay. The women interviewed expressed fears of death, disease, powerlessness, and mutilation, and the resulting loss of respect and relationships. They voiced a good deal of fatalism with regard to personally contracting the disease, feeling that God's will ultimately determined whether any given individual would experience it. They were not convinced of the benefits of prevention and had uneven knowledge of the warning signs of breast cancer. Beyond the issue of cancer itself, the idea of single mastectomy was particularly troubling to them because of traditional health beliefs emphasizing balance.

Like the women whose experiences are represented in essays earlier in the volume, their discussions emphasized the central importance of women's networks and the extended family, and recognition that the disease would affect all family members, not only the person with cancer. Hispanic women expressed great concern about what their illness might mean to their families. This too, was conceived of in terms of loss of social balance or equilibrium. Saint-Germain and Longman urge recognition of this social (rather than individual) concept of health by health professionals, who should encourage

Hispanic women to have a relative or other person close to them accompany them to a breast cancer screening, emphasizing the benefits of early detection not only for the individual but for her family and friends.

Writer Lois Lyles' "Cancer in the Family" concludes Part Four. Lyles' personal narrative explores her own family's response to her mother's breast cancer. Like so many women of color, Lyles' mother's cancer was not detected until it was at an advanced stage. For her mother, coping with the cancer meant not only dealing with the severity of illness, her unfamiliar dependence, and the drastic changes in her body, it also tore open wounds within the social fabric of the family, altering her relationship to her husband, her daughter, and other family members. As the concerned adult daughter who finds herself helping and looking on, Lyles observes her mother's scarred body and thinks that "she has been a soldier in some dubious battle." For the daughter occupying both caretaking and familial roles, the cancer brings its own crises, raising to the surface feelings and passions long repressed. The struggle she experiences ends with a note of self-discovery and hope.

In her own struggle with cancer, Audre Lorde has done a great deal to heighten women's awareness of their own risk and to open debate about the feelings that having cancer arouses and the meanings that we attach to it. Her *The Cancer Journals* (1980) and part of her latter collection, *A Burst of Light* (1988), chronicle her experience, decisions about treatment, and responses. The quote from "A Burst of Light: Living with Cancer," that serves as an epigram to the main introduction to this collection speaks especially to the issue raised in this section of the book. In the essay Lorde urges women to break the code of silence surrounding the issue of cancer, to question the sense of powerlessness and stoicism that characterizes women of color's response to disease, and to confront the risks and speak out about them. That call to empowerment is also the message of the essays in Part Four.

Information and instruction about breast self-examination can be obtained from local chapters of the American Cancer Society, as well as from health practitioners and women's health clinics.

Breast Cancer, Breast Self-Examination, and African-American Women

TERESA C. JACOB, LESLIE E. SPIETH, AND NOLAN E. PENN

Introduction

Death from breast cancer is the leading form of cancer mortality among African-American women (USDHHS 1986a). The American Cancer Society (1990) reports that approximately one in every ten women in the United States will develop breast cancer at some time. The American Cancer Society also estimates that there will be 150,900 new cases of breast cancer in 1990, and of these new cases, approximately 44,300 will result in death. The age-specific mortality rate (per 100,000) for all cancer sites combined is higher for African-American women aged thirty-two to seventy-four than for white women within the same age group. Although African-American women are less likely than white women to develop breast cancer, once cancer has occurred their survival rates are much lower than among whites. One of the real tragedies in these statistics is that the breast cancer mortality rate could be dramatically reduced through behavioral changes and greater access to quality health care. In fact, the American Cancer Society (1988) estimates that in 1988 approximately 174,000 of all the deaths related to malignancies, including breast cancer, might have been prevented by earlier diagnosis and prompt treatment.

Because the exact cause of breast cancer remains unknown, the only effective means of reducing the breast cancer mortality rate and increasing the chances of a complete recovery from this disease is early detection. Secondary

244

prevention measures—that is, early detection measures—must be employed to decrease breast cancer mortality rates, since a method of primary prevention is not presently available. Secondary prevention measures for breast cancer are: mammography—a breast x-ray technique; a clinical breast examination by a health professional; and breast self-examination (BSE). Unfortunately, these measures are under-utilized by American women, and performance rates of BSE are especially low. Various surveys conducted during the past ten years indicate that whereas about 61 percent of all American women reported performing self-examination sometime within the previous year, only 38 percent reported performing a monthly BSE (American Cancer Society 1978, 1980; Costanza and Foster 1984; Dickson et al. 1986; EVAXX 1981; Holtzman and Celentano 1983; Huguley et al. 1988; and National Cancer Institute 1980). Although breast cancer is a risk faced by all women, it appears that very few take the necessary steps to reduce their chances of mortality from this disease.

Risk Factors Affecting African-American Women

Not all women are equally at risk for developing breast cancer, nor do they have equal chances of surviving it. Both age and race affect breast cancer incidence and survival rates. Premenopausal African-American women have a higher *incidence* of breast cancer than premenopausal European-American women, whereas postmenopausal African-American women have a lower incidence than postmenopausal European-American women. Across all age groups, African-American women have lower *survival* rates than their European-American counterparts. In addition, African- and European-American women under thirty-five have lower breast cancer *survival* rates than older African- and European-American women (Baquet and Ringen 1986; Ries, Pollack, and Young 1983; USDHHS 1986a).

Three community medicine physicians in Southern California, G. E. Gray, B. E. Henderson, and M. C. Pike (1980), have suggested that the differences in breast cancer *incidence* between African-American and European-American women correlate with: (1) early age at menarche, which increases the risk of breast cancer in premenopausal women; (2) late age at menopause, which increases the likelihood of breast cancer in postmenopausal women; and (3) late age at the birth of a woman's first child, which increases the likelihood of breast cancer in postmenopausal women. African-American women have a higher incidence of premenopausal breast cancer because they begin menstruating approximately six months to one year earlier than European-American women. A lower incidence of postmenopausal cancer among African-American women occurs because, on average, their first full-term pregnancy and their onset of menopause both occur at an earlier age than among European-American women.

Differences in *survival* between African-American and European-American women are attributed to many factors. Several studies have documented a tendency for African-American women of all ages to have their breast cancer detected at a later stage than women of other racial groups (e.g., Bain, Greenberg, and Whitaker 1986; Polednak 1986; Satariano, Belle, and Swanson 1986; USDHHS 1986a). It has also been reported that single African-American women under the age of sixty have the highest proportion of regional and metastatic (non-localized) cancer (Polednak 1986). Moreover, a higher proportion of African-American women with advanced disease do not receive surgery (Bain, Greenberg, and Whitaker 1986).

Underlying the differences in stage at diagnosis and treatment may be a difference in socioeconomic level. Lower socioeconomic levels have been correlated with lower survival rates (Dayal, Power, and Chiu 1982), and African Americans are over-represented in the lower socioeconomic levels (USDHHS 1986b). Differences in socioeconomic status influence access to state-of-the-art treatment, quality of medical care, delay in treatment, access to screening, nutritional status, dietary patterns, and state of the immune system. Finally, differences in education may be responsible for a lack of awareness of breast cancer warning signs and insufficient knowledge of the guidelines for early detection of breast cancer (e.g., Bang, Perlin, and Sampson 1987; Polednak 1986).

In addition to the foregoing sociological factors, biological differences have also been shown to exist between African- and European-American women. A higher proportion of malignant tumors in African-American patients do not have estrogen receptors (e.g., Beverly et al. 1987). The presence of estrogen receptors is associated with improved prognosis because of a better response to hormonal therapy, slower tumor growth, and more differentiated tumors. Thus the type of tumors found more frequently in African-American women are associated with a worse prognosis. Whether this biological difference is due to racial differences and/or environmental factors has yet to be determined.

Three Methods of Early Detection of Breast Cancer

Regardless of the reasons for the varying incidence and survival rates between racial groups, the fact remains that the excessive mortality from breast cancer among African-American women could best be decreased by placing an emphasis on early detection of this disease. For treatment to be maximally effective, the detection of breast cancer should occur when the malignant tumor is at its smallest detectable point. Because the size of a cancerous tumor is a function of time, the earlier a lump is detected, the smaller it will be, and hence, the better the chances for a complete recovery. Ideally, detection should occur when a woman is free from other symptoms of the disease—that is, before the tumor has spread to the lymph nodes and other structures surrounding the breasts, and while the malignant lump is still discrete and more easily removable.

Using lump size as the most important criterion, mammography is generally considered to be the most effective method of early breast cancer detection because the imaging technique can detect abnormal lumps in breast tissue which are too small to be detected manually. The drawbacks to mammographic utilization are its high cost (estimates range from $60 to $250 per session) and the fact that the American Cancer Society (1988) does not recommend mammography for asymptomatic women under forty years of age, because younger women's breast tissue is often too dense to obtain a useful mammogram. Since mammography is not recommended for women *under* forty, asymptomatic African-American women in this age group (who are at risk for breast cancer) are not provided with the option of obtaining a mammogram as a means of secondary prevention. However, for women *over* forty it is likely that the high cost of mammography is a major impediment to its utilization.

The other two methods available for the early detection of breast cancer are the clinical breast examination performed by a health professional and breast self-examination (BSE). The relative disadvantages of clinical breast examinations are, once again, the cost and the fact that such examinations are usually performed only on an annual basis.

BSE is an early detection technique that can be easily and conveniently performed at home. The examination takes only a few minutes and, when performed correctly, is effective for detecting lumps as small as 3 millimeters (Hall et al. 1980). Several methods of BSE are currently available, including the American Cancer Society method and the MammaCare Method© developed by Pennypacker and his colleagues (1982). These methods generally encompass twelve to fourteen distinct steps which comprise a complete and thorough palpation of the breast tissue. When women are trained to perform BSE competently, using simulated breast models, they are able to detect simulated lumps between 1–2 millimeters in diameter (Adams et al. 1976; Stephenson et al. 1979). It has also been found that when women with no previous experience are trained to perform BSE by using plastic breast models, 65 percent of these women can detect lumps as small as .25 centimeters in human breast tissue (Hall et al. 1980). These results are extremely promising, particularly in light of the fact that some investigators have estimated that the detection of lumps between 1 and 2 centimeters could almost double survival rates (see Adams et al. 1976).

The Efficacy of Breast Self-Examination

There has been some controversy regarding the relative value of BSE. The debate revolves around three issues. First, some physicians doubt whether women can be the guardians of their own health, believing that women may experience excessive anxiety or a false sense of security as a consequence of performing BSE (Cole and Austin 1981; Frank and Mai 1985; Moore 1978). However, no empirical studies have addressed these concerns. A second issue which has been raised suggests that women might not report the findings of their breast self-examinations. However, studies have shown that the interval between detecting a lump and reporting it to a physician is shorter among women performing BSE (Foster and Costanza 1984; Philip et al. 1986). Finally, other physicians question whether BSE has value above and beyond an annual clinical examination (Fletcher and O'Malley 1986). Data relevant to this question will be discussed in the next section of this paper.

A recent review of the literature indicated that the overall evidence for the value of BSE is favorable (Jacob and Penn 1988). Although most of the studies published before 1987 which were relevant to the issue of the value of BSE were reviewed, very few involved African-American women as participants. The studies reviewed by Jacob and Penn compared the stage of malignant tumors found by one of three methods: (1) accidental discoveries, (2) breast self-examination, and (3) clinical breast examination. In general, these studies showed a positive effect of BSE practice: performance of the exam was shown to increase the chances of early detection relative to accident and to be at least as effective as a clinical breast examination. To date, no empirical data demonstrate unequivocally that the sensitivity of BSE is not at least comparable to that of a clinical breast examination.

The most compelling evidence in favor of BSE comes from an empirical study which assessed the value of BSE in directly affecting survival rates—the most relevant outcome measure (Costanza and Foster 1984; Foster and Costanza 1984). This study determined that death as a result of breast cancer was significantly reduced in BSE performers as compared with non-performers. The survival of breast cancer patients five years after detection was 75 percent for breast self-examiners versus 57 percent for non-examiners (Foster and Costanza 1984). Several additional studies found that a significantly higher percentage of BSE performers, as compared with infrequent and non-performers, discovered tumors at an earlier stage of cancer (Feldman et al. 1981; Foster and Costanza 1984; Huguley and Brown, 1981; Owen et al. 1985; Philip et al. 1984, 1986). In one study, for example, 48 percent of those who frequently practiced BSE were diagnosed at an earlier stage of breast cancer, in contrast with only 38 percent of those who rarely practiced BSE and 33 percent who never practiced BSE (Feldman et al. 1981). The size of the tumors discovered by BSE performers were also significantly smaller than those found by non-performers. Specifically, Foster and Costanza (1984) found that the maximum diameter of the tumors found in BSE performers was 2.1 centimeters, whereas the maximum diameter of the tumors found in non-performers was 3.2 centimeters. The size of tumors found by non-performers is an important measure, since the majority of lumps currently detected (70–95 percent) are accidentally discovered by women in their own breast tissue (e.g., Huguley and Brown 1981; Smith and Burns 1985). Most of the lumps discovered accidentally by women in their own breasts are reported to be approximately 3 centimeters in size (Stephenson et al. 1979). Thus, as shown by this evidence, proper BSE training enables women to detect lumps significantly smaller than those found by accident.

The strength of the evidence supporting BSE is influenced by the fact that the results of several recent studies (e.g, Holtzman and Celentano 1983) indicate that the majority of women who perform breast self-examinations do so incorrectly. In one particular study, E. Kenney and her colleagues (1989) measured the proficiency of seventy-three women in performing BSE, and not one performed a complete and correct examination. The reported lack of general competence in women's performance of BSE might have prompted some health professionals to doubt the advisability of relying on women as monitors of their own health in this manner (Cole and Austin 1981; Howard 1981; Moore 1978). Yet two important points should be noted. First, *competent* performance would further increase the benefits of this early detection technique, and second, *the benefits of BSE occur even when the technique is not performed at peak proficiency.* Therefore, if a high standard of training is maintained, the benefits resulting from widespread BSE education and practice should be greatly increased.

A Comparison of Clinical and Self Breast Examination

As mentioned earlier, despite the fact that BSE has been shown to be a valuable technique, disagreement exists within the medical community regarding the extent to which BSE can be used as a primary means of early detection of breast cancer. A commonly held belief is that a clinical breast examination is superior to a BSE. Two methods can be used to test this belief. One method consists of comparing the stage at diagnosis of tumors detected by BSE performers with that of tumors detected by health professionals. The second method consists of directly comparing BSE performers with health professionals in their ability to find breast tumors.

When the first of these methods was used, no difference was found between the clinical breast exam and BSE in the stage of tumors detected (e.g., Greenwald et al. 1978; Owen et al. 1985).

The present authors used the second of these methods. We directly compared the proficiency of women trained to perform BSE competently with the proficiency of health professionals (Jacob et al. 1990a). Proficiency was assessed in terms of number of embedded lumps found in opaque, plastic breast models. A small sample of college students, including African-American and white women, was trained to perform BSE competently using the MammaCare Method©. Their proficiency was then tested and compared to the proficiency of practicing health professionals using the same test models. The results of this comparison indicated that: (1) women can be trained to perform BSE competently, and (2) given this training, they are at least as accurate as health professionals in detecting simulated lumps in breast models. It should be noted that this is the first reported study of its kind, and the fact that only college women participated may affect the generality of the findings. Further research with a more inclusive sample is necessary before it can be concluded that all women, regardless of age and educational level, can be trained to perform a breast examination as competently as health professionals. Our data strongly suggest, however, that this is possible.

Performance Rates and Attitudes of African-American Women

Given the fact that BSE has been shown to be a valuable early detection method, the questions which remain are whether women will practice the exam and, if so, under what conditions. Most of the available data regarding these questions have been drawn from studies in which the majority of participants were European-American women. We recently conducted the first published survey in which African-American women were queried about their practice, attitudes, and knowledge of BSE (Jacob, Penn, and Brown 1989). Participants were 180 African-American women, recruited from churches in Southern California. Our results showed that 89 percent of the respondents reported having practiced the exam at least once during the previous year, and 50 percent reported having practiced BSE at least monthly (Jacob, Penn, and Brown 1989). The monthly practice of BSE in this sample was at the high end of the range of regular practice reported by all American women (25–49 percent). However, consistent with previously reported results from surveys of European-American women (Holtzman and Celentano 1983; Kenney et al. 1989), less than half of our survey respondents indicated performing the exam correctly. That is, the majority (67 percent) of the breast self-examiners reported correctly performing at *most* two of the five examination items included in the questionnaire. In addition, most of the breast self-examiners reported that the duration of their examination was only three minutes or less, an amount of time clearly insufficient to perform a complete exam (Mamon and Zapka 1986). In summary, our survey showed that while the majority of participants perform BSE fairly frequently, most are not proficient. The reported lack of proficiency among the African-American women who participated reflects the previously noted fact that very few women are properly trained to perform a complete and proficient breast self-examination.

Results from the same survey (Jacob, Penn, and Brown 1989) also indicated that the women who reported performing BSE on a regular basis were more likely to have been taught the breast cancer detection method by either a physician or a nurse, as opposed to having learned about it through information booklets or other media sources. A possible interpretation of these findings is that women who have more regular contact with a physician or nurse are encouraged and supported in their practice of the self-exam. In fact, compared to non-performers, breast self-examiners in our sample had more contact with health professionals, obtained other exams for early cancer detection more often, and visited physicians in clinics or private offices more frequently than in hospital emergency rooms. The best predictor of BSE practice among the women in our sample was the type of setting in which medical care was usually sought. Other studies have also shown that person-to-person training, unavailable in emergency room settings, is strongly associated with the frequency of BSE performance (e.g., Champion 1985).

In addition, results from our survey indicated that breast self-examiners were older than non-examiners. This may reflect older women's increased perception of breast cancer risk. The self-examiners in our survey also had higher annual incomes than the non-performers (Jacob, Penn, and Brown 1989). Thus women in higher socioeconomic levels, who are most able to afford an examination by a health professional, are also more likely to perform BSE. These results suggest that women at higher socioeconomic levels have frequent examinations via a variety of methods, while another, larger group of women at lower socioeconomic levels are not examined at all.

Finally, our survey (Jacob, Penn, and Brown 1989) also confirmed the consistent finding of previous studies (e.g., Mamon and Zapka 1986; Zapka and Mamon 1986) that one of the best predictors of regular BSE performance is the confidence a woman has in her ability to perform the examination. Thus if an African-American woman is confident about her ability to perform BSE, she is more likely to do so.

In summary, regular BSE performance occurs among African-American women who are proficient, have a high degree of confidence in their ability to perform the examination, and have regular contact with health professionals. Based on these findings, we believe that personal interaction with a health professional is probably the optimal setting for BSE training, because women who practice the technique in the presence of a health professional are generally given feedback on their performance and are trained to a high degree of proficiency (e.g., Foster and Costanza 1984).

Unfortunately, physicians and other health professionals are often unable or unmotivated to take the time to train their patients to competency. When that is the case, there are three alternatives open to women. First, a woman may schedule an appointment during which a BSE method can be learned. As a second alternative, women may be trained by other women who are proficient in the technique. The critical component of the interaction between a patient and a health care practitioner is most likely the feedback provided to the patient regarding her performance of BSE. This encouragement and support may also be derived from caring relationships among women. Therefore we believe that the transfer of this information between women is a viable option. In fact, it may be the preferred mechanism for women who do not have ready access to health care for economic reasons. The American Cancer Society has implemented such a program, known as the Special Touch program, in which women from various health professions are trained to teach BSE to women within the community (Zoila Escobar, San Diego branch of the American Cancer Society, telephone interview, 5 July 1990). While this is a positive step, to our knowledge no research has been conducted to evaluate the program. Attempts to implement health campaigns of this nature must ensure the competency of BSE trainers and trainees and should be evaluated as a whole. These would be worthwhile topics for future research. As a third option for learning to perform BSE, women may obtain information from non-profit organizations, such as the American Cancer Society. Home-practice kits are also available through the MammaTech Corporation in Gainesville, Florida.

Psycho-social Factors Influencing Breast Self-Examination

A woman's beliefs about illness and health behaviors profoundly affect her practice of BSE, as does her confidence in her ability to perform BSE. One theoretical model which considers health and illness beliefs is the Health Belief Model (HBM). The HBM emphasizes four concepts: perceived susceptibility to a disease, perceived seriousness of a disease, perceived benefits of a health behavior, and perceived barriers to performing a health behavior (Rosenstock 1966; Becker 1974). According to the HBM, an individual will engage in a specific health behavior to prevent or ameliorate the risk of an illness if s/he holds the following beliefs: (1) that s/he is susceptible to that illness; (2) that the illness is serious; and (3) that the specific health behavior will be effective in preventing or ameliorating the illness. In addition, there should not be any actual or perceived barriers which preclude the individual from engaging in the health behavior. It has been postulated that a relationship exists amongst the HBM components and BSE practice (e.g., Champion 1985). Results from our survey (Jacob, Penn, and Brown 1989) indicated that among African-American women the regular performance of the self-exam was associated with belief in its benefits. That is, monthly performers, more often than infrequent performers, believed BSE to be beneficial. In another survey, a separate sample of 159 African-American women in Southern California were asked which factors may have prevented them from performing BSE (Jacob et al. 1990b). Very few of these women reported embarrassment in performing a BSE (5.7 percent), while more than 65 percent reported difficulty in remembering to perform the examination and slightly more than half (54 percent) reported a lack of confidence in their ability to perform the technique. Thus health campaigns which are geared toward increasing the rate of BSE practice among African-American women should enhance their confidence in their ability to perform BSE, enhance their perceptions of the benefits associated with BSE practice, and address their reported difficulty in remembering to perform the exam.

Conclusion

It seems clear that in order to decrease the breast cancer mortality rate, women must take an active role in monitoring their own health. Since the majority of lumps are discovered accidentally by women themselves, it follows that if women were encouraged to palpate their own breast tissue regularly and systematically, the mortality rate from this disease would decrease. The evidence strongly demonstrates that a proficient breast self-examination is a valuable tool which can be used and trusted by all women as a means of becoming more independent with regard to their own health care. In particular, African-American women under forty should be actively involved in early detection practices. Of the early detection measures, BSE seems especially appropriate, because it is a private, non-invasive procedure recommended to asymptomatic women of all ages and socioeconomic levels.

In order to maximize the likelihood that women will practice BSE, women would best be advised to seek personal training either by a health professional or a knowledgeable woman who will train them to proficiency and assist them in developing an increased sense of confidence in BSE performance. These preconditions will enable women to overcome barriers to practicing the exam. Worthy of re-emphasis is the fact that such conditions may be achieved not only by a health professional, but also by women who are proficient in performing the examination. The practice of BSE is very empowering in that it increases a woman's autonomy and control over her personal health. As a means of translating the preceding evidence and theoretical discussion into a practical approach for African-American women, the following guidelines are suggested:

SEVEN STEPS TO EMPOWERMENT
WITH BREAST SELF-EXAMINATION

In order to empower herself, a woman should possess:

1) a realistic knowledge of her individual risk of developing breast cancer;
2) a basic knowledge of the three available methods for the early detection of breast cancer;
3) the ability to perform a breast self-examination proficiently;

4) a belief in the positive value of monthly breast self-examinations;
5) confidence in her ability to detect a suspicious lump and to distinguish between normal and abnormal breast tissue;
6) a commitment to her personal health which motivates her to choose to practice BSE each month; and
7) the willingness to inform and teach her family and friends about the value and practice of BSE.

Early detection is the best hope for reducing breast cancer mortality rates. Given the established value of BSE practice and the threat of breast cancer among African-American women, it is vital to encourage widespread, effective BSE practice.

Works Cited

Adams, C. K., D. C. Hall, H. S. Pennypacker, M. K. Goldstein, L. L. Hench, M. C. Madden, G. H. Stein, and A. C. Catania. 1976. "Lump Detection in Simulated Human Breasts." *Perception and Psychophysics* 20(3):163–67.

American Cancer Society. 1978, 1980, 1988, 1990. *Cancer Facts and Figures.* New York: American Cancer Society.

Bain, R. P., R. S. Greenberg, and J. P. Whitaker. 1986. "Racial Differences in the Survival of Women with Breast Cancer." *Journal of Chronic Disease* 39(8):631–42.

Baines, C. J., A. B. Miller, and A. A. Bassett. 1989. "Physical Examination: Its Role as a Single Screening Modality in the Canadian National Breast Screening Study." *Cancer* 63(9):1816–22.

Bang, K. M., E. Perlin, and C. C. Sampson. 1987. "Increased Cancer Risks in Blacks: A Look at the Factors." *Journal of the National Medical Association* 79(4):383–88.

Baquet, C., and K. Ringen. 1986, "Cancer Control in Blacks: Epidemiology and NCI Program Plans." In: *Advances in Cancer Control. Health Care Financing and Research*, edited by L. E. Mortenson, P. T. Engstrom, and P. N. Anderson, 215–27. New York: Alan R. Liss.

Becker, M. H. 1974. "The Health Belief Model and Personal Health Behavior." *Health Education Monographs* 2:324–508.

Beverly, L. N., W. D. Flanders, R. C. P. Go, and S. J. Soong. 1987. "A Comparison of Estrogen and Progesterone Receptors in Black and White Breast Cancer Patients." *American Journal of Public Health* 77(3):351–53.

Champion, V. L. 1985. "Use of the Health Belief Model in Determining Frequency of Breast Self-Examination." *Research in Nursing and Health* 8:373–79.

Cole, P., and H. Austin. 1981. "Breast Self-Examination: An Adjuvant to Early Cancer Detection." *American Journal of Public Health* 71(6):572–74.

Costanza, M. C., and R. S. Foster. 1984. "Relationship Between Breast Self-Examination and Death from Breast Cancer by Age Groups." *Cancer Detection and Prevention* 7:103–08.

Dayal, H. H., R. N. Power, and C. Chiu. 1982. "Race and Socio-Economic Status in Survival from Breast Cancer." *Journal of Chronic Disease* 35:675–83.

Dickson, G., M. A. Parsons, P. Greaves, K. L. Jackson, J. J. Kronenfeld, W. B.

Ward, and J. R. Ureda. 1986. "Breast Self-Examination: Knowledge, Attitudes and Practice Behaviors of Working Women. *AAOHN Journal* 34(5):228–32.

EVAXX, Inc. 1981. "Black Americans' Attitudes Toward Cancer and Cancer Tests." *Cancer* 31(4):212–18.

Feldman, J. G., A. C. Carter, A. D. Nicastri, and S. T. Hosat. 1981. "Breast Self-Examination, Relationship to Stage of Breast Cancer at Diagnosis." *Cancer* 47: 2740–45.

Fletcher, S. W., and M. S. O'Malley. 1986. "Clinical Breast Examination." *Hospital Practice* 21(54): 80, 82–84, 89.

Foster, R. S., and M. C. Costanza. 1984. "Breast Self-Examination Practices and Breast Cancer Survival." *Cancer* 53:999–1005.

Frank, J. W., and V. Mai. 1985. "Breast Self-Examination in Young Women: More Harm than Good?" *Lancet* 1:654–57.

Gray, G. E., B. E. Henderson, and M. C. Pike. 1980. "Changing Ratio of Breast Cancer Incidence Rates with Age of Black Females Compared with White Females in the United States." *Journal of the National Cancer Institute* 64(3):461–63.

Greenwald, P., P. C. Nasca, C. E. Lawrence, J. Horton, R. P. McGarrah, T. Gabriele, and K. Carlton. 1978. "Estimated Effect of Breast Self-Examination and Routine Physician Examination on Breast Cancer Mortality." *New England Journal of Medicine* 299:271–73.

Hall, D. C., C. K. Adams, G. H. Stein, H. S. Stephenson, M. K. Goldstein, and H. S. Pennypacker. 1980. "Improved Detection of Human Breast Lesions Following Experimental Training." *Cancer* 46:408–14.

Holtzman, D., and D. D. Celentano. 1983. "The Practice and Efficacy of Breast Self-Examination: A Critical Review." *American Journal of Public Health* 73(11): 1324–26.

Howard, J. 1981. "Breast Self-Examination: Some Unanswered Questions." In: Proceedings of the 17th Annual Meeting of the Society of Prospective Medicine, August 31–September 2, 1981, Stevens Point, Wisconsin.

Huguley, C. M., and R. L. Brown. 1981. "The Value of Breast Self-Examination." *Cancer* 47:989–95.

———, R. S. Greenberg, and W. S. Clark. 1988. "Breast Self-Examination and Survival from Breast Cancer." *Cancer* 62:1389–96.

Jacob, T. C., and N. E. Penn. 1988. "The Need and Value of Breast Self-Examination." *Journal of the National Medical Association* 80(7):777–87.

———, and M. Brown. 1989. "Breast Self-Examination: Knowledge, Attitudes and Performance Among Black Women." *Journal of the National Medical Association* 81(7):769–76.

———, J. Giebinck, and R. Bastien. 1990a. "A Comparison Between the Clinical and the Self-Examination of the Breast." Under editorial review; findings available from the first author.

Jacob, T. C., N. E. Penn, J. A. Kulik, and L. E. Spieth. 1990b. "Maintenance Strategies for BSE Practice in Black Women." In preparation; findings available from the first author.

Kenney, E., M. F. Hovell, C. R. Newborn, and J. P. Elder. 1989. "Breast Self-Examination among College Women: Predictors for Cancer Control." *American Journal of Preventive Medicine* 5(1):27–33.

MammaTech Corporation, 930 NW Eighth Ave., Gainesville, Fla. 32601.

Mamon, J., and J. G. Zapka. 1986. "Breast Self-Examination by Young Women: I. Characteristics Associated with Frequency." *American Journal of Preventive Medicine* 2(2):61–69.

Moore, F. D. 1978. "Breast Self-Examination." *The New England Journal of Medicine* 299(6):304–05.

National Cancer Institute. 1980. "National Survey on Breast Cancer. A Measure of Progress and Public Understanding." NIH Publication No. 81–2306. U. S. Government Printing Office.

Owen, W. L., A. F. Hoge, N. R. Asal, P. S. Anderson, A. S. Owen, and A. J. Cucchiara. 1985. "Self-Examination of the Breast: Use and Effectiveness." *Southern Medical Journal* 78(10):1170–73.

Pennypacker, H. S., H. S. Bloom, E. L. Criswell, P. Neelakantan, M. K. Goldstein, and G. H. Stein. 1982. "Toward an Effective Technology of Instruction in Breast Self-Examination." *International Journal of Mental Health* 11(3):98–116.

Philip, J., W. G. Harris, C. Flaherty, C. A. F. Joslin, J. H. Rustage, and D. P. Wijesinghe. 1984. "Breast Self-Examination: Clinical Results from a Population-Based Prospective Study." *British Journal of Cancer* 50:7–12.

Philip, J., W. G. Harris, C. Flaherty, and C. A. F. Joslin. 1986. "Clinical Measures to Assess the Practice and Efficiency of Breast Self-Examination." *Cancer* 58(4):973–77.

Polednak, A. P. 1986. "Breast Cancer in Black and White Women in New York State: Case Distribution and Incidence Rates by Clinical Stage at Diagnosis." *Cancer* 58:807–15.

Ries, L. G., E. S. Pollack, and J. L. Young. 1983. "Cancer Patient Survival: Surveillance, Epidemiology, and End Results Program, 1973–1979." *Journal of the National Cancer Institute* 70(4):693–707.

Rosenstock, I. M. 1966. "Why People Use Health Services." *Millbank Memorial Fund Quarterly* 44 (supplement): 94–127.

Satariano, W. A., S. H. Belle, and G. M. Swanson. 1986. "The Severity of Breast Cancer at Diagnosis: A Comparison of Age and Extent of Disease in Black and White Women." *American Journal of Public Health* 76(7):779–82.

Smith, E. M., and T. L. Burns. 1985. "The Effects of Breast Self-Examination in a Population-Based Cancer Registry: A Report of Differences in Extent of Disease." *Cancer* 55:432–37.

Stephenson, H. S., C. K. Adams, D. C. Hall, and H. S. Pennypacker. 1979. "Effects of Certain Training Parameters on Detection of Simulated Breast Cancer." *Journal of Behavioral Medicine* 2(3):239–50.

U. S. D. H. H. S. 1986a. *Cancer Among Blacks and Other Minorities: Statistical Profiles.* U. S. Department of Health and Human Services. NIH Publication No. 86–2785. U. S. Government Printing Office.

———. 1986b. *Health Status of the Disadvantaged, Chartbook 1986.* USDHHS Publication No. (HRSA) HRS-P-DV86-2. U. S. Government Printing Office.

Zapka, J. G., and J. A. Mamon. 1986. "Breast Self-Examination by Young Women: II. Characteristics Associated with Proficiency." *American Journal of Preventive Medicine* 2(2):70–78.

Resignation and Resourcefulness: Older Hispanic Women's Responses to Breast Cancer

MICHELLE SAINT-GERMAIN AND ALICE LONGMAN

Introduction

The United States has the sixth largest concentration of Hispanics in the world (16.9 million), and their numbers are expected to double every five years (Texidor 1987). Hispanics over sixty-five years of age are the fastest-growing segment of the elderly, and women outnumber men (Cubillos 1987). Yet the health care beliefs of older Hispanic women are largely unknown to most health care professionals (Kosko and Flaskerud 1987).

Breast cancer is one of the most commonly diagnosed forms of cancer in older women and a major cause of death. While there is no known way to prevent the disease, survival is enhanced by early detection and treatment. Breast cancer occurs less frequently in women, including Hispanics, of low socioeconomic status (SES), but such women are also more likely to be diagnosed at a later stage, with poorer prognosis for survival (Farley and Flannery 1989; Frunch 1986; Newell and Mills 1986). Hispanics are more likely to have late stage diagnosis than Anglos, due to irregular screening and the failure to detect and respond to breast cancer symptoms (Richardson et al. 1987). Most research has found socioeconomic factors to be more important than cultural or other factors in access to health care (Lee 1976; Marks et al. 1987; Saint-Germain and Longman 1990). For Hispanics, health care is often a luxury, as food, clothing, and shelter come first. In our study, the average three-person household income was only $500 to $1,000 per month.

Thus removing barriers to access (cost, availability, transportation) should be the first plan of action. Convincing physicians to recommend breast cancer screening for their older patients is another barrier that must be overcome (Cohen et al. 1982; Fox et al. 1988). Even with free or low-cost screening, however, not all women will choose to participate (Grady et al. 1983; Lurie et al. 1987; Rimer et al. in press; Taplin et al. 1989). With the incidence of breast cancer on the rise, it is increasingly important to understand the perceptual and motivational factors that influence women's screening decisions (Fink et al. 1968).

Previous research with Anglos has found that women do not participate in breast cancer screening because of various fears: fear of finding something, like cancer or an incurable disease; fear of mutilation, of losing one or both breasts; fear of radiation or other technology; and embarrassment from exposing their breasts (Crooks and Jones 1989). But Marjorie Kagawa-Singer (1987) points out that "consideration of cultural differences" has been largely ignored in the field of cancer research.

Methodology

In order to address these concerns we conducted a study of 409 Hispanic women over age fifty living in Tucson, Arizona. The sample was selected using random cluster sampling from ethnically heterogeneous as well as ethnically homogeneous neighborhoods and from a wide range of income levels. A sixty-three-item questionnaire was developed and pre-tested on a pilot sample that resembled the target population. The questionnaire was translated into Spanish and back-translated into English to ensure comparable meaning in both languages. A group of trained bilingual women from the community with previous experience in health surveys conducted interviews lasting from thirty to ninety minutes in the respondents' homes, in the language of their choice.

We asked each respondent a series of questions about social and demographic characteristics, acculturation, access and barriers to health care, knowledge and beliefs about breast cancer, past medical history, and what it would mean to get breast cancer. The Hispanic women we interviewed reported fears of death, disease, and mutilation, as well as loss of sexuality, relationships, control, social support, and respect; this was consistent with reports from other ethnic groups (Magarey 1988). In the following pages, however, we compare our findings specifically with extant literature on Hispanic health care beliefs. We report what the women in our sample say they know about breast cancer, how they perceive it, and the wide range of responses they give to the possibility of the disease, using their own words as often as possible. Finally, we draw some conclusions and implications for health care practitioners and for further research.

Health and Illness

The Hispanic population in the United States exhibits a "wide range of variability in cultural characteristics" (Kranau et al. 1982), for example in terms of country of origin, language preference, acculturation, socioeconomic status, and so forth. Nevertheless there are some broad themes running through the literature on Hispanics and health. The Hispanic view of health and *enfermedad* is "holistic" (Giachello 1985), and it includes "spiritual, moral, somatic, physiological, psychological, social, and metaphysical" dimensions (Kosko and Flaskerud 1987). The Spanish word *enfermedad* refers to the English concepts of disease (internal "bodily events and processes") and illness (a person's "socio-culturally structured behaviors and interpretations" that are "a response to these processes") (Kay 1972). Health is often seen as good fortune, luck, or a gift from God, and *enfermedad* as a punishment for sins (Kosko and Flaskerud 1987). One woman in our study said, "I have faith in God that I won't get sick," while another said, "I beg God not to let it happen to me." One woman believed that she wouldn't get breast cancer because "I don't do anything wrong." For others, God represents a source of strength. "I would ask God to guide me," said one.

Estar conforme (to conform to God's will) is another theme. Disease may be accepted as God's will, "about which little can be done" (Moustafa and Weiss 1968). One woman in our sample saw breast cancer as a "mortification" that she would have to "suffer with patience." Others said they would prepare or wait for death, or "just ask God to take me away." "I would have to get along with it if this is what God sends me," said another. But some of the women in our study wondered why God would have sent this disease. "I suffer enough in my case," said one woman. Others said they would accept it, but they wouldn't like it. One woman concluded, "I guess the hardest thing is to accept it."

Another often-mentioned cause of disease is an imbalance, either within the individual (e.g., the dislocation of internal organs) or between the individual and the environment (e.g., jumping into a cold pond when a person is hot and sweating) (Moustafa and Weiss 1968). There are a number of words in Spanish (e.g., *manco*, *tuerto*, which have no English equivalents) that describe people with imbalances (e.g., one arm, hand, leg, eye, and so on). Thus the possibility of losing a breast is very troubling. "I wouldn't like to look at my body," said one woman. "It would be very weird to go out with only one breast," remarked another, "like only having one arm or one leg." Another said she wouldn't want to be operated on because "then you would lean to one side." "I wouldn't be a complete person anymore," declared one; *"fregado"* (broken; out-of-order) was the term used by another; a third remarked that afterward she "wouldn't go out of the house" if she only had one breast. But others dealt with the possibility of losing a breast by joking. "Then I would be broke *and* flat-chested," said one, while another laughed that "my breasts are too small as they are—I couldn't afford to lose any more."

Some authors cite magical causes of disease, such as witchcraft, evil eye, and casting spells. Sustained emotional states such as *susto* (fright), "anger, desire, rejection, embarrassment or shame, disillusion, and sadness" can also be causes (Clark 1970). While none of the women we interviewed made allusion to witchcraft or magic, some did mention strong emotions. "*Que susto!*" was a common expression, or "I would die of *susto.*" Another remarked that it would be *penoso* (shameful) and *triste* (sad). Others said they would become agitated, "cry every day," or "*volver loca*" (go crazy). Others said they would be frightened, get an attack of *nervios* (nerves), or die from "*pura pena*" (pure shame).

"Scientific" explanations, such as germs, "microbes," or contagion, are also accepted as causes of disease, as is a disregard for hygiene rules (Kay 1972). Cancer was characterized by our sample as a dirty disease that one could get from being in a hospital, or from being around other people with cancer or corpses of people who had died from cancer. "*Que feo!*" (how ugly) was a common response. "I would rather die of anything than cancer," was another. One woman called cancer *cochinada* (filth), and said that "when it gets inside you, you die quicker." Another remarked that "it is rotten—people suffer and can't eat." Other women said they would not let anybody touch them, and another said "my husband couldn't touch me."

Officially recognized signs and symptoms of breast cancer are a lump in the breast, scaly skin, heat or swelling, differences between breasts, puckering, ache or pain, and unusual nipple discharge. Most women in this sample could name only one or two of these official signs, most commonly a lump or an ache.[1] A number of erroneous symptoms were also frequently cited as signs of breast cancer, such as hot flashes, fever, itching, rash, dizziness, back pain, bruises, sores that won't heal, inverted nipples, and general nausea.

There was also scant knowledge of the risks for breast cancer. While the incidence of breast cancer cannot be predicted with any certainty, there are some factors associated with the disease. Increasing age, family history of breast cancer, never giving birth, first birth after age thirty, extended fertility (early menstruation and late menopause), and obesity are thought to be risk factors for breast cancer. On the average, the women in this sample could name only one—family history. Other behaviors they often erroneously identified as putting women at increased risk for breast cancer included smoking and drinking, using drugs, non-traditional lifestyles, using underarm deodorant, stress, breast feeding too much or not enough, excessive fondling of the breasts, jogging, and wearing "modern bras."

The Hispanic women in our sample thought that only about one of every twenty women develops breast cancer in her lifetime, although the current national average is one woman in nine. Neither did most of the women in our sample know that they are in the prime age range for breast cancer (over fifty). Many agreed that *some* women are more likely to get breast cancer than others (as a result of engaging in the risky behaviors named above), but only 8 percent rated their *own* chance of getting breast cancer as higher than that of other women. The others thought they had either the same chance as other women (41 percent) or less chance (47 percent); some could not answer the question (4 percent).

Disease prevention is not a well-understood concept among some groups, including older Hispanics. If disease is something that is natural or caused by supernatural factors, it is hard to see how it can be prevented (Moustafa and Weiss 1968). As one woman explained, "I would accept it because it is a natural cause, and prepare for death." Preventive medicine is thus a strange concept, one that is resisted unless it can be shown to produce observable changes (Rose 1978). In our study, going to the doctor without feeling ill was seen not only as a waste of scarce resources, but as "just asking for trouble," since "doctors are sure to find something wrong with you" and "you can't trust tests." Only half the women in our sample thought that there was a very good chance of a cure if cancer is discovered at an early stage.

We asked women if they knew of any traditional or alternative (folk) remedies for preventing or treating breast cancer. Only a handful responded, and these gave generally vague references to herbs, cactus, or vitamins. Belief in alternative folk medicine or traditional remedies, however, does not necessarily lead to resistance to or rejection of the formal health care system. Folk medicine deals with the more interpersonal aspects of illness, while "scientific" medicine deals with the more "objective" aspects of disease (Rose 1978).

Illness and the Family

The literature on Hispanic women has generally assumed that whatever happens to women happens within a family context (Cotera 1976; Lindburg and Ovando 1977). Depictions of the Hispanic family have ranged from romanticized portrayals of the extended family as a haven in a hostile world (Keefe 1979; Lindburg and Ovando 1977) to condemnations of the *macho* role of the male and the "weak, . . . submissive, exploited, physically abused . . ." role of the female (Cotera 1976).

Empirical research has shown that Hispanics tend to live in nuclear family households but maintain close social relationships with an extended network of real or fictive kin, e.g., *comadres* (the godmother of one's child who becomes like a sister) (Rose 1978; Keefe 1979). Members of this network live near one another and provide primary social contacts as well as a reciprocal mutual aid system. Commonly exchanged services include baby-sitting, financial aid, help during illness, transportation, translation, and interaction with doctors or other authorities (Keefe 1979). Within this network, Hispanic families "rely almost exclusively on women as sources of advice and help in health matters" (Markides et al. 1986).

In this context illness encompasses interpersonal responses to disease. Because illness can represent a crisis for the family (Clark 1970), one of the tasks of the extended network is the interpretation of symptoms manifested by individual members. Since there are many illnesses that share symptoms, labeling is often done by the kin group. A person is not sick until it is validated by the extended family (Rose 1978). Once validated, however, the person can count on the group for support. One respondent noted that cancer would be a "financial burden on the family"; another expected that the "family would need to help out more at home."

Health and illness are evaluated not only through external cues such as symptoms, but also in light of the person's ability to carry out usual duties. Health is measured by the "absence of pain, a well-fleshed body, and a high level of physical activity" (Rose 1978). If a person is not in pain or otherwise visibly affected, then she is not ill. Consistent with this social definition of illness, two-thirds of the women interviewed in our study thought it was possible for someone to have breast cancer and not feel ill; however, since 92 percent could name things they thought were symptoms of breast cancer, they may have meant that a woman could have breast cancer but not have it acknowledged as illness by the family as long as she could still function. "So long as I don't get too sick, it wouldn't bother me," said one woman.

For Hispanics, illness is clearly accompanied by such signs as dizziness, pain, and loss of normal functioning (Kay 1972). Cancer was described by one woman we interviewed as marked by "pain that is strong and sharp." Illness is experienced by the individual as distinctly unpleasant, both because it is personally painful and because it is accompanied by the fear of loss of certain social privileges and respect from family and friends (Clark 1970) who will be required to fill in for the ill member. But the women in our sample also said they would rely on their own individual good health, strength, and natural ability to overcome such adversity. Some named concrete actions, such as going on a diet, giving up fats, quitting smoking, or "start taking better care of myself." "I would fight against the cancer," responded another. Others pointed out that they had been or were likely to be the caregivers in the event that a female relative had cancer and that they would take on this task as part of their family obligation.

Effect on the family was of considerable interest to the women in our sample: "When something happens to a member of the family, everyone is worried and concerned." "The family would be disrupted," or, "it would affect the whole family," were frequent responses. "I know we would just take it one day at a time, like other things," said one. "I have some adorable granddaughters who would cry for me," said another. Pragmatically, one woman commented that, "I'd move to Denver where my son could afford to bury me." Although the family could be counted on to provide support, some women voiced a fear of loss of independence; one said, "I would rather die than become bedridden." Many women were concerned about becoming a burden, and they wondered how they would accomplish their domestic responsibilities. "I would be limited," said one woman; "it would be hard to do daily chores," commented another; a third worried whether she "could still baby-sit." Another said, "I would want to die quickly, not suffering long term and burdening my family and friends."

As in many cultures, these norms may come into conflict or give rise to contradictory feelings. On the one hand, life is full of countless minor pains and traumas—cold, hunger, fear—that should be borne with dignity and courage, following the norm of *sacrificio* (sacrifice for the family). Women should make the effort to continue regular activities and duties as long as possible, for giving in to illness is an admission of (perhaps moral) weakness (Clark 1970). On the other hand, since the extended kin group is the final arbiter of health and illness, women often discuss their symptoms aloud as a way of seeking validation of their health status and to confirm that they are making sacrifices for the family.

Just as the extended group makes decisions about whether one is well or ill, the individual is not free to make decisions about treatment for illness (Clark 1970). Treatment decisions are undertaken within the family unit. And since disease can be caused by an imbalance in the body or an upset in social relations, treatment may aim to correct the bodily or social imbalance as much as it aims to alleviate symptoms (Rose 1978).

Effects of Breast Cancer

We asked our respondents an open-ended question about how they thought having breast cancer would affect their daily life or the way they live now. In order to get a sense of the distribution of these attitudes and feelings among our sample, we further categorized their responses along six dimensions often expressed by people with cancer. These scales were derived from Weissman's *Coping with Cancer* (1979), which is based on interviews with cancer patients.[2] The six Likert-type scales used in this study are: hopelessness, turmoil, powerlessness, denial, abandonment, and limited time perspective. Coding ranged from a score of 1 for weak or mild manifestations of the concept, to a score of 4 for strong or severe manifestations.

The most often-mentioned effect in our study was turmoil, with scores averaging 3.2 on a scale of 1 to 4. Three-quarters of the sample (N=304) gave some response that could be classified on the turmoil scale. Over half of those reporting turmoil fell into the most severe category, making statements such as "I would be devastated." Still, some responded with considerable equanimity.

Denial figured in the statements of about half the women (N=177). Again, many of those expressing denial made strong statements, such as, "I won't get it" or "I wouldn't want to know if I had it." The average score on denial was also strong (just under 3 on a scale of 1 to 4). Others were more realistic in considering just what arrangements would have to be made in the event they did get breast cancer.

The next most commonly mentioned effect was powerlessness (N=156). As opposed to the two scales mentioned above, however, as many women scored at the very lowest end of this scale as at the highest level (with the average score falling in the middle at 2.4). That is, about one-third of the women indicated they did not feel powerless to deal with the situation, exemplified in their action statements; "I would see a doctor" or "I would get chemotherapy." Another third felt severe lack of power, saying such things as "I would not be able to cope" or "It would just eat me up." The remaining third fell between these two extremes. One woman covered all bases by saying, "I would put myself in the doctor's hands and God's."

About one-third of the sample (N=129) made statements that fell along the dimensions of the hopelessness scale, with the average score falling just about in the middle of the scale (2.6). There was a fairly even spread of responses in all the categories, ranging from statements by women who named specific treatments or said matter-of-factly that they "would just get over it," to more severe statements, e.g., "I would surely die."

Three of every ten women in our sample indicated that the thought of breast cancer provoked some concern about time (N=121). Again there was a fairly even spread among the responses (with the average score falling just in the middle at 2.5), ranging from "I would take care of it and go on," to "I would have to live every day as if it were my last."

Only about one in ten women in this sample expressed feelings of abandonment; on the contrary, there were many positive affirmations of support, such as "My family would help me." Those who lived alone or in the household of another family were more likely to express doubts or concerns. "I'm alone so I don't know how I'd live," said one. "I live with my sister's family so I would try to leave so they wouldn't have to take care of me," said another. We assume that women who did not specifically mention family took it for granted that they would have support, since the average score on abandonment was a low 2.2 on a scale of 1 to 4.

In order to find out more about the attitudes of women in our sample, we then explored the relationship of demographic, cultural, medical history, knowledge, and other variables to scale scores. In nearly all cases, the variables we looked at maintained a constant positive or negative correlation across all the scales. In the following sections we focus the discussion on those associations which reached the .05 level or more of statistical significance.

The older women in this sample gave more severe responses on all six scales. They were significantly more likely than younger women to feel more hopeless, to deny more strongly that they could get breast cancer, and to have a shorter time perspective in the event they did develop the disease. More highly educated women were significantly less likely to deny strongly that they might get breast cancer, as were women who worked outside of the home. Level of household income was also inversely related to strength of denial.

Level of access to formal health care was not related to how Hispanic women reacted to the question of impact, except that those with less access had shorter time perspectives. Similarly, women who reported experiencing more barriers to health care expressed significantly more severe levels of turmoil than women with fewer barriers. Women with some type of health insurance felt less powerless at the thought of having to deal with the impact of breast cancer, but they also expressed more severe turmoil at the thought.

The women in this study all identified themselves as belonging to an ethnic group other than Anglo-Saxon. Women who said they were Latin, Central, or South American, or who named a specific national group (e.g., Mexican) were significantly more likely to feel more severe degrees of hopelessness, powerlessness, and curtailed time perspective than women who were more acculturated (e,g, Mexican-American or American of Hispanic descent). Spanish-speakers tended to have more severe scores on powerlessness and denial than English-speakers.

Interestingly, there were no significant differences in reaction to the possibility of developing breast cancer between women who rated their health as excellent, good, fair, or poor, except that healthy women were more likely to feel less turmoil. Women who get regular preventive care (physical exams, gynecological exams, dental checks, and tests for colon cancer) had a significantly longer time perspective than other women. In fact, women who believed there was a good chance that breast cancer can be cured if detected early felt less hopeless about their ability to deal with the disease and had a longer time perspective of life after breast cancer.

Surprisingly, women who had been seen by a doctor within the past year expressed more severe turmoil at the thought of developing breast cancer than women who had not seen a doctor. Some women viewed breast cancer as a "death sentence." "It is like being told, 'tomorrow you will die,' " said one woman. Women who had seen a doctor more recently knew more about breast cancer and its treatment. Other comments made by our respondents, however, indicated that they were more threatened than reassured by knowledge of the treatments available for breast cancer (i.e., surgical breast removal, chemotherapy, radiation therapy, male hormone therapy, and so on). "I don't like to read or hear about breast cancer . . . it scares me," said one; and "my sister had her breast removed—it's scary" said another. "Everyone knows that cancer means pain, surgery, difficult therapies," one commented. "I would be afraid of suffering too much from hard things to go through like surgery and therapies," declared another. Respondents regarded treatment for breast cancer as "very powerful, very serious"; one woman commented that "no one in my family has ever been *that* sick." Some thought the treatment would be worse than the disease. "I'd kill myself first," said one; "I would die: nothing more, nothing less," said another. Others mentioned chemotherapy as particularly frightening. "People suffer with chemical therapy [*sic*] because food makes you sick to your stomach," said one, while another remarked that "for people with chemotherapy, their relatives suffer a lot."

Still, most respondents of first-hand experience with breast cancer tended to have more positive attitudes, such as the woman who said, "my aunt did OK with the treatment." Women who knew about family history as a risk factor were less likely to deny that they could get breast cancer and less powerless in their approach to the disease.

Surprisingly, having been tested for breast cancer by having a mammogram, having a clinical breast examination (CBE), or doing breast self-examination (BSE) did not generally result in a reduction in turmoil, powerlessness, or hopelessness. In fact, women who had ever had their breasts examined expressed more turmoil. Furthermore, women who are nervous at the thought of having their breasts examined by a health professional reported more severe feelings of powerlessness. It is troubling to think that information about the good results that can be obtained with early detection and treatment of breast cancer is not reaching women who have regular contact with the formal health care system. Perhaps having more female and Spanish-speaking health care professionals would alleviate this situation, as many of the women in our sample expressed a preference for female practitioners.

Women in this study who said they might have a mammogram in the future, however, were an optimistic group, as they were more hopeful, less powerless, less likely to engage in denial, and had a longer time perspective in relation to surviving the disease. This is consistent with other research that has found that making a public commitment often increases the likelihood that people will engage in a desired behavior (Sensenig and Cialdini 1984).

Women who said they regularly perform breast self-examination expressed both more turmoil and a longer time perspective than women who did not do BSE. This is because there were really two groups of women: the minority, who perform BSE correctly, and the majority, who do not. Women who performed the procedure correctly did not experience more turmoil and had a longer time perspective, while the obverse was true for those doing the procedure incorrectly.

Women who were less knowledgeable about breast cancer, its signs and symptoms, risks for the disease, and its incidence in the population were significantly more likely to deny that they could get the disease. Thus general knowledge seems to help women be prepared to think about how they would deal with breast cancer. Knowing that there are ways to check for breast cancer (mammography, CBE, BSE) seems to help women to have more positive responses to the possibility of developing the disease. Women who knew about mammography had a longer time perspective and were less apt to deny that they might get breast cancer; women who knew about BSE were more hopeful, less powerless, and had a longer time perspective.

We also asked women how they learned about breast cancer. Many mentioned reading and television; fewer mentioned radio; and fewer still named family, friends, or neighbors as sources of information. Those women experiencing more cues from the environment to engage in breast cancer screening felt significantly more hopeful and more powerful about dealing with the disease and took a longer time perspective in relation to it than women who had not had such cues.

Lack of health insurance and inability to pay for care were the two most often cited socioeconomic barriers to obtaining mammograms. One third of the Mexican-American women in our sample between the ages of fifty and sixty-four had no health insurance at all. This is compounded by Mexican-American women's lower average household and per-capita incomes, so they are less likely to be able to pay for out-of-pocket expenses for health care not covered by insurance. Uncertainty about the cost of a mammogram was also a deterrent for some women. Fifty-five percent of the women in the study had no idea what a mammogram cost, and their estimates ranged from $5 to $1,000. Other studies have shown that when people must pay or co-pay for health care, they tend to use fewer services; however, even with free care, not all those entitled to care will use it (Lurie 1987).

Interestingly, some women who had not had screening reported that no one in their family had ever discussed it with them; that is, it had not been validated within their social circle. The family is an under-utilized resource for promoting preventive breast cancer screening for older Hispanic women. For example, a woman's siblings or adult children could play a role in convincing her that screening for breast cancer would be good both for her and for the family.

Conclusions

The cost in terms of years of life lost due to cancer is greater for women than men, and the most costly cancer for women is breast cancer. In 1984, 760,000 years of life were lost among the 39,470 women who died of the disease in the United States. If mortality could be reduced by

30 percent through the use of breast cancer screening, early detection, and prompt treatment, 11,800 deaths could be avoided and 227,000 fewer years of life would be lost (Horm and Sondik 1989). Thus breast cancer remains a serious challenge to women's health and quality of life.

Older women in general are not convinced of the benefits of prevention and have only vague notions of the warning signs and risks for breast cancer. In addition, they have erroneous notions about the causes and manifestations of breast cancer which affect their decisions about screening behavior. For most women, breast cancer screening is perceived as risky behavior, because the fear of finding something predominates over the fear of not finding cancer if it is present (Meyerowitz and Chaiken 1987). But prevention remains an important goal for older women, as 50 percent of all cancers occur after age sixty-five, and more women over fifty-five have late-stage diagnosis than do younger women (Welch-McCaffrey and Dodge 1988).

Socioeconomic status remains an important influence on how older women perceive breast cancer. Higher levels of education, income, health insurance, and access to health care reduce feelings of powerlessness, denial, and turmoil. But more research needs to be done on cultural variations in response to breast cancer. According to one study, a typical Hispanic response is shame or repentance, rather than anger (Kagawa-Singer 1987). Yet the absence of hostility or the presence of a stoical or helpless attitude has been associated with shorter survival rates for breast cancer patients (Magarey 1988). While only one respondent in our study said she would get angry if she got breast cancer, many others emphatically indicated that they would fight, resist, or overcome the disease.

Breast cancer represents a threat to both a woman's individual sense of balance (i.e., loss of a breast) and her equilibrium in terms of relationships with significant others. To address this situation, programs must work with existing Hispanic cultural values. As the examples given in this chapter show, however, resourcefulness is as typical a response as resignation to the possibility of breast cancer. Education programs should incorporate such traditional values as respect, *sacrificio*, and *ejemplo* (exemplary behavior) (Solis et al. 1985), but in novel ways. For example, older, well-respected members of the Hispanic community could set an example for middle-aged women by getting breast cancer screening themselves. The embarrassment or indignity of breast cancer screening could be acknowledged as a short-term sacrifice on the woman's part in order to safeguard her health for her family's sake in the long run.

New studies on social networks suggest that education about breast cancer is well received when undertaken in small, kin-based or church-based groups (Eng et al. 1985; Gottlieb 1985; Israel 1985). Another study shows that close social networks that approximate the kinship model can develop among working Hispanic women (Zavella 1985). These networks could provide the basis for a work-based intervention program. Ideally such campaigns would be conducted by older women who have had first-hand experience with breast cancer. It would be imperative to give Hispanic women ample opportunity to work through the illness (interpersonal) aspects of breast cancer, rather than to simply focus on the technical (disease-related) aspects, manifestations, and treatment.

This is supported by our finding that powerlessness, hopelessness, and curtailed time perspective were strongly related in this sample. Giving women the knowledge that they can detect breast cancer, that it can be treated, and that there is life after breast cancer is one important part of the message. This would be the approach to take with the "objective" aspects of the disease. Likewise, denial, turmoil, and abandonment were also closely related. These are the interpersonal, social manifestations of breast cancer as an illness. Thus it is important to pay attention to both the internal and the interpersonal feelings that the possibility of breast cancer arouses, especially in relation to significant others, where it is easier to deny that one will get the disease than to contemplate the perceived disaster it would create in the woman's individual and social life.

In accordance with the familial aspect of health care decision making, women should be urged to have a relative accompany them when they go for breast cancer screening. As a doctor's recommendation is one of the most commonly mentioned reasons for getting a mammogram, it would be important for the doctor to explain to all family members together (rather than just to the woman herself) the importance of preventive screening in preserving the woman's health—for her own sake and for the sake of the family (Kruse and Phillips 1987).

Culturally appropriate cues that prompt Hispanic women to get breast cancer screening are needed in order to break down the barriers of myth, silence, and resignation and to encourage resilience and resourcefulness as acceptable responses to the challenge of conquering breast cancer.

Notes

This study was funded by a grant from the AARP/ANDRUS Foundation.
1. There is very little cross-cultural research on women's knowledge about the signs and symptoms of breast cancer. Our own comparative research (Saint-Germain and Longman, 1990) has demonstrated no significant differences between Hispanic and Anglo women over age 50 on knowledge variables, and the small differences that do occur are explained by level of education and socio-economic class rather than cultural factors.
2. We were unable to find any studies that focused specifically on how Hispanic women would cope with the possibility of breast cancer, as most previous research has been conducted with people who already have cancer.

Works Cited

Clark, Margaret. 1970. *Health in the Mexican-American Culture.* Berkeley: University of California Press.

Cohen, David, Benjamin Littenberg, Cheryl Wetzel, and Duncan Neuhauser. 1982. "Improving Physician Compliance with Preventive Medicine Guidelines." *Medical Care* 20:1040–45.

Cotera, Martha P. 1976. *Diosa y Hembra: The History and Heritage of Chicanas in the U. S.* Austin, Tex.: Information Systems Development.

Crooks, Catherine E., and Steven D. Jones. 1989. "Educating Women about the Importance of Breast Screening: The Nurse's Role." *Cancer Nursing* 12:161–64.

Cubillos, Hermina L., with Margarita M. Prieto. 1987. *The Hispanic Elderly: A Demographic Profile.* Washington, D. C.: National Council of La Raza.

Eng, Eugenia, John Hatch, and Ann Callan. 1985. "Institutionalizing Social Support through the Church and into the Community." *Health Education Quarterly* 12:81–92.

Farley, Thomas A., and John T. Flannery. 1989. "Late-Stage Diagnosis of Breast Cancer in Women of Lower Socio-Economic Status: Public Health Implications." *American Journal of Public Health* 79:1508–12.

Fink, Raymond, Sam Shapiro, and John Lewison. 1968. "The Reluctant Participant in a Breast Cancer Screening Program." *Public Health Reports* 83:479–90.

Fox, Sarah, Dennis Klos, and Carole Tsou. 1988. "Underuse of Screening Mammography by Family Physicians." *Radiology* 166:431–33.

Frunch, Donna P. 1986. "Socioeconomic Status and Survival for Breast and Cervical Cancer." *Women and Health* 11:37–54.

Giachello, Aida L. 1985. "Hispanics and Health Care," pp. 159–94, in Cafferty and McCready, *Hispanics in the United States: A New Social Agenda.* New Brunswick, N. J.: Transaction Books.

Gottlieb, Benjamin H. 1985. "Social Networks and Social Support: An Overview of Research, Practice and Policy Implications." *Health Education Quarterly* 12: 5–22.

Grady, Kathleen, Stephen Kegeles, Adrian Lund, Claudia Wolk, and Niel Farber. 1983. "Who Volunteers for a Breast Self-Examination Program? Evaluating the Bases for Self-Selection." *Health Education Quarterly* 10:74–94.

Horm, John W., and Edward J. Sondik. 1989. "Person-Years of Life Lost Due to Cancer in the United States, 1970 and 1984." *American Journal of Public Health* 79:1490–93.

Israel, Barbara A. 1985. "Social Networks and Social Support: Implications for Natural Helper and Community Level Interventions." *Health Education Quarterly* 12:65–80.

Kagawa-Singer, Marjorie. 1987. "Ethnic Perspectives of Cancer Nursing: Hispanics and Japanese-Americans." *Oncology Nursing Forum* 14:59–65.

Kay, Margarita. 1972. "Health and Illness in the Barrio." A dissertation submitted to the faculty of the department of Anthropology for the Ph.D., University of Arizona.

Keefe, Susan E. 1979. "Urbanization, Acculturation, and Extended Family Ties: Mexican-Americans in Cities." *American Ethnologist* 6:349–65.

Kosko, Debra A., and Jacquelyn H. Flaskerud. 1987. "Mexican-American, Nurse Practitioner, and Lay Control Group Beliefs about Cause and Treatment of Chest Pain." *Nursing Research* 36:226–31.

Kranau, Edgar, Vicki Green, and Gloria Valencia-Weber. 1982. "Acculturation and the Hispanic Woman." *Hispanic Journal of Behavioral Sciences* 4:21–40.

Kruse, Jerry, and Debra M. Phillips. 1987. "Factors Influencing Women's Decision to Undergo Mammography." *Obstetrics and Gynecology* 70:744–48.

Lee, Isaiah C. 1976. *Medical Care in a Mexican-American Community.* Los Alamitos, Calif.: Hwong Publishing.

Lindburg, Kristina, and Carlos J. Ovando. 1977. *Five Mexican-American Women in Transition: A Case Study of Migrants in the Midwest.* San Francisco: R & E Research Associates.

Lurie, N., et al. 1987. "Preventive Care: Do We Practice What We Preach?" *American Journal of Public Health* 77:801–04.

Magarey, Christopher J. 1988. "Aspects of the Psychological Management of Breast Cancer." *Medical Journal of Australia* 148:239–42.

Markides, Kyriakos S., Joanne S. Boldt, and Laura A. Ray. 1986. "Sources of Helping and Intergenerational Solidarity: A Three-Generation Study of Mexican-Americans." *Journal of Gerontology* 41:506–11.

Marks, Gary, Julia Solis, Jean L. Richardson, Linda M. Collins, Lourdes Birba, and John C. Hisserich. 1987. "Health Behaviors of Elderly Hispanic Women: Does Cultural Assimilation Make a Difference?" *American Journal of Public Health* 77:1315–19.

Meyerowitz, Beth E., and Shelly Chaiken. 1987. "The Effect of Message Framing on Breast Self-Examination Attitudes, Intentions, and Behavior." *Journal of Personality and Psychology* 52:500–10.

Moustafa, A. Taher, and Gertrude Weiss. 1968. *Health Status and Practices of Mexican-Americans.* Los Angeles: University of California Press.

Newell, Guy R., and Paul K. Mills. 1986. "Low Cancer Rates in Hispanic Women Related to Social and Economic Factors." *Women and Health* 11:23–36.

Richardson, Jean, Gary Marks, Julia Solis, Linda Collins, Lourdes Birba, and John Hisserich. 1987. "Frequency and Adequacy of Breast Cancer Screening among Elderly Hispanic Women." *Preventive Medicine* 16:761–74.

Rimer, Barbara, Sharon Davis, Paul Engstrom, Ronald Myers, Jay Rosan, Laurie Fox, and Robert McLaughlin. In press. "An Examination of Compliance and Noncompliance in an HMO Cancer Screening Program," in *Advances in Cancer Control V: Cancer Program Product Line Management.*

Rose, Linda C. 1978. *Disease Beliefs in Mexican-American Communities.* San Francisco: R & E Research Associates.

Saint-Germain, M. A., and Alice J. Longman. 1990. "Older Women and Preventive Health Care: Final Report." Submitted to the AARP/Andrus Foundation, February 28.

Sensenig, P. E. and R. B. Cialdini. 1984. "Social Psychological Influences on the Compliance Process: Implications for Behavioral Health." In J. Matarazzo, N. Miller, S. M. Weiss, and J. A. Herd, eds., *Behavioral Health: A Handbook of Health Enhancement and Disease Prevention*, pp. 384–92. New York: Wiley.

Solis, Julie, Jean Richardson, John C. Hisserich, Fernando Torres-Gil, Gary Marks, Lourdes Birba, and Norma Alicia Pino. 1985. "Cancer Screening Behavior among Elderly Hispanic Women." Keynote address at the Second International Conference on Cancer and Hispanics, Nogales, Arizona, November 21–22.

Taplin, Stephen, Carolyn Anderman, and Louis Grothaus. 1989. "Breast Cancer Risk and Participation in Mammographic Screening." *American Journal of Public Health* 79:1494–98.

Texidor del Portillo, Carlota. 1987. "Poverty, Self-Concept, and Health: Experience of Latinas." *Women and Health* 12:229–42.

Weissman, Avery D. 1979. *Coping with Cancer.* New York: McGraw-Hill.

Welch-McCaffrey, Deborah, and Jan Dodge. 1988. "Planning Breast Self-Examination Programs for Elderly Women." *Oncology Nursing Forum* 15:811–14.

Zavella, Patricia. 1985. "Abnormal Intimacy: The Varying Work Networks of Chicana Cannery Workers." *Feminist Studies* 11:541–57.

Cancer in the Family

LOIS LYLES

Waiting for New Year's: The Hospital

"Lois, I guess you'd better not look at this," my mother says. Humped over and sitting on the edge of the hospital bed, she begins unbuttoning her pajama top. The nurse is already drawing the green, floor-length curtain that makes a cubicle of the area around each bed in the double-occupancy room. Now the bed next to my mother's is temporarily vacant, so she has the luxury of sleep undisturbed by the groaning of the miserably ill women who, on various occasions during my mother's stay, have been bedded in the room.

"All right," I agree. I swing the massive wooden door shut, and leave the nurse alone with my mother to begin the examination of my mother's chest. Standing at the picture window at the corridor's end, I let the sun's rays burnish my face. The corridor is sticky with the caramel tones of high-volume Spanish. I turn and see, for the first time, the inhabitant of the room which has a pink "Special Precautions" warning placard protruding from its doorway. At the comfortable distance of six feet, the patient is chatting with his guard. The AIDS victim is young—no older than twenty-five, surely. He wears five-and-dime slippers of brown corduroy, and his slight body is clothed in pajamas too thin for December. In a lemon-yellow face, brown eyes and cherry lips move with animation as he speaks. I wonder at his apparent vitality, at his so terribly menaced youth, and at the fierce voracity

273

of the disease which will snap up his life—more quickly, perhaps, than my mother's illness will consume hers.

Several mornings later, as my mother is dressing herself in preparation for her discharge from the hospital, I speak with a nurse outside my mother's room.

"Is there any special care my mother will require once she is home?"

The nurse gazes at me questioningly, pityingly. "No. One of Mrs. Lyles' main difficulties is coming to terms with her illness. For example, I tried to get her to look at the mastectomy scar in the mirror while I was with her, and she refused."

What can I do but nod? How does one "come to terms" with the loss of a part of one's body? How does one "come to terms" with the loss, creeping closer and closer, of one's life?

Cousin David is with Dad and me this New Year's Day, helping to pack Mama's things so that she can be brought home. The checkout time was to be eleven a.m., but because I had misunderstood this and had not gotten Mama dressed on time, we are late. Dad is bullying Mom and the nurse about the difficulty of finding a pharmacy open to fill Mom's prescriptions on a holiday; about her unreadiness to leave; about everything. He is a tall, husky man barking at a trembling, shrunken rag of a woman. Standing, he leans over her and shouts at her bowed head as she sits wearily on the hospital bed.

Dad and David load the steel hospital trolley with Mama's belongings, and the two men are off down the hall. Mama tells me she needs her glasses, stockings. I run down the hall and tell Dad.

"Your mother is crazy," he declares. "She's got everything she needs."

"You're rushing her!" My head is blazing.

He retorts that she is off her head. Then he shambles off with the triple-shelved trolley, packed with cardboard boxes of pajamas, underwear, toiletries; with the greeting cards and potted plants of well-wishers.

"Stop, let me look just a minute!"

On the middle shelf, I find her glasses, shoved in a corner beneath a piece of embroidery tightened over a small hoop. Next my hands dive into a blue nylon duffel bag and rescue her balled-up stockings.

Back in her room, I help her finish dressing. Her legs, eased with painful slowness into the stockings, are shriveled tan sticks. An orderly comes, helps her into a wheelchair. He rolls her slowly into the corridor and down the hall.

Now missing is the pink sign that has flagged the door on the right-hand side of the hall, not far from my mother's room. "Precautions Warranted in Handling Blood and Body Fluids," the sign had read. The young Latino AIDS victim, whose room has been guarded by blue-uniformed men, is gone—where?

I walk a few paces behind my mother. Her pigeon-like, hump-shouldered, wasted body is garbed in a cardinal-red coat, which is new, and of plush wool. A cheap white knitted cap covers her head. Her clothing combines a main theme of jaunty, coruscatingly vivid color with pallid off-notes suggesting poverty and defeat. She is a picture which seems to corrade all my senses. Midway down the hall, in the room occupied by two middle-aged black men, a radio belts out the blues.

New Year's Night: The House

Sound the alarm! Raise the windows high—our screams should rocket into the silent night. Let the hue and cry tear like wildfire through the streets where Christmas lights still festoon the houses, warmly painting the dark. Get the neighbors up from their peaceful beds. Cry what I cry—come by here, somebody! Why should we, as though disgraced, keep our hands over our mouths, conceal my mother's suffering and our grief, tell friends and neighbors all is well? Why should we lock our doors, and keep still within, while we burn alive from this invisible conflagration? Help! Cancer! Cancer! Cancer!

Eating

And what will the cancer have to eat, of my mother's sparrow body? My mother is so little, five feet five, flesh dwindling before our eyes; ninety, it looks like she weighs—what will the cancer have to eat? Her feet, size six and a half; give my shoes to the Goodwill, she says, nobody but Jean got feet little as mine, and Jean's so glamorous, she'd never wear 'em.

Mama's face is gaunt and her eyes are huge and frightened—brown squirrel eyes. The only big thing on her is her hips. When she is bedridden, I look at her hips and think, *I came from there.* We have the same shape, she and I: small-breasted, big-hipped. She is so little, haggard, and frightened; what will the cancer have to eat?

Cancer eats us all. Dad cooks cheeseburgers with a crisp bacon garnish one night. The cold meat sits out after the meal, a white grease congealing on each patty. The meat is left on the kitchen counter two days. There is little time to cook, and to monitor the storage of food. I ask Mama if the hamburgers are safe to eat, if Ahmed can have them for dinner on the third day. She always knew such things, I could always ask. Who will I have to ask after she is gone?

She says yes, let him have one. With misgivings, I feed it to my son, twelve-year-old Ahmed; there is nothing else for supper. Early the next morning I hear him vomiting behind the closed bathroom door.

When the ambulance comes the first time the pork chops for dinner are thawing on the kitchen counter. No time to put them away. When it comes down to cooking them, hours and hours later, after the crisis (the stroke Mama suffered), I am scared the meat is spoiled.

Dad stops at the Burger King when we are on the way back from the emergency room, Mama wrapped up in a white blanket on the front seat. At the house, I put Mama to bed while Ahmed and Dad sit in the kitchen, eating burgers and fries. I don't eat. Ahmed soon stops eating and goes to bed. I whisper to him in the dark of his room: "What's wrong?" He says the night in the emergency ward waiting room put him off his food.

Sometimes, at night, from my own bedroom (across the hall from Ahmed's), I hear peculiar sounds, human, coming from the darkened room of the child.

Sleep

Cancer hath murdered sleep. I wake three or four times per night, remembering there is no reason I should arise the next day to another dawn of grief.

Cancer hath murdered sleep. Mama is plagued by insomnia. And even if she were not, her sleep would be destroyed—at her physician's orders. Even if she is asleep at midnight, or at two a.m., or at five a.m., or at ten a.m., I must wake her—not for just one medication at each of these times, but sometimes for two, three, or four pills. The hard, round, shiny pill (Slow-K) is my particular enemy; it sticks in her throat. When I try to stab its shell with a fork, to shatter it into manageable fragments, it dances around its nest, a china saucer. Ampicillin, a white gritty substance encased in a gelatinous red capsule which easily breaks apart, is more friendly. But there are others, some of which must be taken with food; and it is an additional agony for her to eat a cracker, or to drink a glass of milk, at one of the wolf hours. After her second stroke, I must try to mash the pills and get her to lick the crumbs of medicine from my fingers.

When she cries at being awakened, I (and sometimes Ahmed, who is always concerned, always ready to enter the room and help) tell her firmly, "Do your job. Take your pills." My heart blisters as I deliver this instruction. Sometimes she moans, "I'm so tired. I just want to rest, forever."

Scar Tissue

Tap, tap, tap. Lightly my knuckles meet the smooth blond wood of the door to the master bedroom.

"Mom, the nurse is here." I make my voice soft.

"All right, Lois. Come in."

I enter, followed by the heavy-set, ebony-skinned nurse. "Mom, this is the visiting nurse, Mrs. Hutchins."

"Call me Elizabeth, please." She smiles, opening her large mouth wide and showing the gap between her front teeth. Did the gap-toothed Wife of Bath look this robust, friendly, hearty? I hope so.

My mother smiles back from her perch at the head of the bed. She is sitting up, ready, involved.

"I want to check the scar on your breast to see that the flesh is healing properly and the sutures are intact," Elizabeth says.

"Lois, perhaps you had better go out while she does this," my mother says. I note the "perhaps," the question in her tone. I am guessing that she wants me to look, to know, to accept. To accept her.

"Mama, I don't have to leave, unless you are certain you want me to," I maintain. I put my hands on my hips and stand at the foot of the bed, facing her.

"All right. Stay." She nods, and begins unbuttoning her out-of-style polyester knit shirt with garish ribbons of chartreuse and neon orange twirling across a solid black background.

Shirt and brassiere fall to the bedspread, and I am seeing. A raw wind batters the inside of my chest and threatens to stop my breath. But I try to make my voice low and calm when I speak. With the nurse, I look, I point. Elizabeth says, "Healing nicely. Look—no pus, no bleeding, no infection. Those are the danger signs to watch out for."

"Yes, the tissue looks clean and healthy," I say. I nearly gag on the last word. Healthy? My mother is dying!

I wanted to say something positive, to help her. Something positive, to strike down in myself, the fright that rose like nausea to the throat, at the sight of that scar.

It is a good scar. No traces of infection. But what a mutilation! Not the loss of the breast, merely. At her age, when the breast has lost its apple-like roundness, its suppleness and firmness, it is no longer a symbol of beauty and eroticism, anyway. (I suppose not—not being a woman of sixty, how would I know? And who is to say what makes a body beautiful?) My mother's remaining breast is an elongated, soft cone, not a globe. And with the removal of the other breast, something more than beauty, however it might be defined, has been cut away. Maybe the loss has been of self-respect. When she was a girl, she was unquestionably beautiful. In middle age, she still carried beauty—the idea of beauty—about her eyes and mouth, like a flame—and her body at least was whole. But *now. . . .*

Much of the muscle near the armpit has been excised, so that a crater, in shape and texture, lies where her breast was. Instead of the smooth, parchment-colored skin which is properly hers, she must view a brown, waffled crust, edged all around by tiny black threads. She is held together with the kind of stitch which she, who taught me sewing when I was about age ten, would have called "over and under."

Nurse Elizabeth examines the skin graft on my mother's right thigh. The thigh scar is not yet actually a scar. The plastic surgeon took a patch of skin about ten inches long by six wide to cover the hole left by the missing breast. Now the graft, a raw, furious pink, gleams under its clear plastic dressing.

I am pleased that my mother seems cheered by my calm, objective appraisal of the results of her surgery. But I am quivering inside, with an ague I cannot still, as I look at her and think, *She has been a soldier in some dubious battle.*

My mother had a lump in her breast for over a year and told nobody until the lump was the size of a tennis ball and the pain became unbearable. She was reared during the Depression, when maladies of all kinds went untreated because sick people had no money to pay the doctor. Her life has been a long struggle to amass enough money to enable her family to live with dignity. Her general rule has been: Don't waste money on doctors. If you are sick, try to bear up and last the sickness out.

Recently I asked Mama, "Why didn't you tell a doctor about the lump in your breast?"

She replied, crying, "I thought it would go away!"

Nurse is winding up. "Mrs. Lyles, you got your wig yet?" she kindly asks. "You know when the radiation treatments begin, your hair's gonna fall out. Plus, the chemotherapy will often make you very sick, just like the radiation. There is a nausea medication you can get in suppository form. You will need that because sometimes you will not feel like eating, and other times you will not be able to keep anything in your stomach."

I cringe inside. What was it Dad said? *Minnie's got a long, hard road to travel, and she knows it.*

The nurse folds her hands as she stands at the foot of the bed, giving more quiet, kind forewarnings to my mother, who now buttons her blouse.

"You will have good and bad days. Sometimes you'll feel O. K. Other days you'll be so low you want to cry all the time. If you want to cry, cry. But remember, I'll want to see you smile, sometimes, too. I can't take too much of that crying." Elizabeth grins, and my mother grins back.

Elizabeth and I walk toward the kitchen, just down the hall from the master bedroom. She tells me, "One thing to remember about the cancer patient is the importance of attitude. Your mother will get depressed at times, but try to encourage her to have hope. After all, who knows? There may be a cure."

I nod, definitely in agreement about the importance of hope; nevertheless, I feel glum about where to look for it. What cure could fly here in time to save Mama?

"Respect is important, too. Always listen to the patient and respect her needs."

I nod vigorously.

A woman's face, sporting glasses, pops around the corner of the doorway to the kitchen. The woman is middle-aged and elegantly coiffed; her hair is short, tightly-curled, and of an improbable shade of brown not much darker than that of her light, reddish-brown complexion.

"Lois?" she says, in a high-pitched, florid voice. Seeing my amazed stare as she enters the kitchen, she gives my name the inflection of a question, rather than a greeting.

"Yes?" I ask coldly.

"Don't you know who I am?"

I shake my head. Who is this? And upstairs, too, where Mama is expecting nobody!

"I'm *Norma*!" she remarks emphatically, as though there is no reason I should not know; no reason anybody alive should not know.

"Oh." My voice, dull, offers no welcome.

It is a cousin, on my father's side—second cousin? third? I cannot recall. In any other circumstances I gladly would have thrown her the "long time no see" bit; would have exchanged familial inquiries and traditional courtesies with her. But now, all courtesy is blotted out by the question mounting large in my head: Why did he let her come up here? Mama doesn't want anybody to know she has cancer! My nerves are on fire.

"Perhaps you'd better go back downstairs awhile,"' I tell Norma, as I unceremoniously grasp her forearm and propel her toward the stairs. Over my shoulder I tell the nurse, "Let's talk again next time you come. I'll see you out. Thanks for your help."

Elizabeth smiles. The three of us go downstairs and I let the nurse out. Norma, looking befuddled, sits down on the couch adjacent to Dad's recliner. As soon as the nurse is gone I turn on Dad. His feet are on a level with his head as he lies back in the chair, but when I start screaming, the thick carpet sounds the thump! of his stockinged feet as he sits upright.

"So Norma is here, is she? Why did you send her upstairs? You knew the nurse was up there, looking at Mom! Don't you have any respect? You know how sick she is! Why would you do that?"

He gapes, then leaps to his feet.

"What's happening up there? Has she had a relapse, to make you carry on like this? Norma, something terrible must've happened to Minnie, to send Lois off."

"Oh, no!" With my index finger, I stab at him repeatedly. "Nothing terrible's happened, and I haven't gone off. But I'll tell you one thing. And I'm a tell it right here, in front of your kin. I'm a tell you 'bout yourself." I am panting with the rage that has flamed up in me from my entrails to my head and that has brought me a terrific release from the fear of him I have known practically my whole life. I am about to do what, in our family, is unforgivable—put the family business in the street.

"You're a terrible person!" I shout. "You don't respect Mama, and you never have. I hate your guts!" My final shout carries me out of the livingroom, back up the stairs, and into my mother's room.

"You know what he did? Norma was up here, on her way back into your room! And the nurse not even gone yet! I am so angry!" Waves of blood assault my brain. My breathing comes fast, fast, fast. "I've never been so angry in my life." Pant, pant, pant. "I told him, too! I said I hated his guts!"

"Lois, Lois." My mother lies back on the bed. Her voice is low: soothing and reproachful simultaneously. "You told him that?"

"Yeah, I told him. And I needed to have told him a long time ago." My stomach feels hot, but my head feels light and free.

I have spoken my mind to him at last. My mother is going, and with her the standard of conduct that has kept a vise on my lips. If she is going to die, I need not try to act quiet, tame, and ladylike any more; I need not try to keep peace in the family for her sake any longer. I need not be afraid of my father any longer, as she has been afraid, and has taught me to be afraid, of the man who for decades has raged and bullied us all into silence. I am miserable at my mother's dying, but fiercely content at the realization that with that terrible event, my deepest self has begun to be born.

PART 5

COMMUNITY ACTION AND PUBLIC HEALTH POLICY

Introduction

The final section of this collection focuses on four interlocking issues affected by federal and institutional health policy: rape and domestic violence, reproductive rights, substance abuse, and sexually transmitted disease.

Community activists and social workers Beth E. Richie and Valli Kanuha address the issue of violence against women as more than individualized acts by perpetrators against victims. They examine the demeaning attitudes about race and women that have shaped institutional responses to victims of domestic violence, and they posit that battered women suffer a two-tiered process of abuse: first from the person who physically hurts them, and second from the agencies to which they turn for help. They explore women of color's own attitudes toward violence, including priorities of racial and family loyalty and the acute awareness of racist discrimination that may face a batterer of color who is turned over to white authorities. Fear of criminalizing the behavior of a significant other makes it more likely that battered women will report incidents to a health care professional rather than to the police. The response of those health professionals is thus crucial to the well-being of abused women, yet studies show that few offer intervention, counseling, or safety information to women who present evidence of abuse. Richie and Kanuha offer composite examples from case studies of women of color's experiences in the health care system. They conclude that community-based crisis intervention services provided by other women of color are essential

281

to changing conditions of hopelessness and unresponsiveness. They cite the success of grassroots, women-centered programs already in existence and recommend new publications by women of color on the issues of violence.

Continuing the theme of the attitudes of providers in health care institutions and of women of color who decide whether or not to use existing health care centers, Katherine Fennelly examines barriers to birth control use among urban Hispanic (primarily Dominican and Puerto Rican) teenagers in New York City.

Among Hispanic and African-American young girls, there is much value placed upon motherhood as a signifier of adult womanhood and upon the value of children and the important role childbearing can have in insuring the continuity of communities of color. Hispanic and African-American young women are less likely to engage in sexual activity as adolescents than young white women, but they are more likely to become pregnant because of the lack of use of contraception. There is general naivete among teenagers about sexuality, sexually transmitted diseases, and the realities of raising children; there are also expectations that one's own mother or other older family members will help care for a new grandchild. Religious as well as community values honor motherhood while rejecting the use of contraception. Young people feel alienated and search for connection and feelings of self-worth. Mass media exalt sex while political and religious authorities place taboos upon its discussion and upon the abilities of health care providers to present a full range of service options to pregnant women. In these circumstances rates of teenage pregnancy have increased significantly among all racial and ethnic groups. There is evidence, however, that birth rates among African-American teenagers have begun declining.

About one-quarter of all children of color are born to teenage mothers. As Faye Wattleton has often pointed out in her speeches as head of Planned Parenthood, the problems of poverty faced by women of color, wherein approximately half of children of color live impoverished, are perpetuated and further complicated by the high rate of teenage maternity. Poverty in turn limits women of color's options with regard to reproduction. Recent federal policies limiting the application of federal funds to provision of abortion services—or other kinds of reproductive services provided by clinics that also conduct abortions—effectively limit women without private financing or personal physicians from exercising the option of legally terminating their pregnancies. These changes disproportionately affect women of color, who are least likely to possess private financial means.

Using a research model that began with the question of why Hispanic teenagers do not utilize birth control services available to them (rather than asking, as Richie and Kanuha do, what structural and attitudinal limitations institutions and health care providers exhibit that prevent them from providing quality care to clients of color), Katherine Fennelly studied data from surveys conducted with authorities who work with Hispanic teenagers in a variety of settings. The questionnaires asked these persons about the motivating factors that would lead some youths to seek and use contraception and others to avoid its use. Fear of exposure to parental and community disapproval, lack of funds, the association of clinics with care for acute illness rather than with preventive services, and the cultural insensitivity and lack of Spanish language skills of providers were among the identified barriers to clinic and contraceptive use. Fennelly also discusses male attitudes toward birth control, notions of manliness, dislike of condoms, and sexual inexperience and embarrassment as deterrents to male use of contraception. Fennelly's respondents emphasized that family support was critical in a teenager's decision to seek clinic care and that young people's lack of knowledge about sexuality was a major factor in teenage pregnancy.

The availability and use of contraception is a key issue not only with regard to women of color's reproductive options, but in their protection from sexually transmitted disease. Issues of naivete about sexuality, the lack of discussion of sex, attitudes that place responsibility for birth control use upon women or limit that use become all the more dire in the context of the AIDS (Acquired Immune Deficiency Syndrome) epidemic.

Until recently, AIDS has been popularly viewed as a disease striking predominately white homosexual males. However, public awareness of the threat to people of color, heterosexuals, drug users, and women has been growing. The sympathetic public reaction to the announcement by basketball superstar Magic Johnson that he is HIV-positive has done a great deal to increase this awareness, particularly among young heterosexual men of color. To use Sonia Sanchez's metaphor of a rapid change of perspective and racial awakening, Magic Johnson's revelation has "cracked the skull" of consciousness about AIDS, broken through old notions of invulnerability and ideas among people of color that AIDS was a problem for someone else. It has also helped some to begin rethinking prior reactions to the disease that were based on homophobic prejudices and to question federal commitment to AIDS care, outreach, and research. Unfortunately, it has yet to focus concern on AIDS as an issue for women. Almost half of the adults identified as infected with the virus worldwide in 1992 were women. The illness is affecting a growing proportion of adolescent girls, and females are biologically more likely than males to contract the virus from heterosexual intercourse with an infected partner.

AIDS is of central importance to people of color. AIDS is killing people of color at much higher rates than whites. The World Health Organization reports that of the ten- to twelve-million adults infected with the disease, the overwhelming majority are in Africa and Asia. In the United States, AIDS is now the number one killer of African-American women in their twenties and thirties. Over half of women who are HIV-positive or who have contracted

AIDS are women of color, and a large percentage of infants born with the AIDS virus are born to women of color.

The dire impact of AIDS on women of color is heightened when one considers that women are also the primary caretakers of the chronically and long-term ill, both within their families and as nurses' aides and nurses in care facilities. Thus the AIDS epidemic strikes women of color as lay and professional providers of care as well as direct victims of the disease. The burden is great, and public health policy grossly inadequate. Little attention has been given to AIDS education, outreach, and treatment for women of color.

Part Five ends with four essays about women of color and AIDS. Women of color are most susceptible to AIDS through intravenous drug use or heterosexual sex with men who are bisexually active or who are intravenous drug users. Diane K. Lewis and Michael C. Clatts both focus on African-American women intravenous drug users, their life experiences, self-perceptions, and attitudes about AIDS. Gloria J. Romero, Lourdes Arguelles, and Anne M. Rivero focus on Latinas' reactions to AIDS, and Mary Romero offers an example of a woman-centered urban intervention program that signals ways in which public health practice can change to more effectively meet the needs of minority women at risk for contracting AIDS.

Lewis, an anthropologist and public health expert who is active in programs to supply services for women at high risk for AIDS, offers profiles selected from in-depth, life-history interviews conducted with twenty-three black women drug users in San Francisco. The women are susceptible to AIDS through needle sharing and unprotected sexual intercourse. Lewis presents case histories of three women, all in their thirties, who began drug use in their teens. Despite their addiction and the risk of AIDS, the women feel that they are in fair to very good health. Lewis suggests that this self-perception of good health may help explain why so few addicted women seek aid from drug treatment programs. Preventive education with regard to sterilization of needles (cleaning with bleach) and changing needle-sharing habits has proven successful in these women's lives. Changes in sexual practices have not been as forthcoming. The women interviewed still engaged in unprotected sexual intercourse, despite knowledge of its risks.

We have seen in other contexts earlier in this volume that many positive aspects of health awareness and care come from the involvement of friends and family members. Lewis supports this view, but shows us that negative health consequences are also relational. Just as other women we have considered were supported in their illnesses or in preventive behavior by their families and friends, so the majority of women interviewed by Lewis were drawn into drug-use networks by people they trusted—family members, friends, or lovers. However, the women all felt that they had at least one family member they could turn to for help if they needed it. Just as other authors in this volume have concluded, Lewis recommends that significant family members be included in treatment strategies and she suggests that the very kind of networking that women engage in to further their drug use can be adapted to help them overcome their addiction.

Like Lewis, Clatts is an anthropologist who has worked with an AIDS intervention program in a major American city. Also like Lewis, he offers us three case studies of female African-American intravenous drug users. Clatts's interviews with women drug users in Harlem show that the women's knowledge of AIDS risks are very high, but that this knowledge does not regularly lead to risk modification behavior. Clatts's essay raises the issues of the prevalence of street prostitution as a way of making a living and the exchange of sex for drugs by women addicts. Like Cummings, Robinson, and Lopez's study in Part One, Clatts's essay emphasizes that the health behavior of many African-American women exists within a nexus of socioeconomic deprivation, homelessness, and memories of racial discrimination, loss, or abuse. Women drug users' lack of action to protect themselves in sexual encounters, despite their fears and preventive knowledge, indicates a sense of fatalism, a paucity of options. Clatts concludes that drug rehabilitation and AIDS awareness programs are unlikely to succeed if they operate in isolation from broader policies designed to provide women with opportunities for equitable employment and decent housing.

In their study of Latinas in Los Angeles County, Romero, Arguelles, and Rivero demonstrate a shared perspective with Lewis and Clatts. They argue, as do Clatts and Lewis, that prevention programs have failed to consider the racial and socioeconomic dynamics of illness and well-being or to incorporate women of color's beliefs or their patterns of reciprocity into prevention campaigns. Like Fennelly, Romero, Arguelles, and Rivero remind readers that the category "Latina" embraces a wide variety of cultural and social backgrounds, and they caution against extrapolating findings from one Latina group and applying them to another. Latinas whose experiences and attitudes are the subject of the Romero, Arguelles, and Rivero study are primarily Chicanas (of Mexican origin) or more recent immigrants from the Caribbean.

Little research has been conducted about Latino/Latina sexuality, an area of understanding that is critical to the formation of effective public health policy with regard to AIDS. Existing studies of Latino sexuality have excluded women; similarly, discussions of Latina sexuality usually focus on heterosexual practices and exclude homosexual ones. Denial of the prevalence of Latino homosexuality or bisexuality is a factor in Latinas' beliefs that they are personally at low risk for HIV infection. The women interviewed stated that they believed they were largely invulnerable to the disease because they assumed primary risk would come through sexual contact with men who had engaged in intravenous drug use. Latinas' feelings of personal remoteness from the AIDS issue testify to the fact that Latina lives are so filled with day-to-day survival issues that risk from AIDS does not carry priority in their minds.

Nevertheless, sexual partners of male intravenous drug users, Latina sex workers, wives or lovers of bisexual men, and women who have difficulty ensuring condom use by a male partner are at high risk. Latinas who do become HIV-positive face rejection and avoidance in their communities because of assumptions of promiscuity or fear of the disease. Additionally, many older Latinas may find themselves caring for an infected young-adult son or daughter. The grief and stress experienced by mothers faced with this kind of caretaking receives little official recognition. Peer support groups for Latinas help facilitate greater knowledge about AIDS, discussion of perhaps unadmitted male bisexuality as a risk factor, and ways to confront domestic violence and issues of communication that make talk of "safe sex" practices seem like wishful thinking.

The final essay on the AIDS issue is Mary Romero's account of the formation of a women's task force that used women's culture techniques to implement street-based preventive behavior among non-drug-using, female, low income, African-American and Latina sexual partners of men who used intravenous drugs. The task force dealt with the difficult issues demonstrated in the experiences of women interviewed in the Clatts and Lewis studies: while outreach to teach the use of bleach to clean needles and other drug paraphernalia had proven readily adaptable, safe sex practices were a much more complicated affair, involving not just the introduction of a relatively value-free physical modification (use bleach, use condoms), but also the modification of deeply entrenched patterns of gender relations, male dominance, and female socioeconomic need. Different outreach methods and sensibilities were clearly needed to address the situations of women at risk through sexual relations with infected male sexual partners.

Romero points out both the limitations and the potential flexibility in the grassroots formation of policy. When the women's task force was planned, local prevention programs already in operation for intravenous drug users were believed to be interchangeably useful either for women or for men. The primary construct of a drug abuser was male and heterosexual. New outreach supposedly designed specifically for women was thus targeted to reach female sexual partners of male drug users. The existence of male sexual partners of drug-using men was not considered, nor were women included in the plan who were themselves drug users or sex workers. Once in the field, the task force members soon discovered these weaknesses in conceptualization and adapted to them.

The community health outreach workers chosen to implement the sexual partners program were African-American or Latina women. Some were lesbians, others heterosexual. Turning away from training based on male-oriented models, these community workers developed their own techniques for organizing their team and beginning outreach to women. A women-only clientele policy was adopted by workers in the sexual partners unit. Workers sought to build bonds with women by recognizing that precedence had to be given to the clients' own ideas of life priorities, including the need for food, housing, and clothing, before a context could be created in which AIDS could be effectively discussed. They helped women by contacting public assistance agencies and by walking them through the assistance system. They rented a room in a hotel where women could gather, find food, relax, and talk. The atmosphere and trust created in this all-female setting was a kind of "homeplace" that opened the door to discussions of sexual behavior and of problems the women faced in practicing safe sex.

Romero's work ends Part Five and the discussion of AIDS on a note of optimism, emphasizing the possibility of changing localized policy to recognize women of color's needs, of implementing new techniques that build from women's own sense of priority and ways of relating to one another, and of making a difference in the level of health risk minority women face in their daily lives.

Battered Women of Color in Public Health Care Systems: Racism, Sexism, and Violence

BETH E. RICHIE AND VALLI KANUHA

Introduction

The problems of rape, battering, and other forms of violence against women have existed throughout history. Only recently have these experiences, traditionally accepted as natural events in the course of women's lives, received significant attention as major social problems (Schechter 1985). For many years there was a tendency for both human service providers and public policy research to focus only on the individual lives of women, children, and men who are damaged or lost due to domestic violence. This narrow focus on individual victims and perpetrators involved in domestic violence rather than on an examination of the role social institutions play in the maintenance of violence against women represents one of the major gaps in our analysis of this pervasive social issue. Paradoxically, the very institutions which have been constructed for the protection and care of the public good—such as the criminal justice system, religious organizations, hospitals, and health care agencies—have long sanctioned disparate and unequal attention to women in society (Lewin and Olesen 1985). Only through a critique of these historically patriarchal and often sexist institutions will we comprehend domestic violence as more than individual acts of violence by perpetrators against victims.

Another equally problematic gap in contemporary analysis and study of violence against women exists with regard to race and ethnicity, i.e., how individual and institutional racism affects the lives of women of color who are battered. With a few notable exceptions, there is very little research on the ways that traditional responses of societal institutions to violence against women are complicated by racism and, therefore, how battered women of color are systematically at a disadvantage when seeking help in most domestic violence situations (Rios 1985). The result is that battered women who are African-American, Latina, Asian/Pacific Islander, East Indian, Native-American, and members of other communities of color are vulnerable to abuse not only from their partners, but from insensitive, ineffective institutions as well.

This chapter will address an important factor which is often ignored in our understanding and analysis of domestic violence. While our increasing knowledge of battered women is usually applied in the context that "all women are vulnerable to male violence," the emphasis of this discussion will be on those differential social, economic, and cultural circumstances that render women of color, in particular, vulnerable to male violence at both individual and institutional levels. In addition, this article will focus specifically on the experiences of battered women of color within the health care system, including hospitals, clinics, and public health agencies. As will be described in later sections, many women of color rely significantly on public health institutions not only for ongoing preventive health care and crisis intervention services, but, more importantly, as a viable access point for other services and institutions, e.g., public welfare, housing assistance, legal advice, and so on. Thus the emphasis of this chapter is on the relationship between health care institutions and battered women of color, although similar critiques could be made about the inadequate response of other public institutions (such as religious organizations or the criminal justice system) to battered women of color. Finally, this essay will discuss some effective strategies and programs which address the unique and complex issues affecting women of color who are battered.

Balancing Our Multiple Loyalties: Special Considerations for Women of Color and Victims of Domestic Violence

In order to understand the special circumstances and tensions experienced by battered women of color it is important to understand the interface of gender inequality, sexism, and racism as they affect women both in their racial/ethnic communities and in society at large. Because of the powerful effects of a violent relationship, many battered women are required, either overtly or covertly, to balance the often conflicting needs and expectations of their batterers, their communities, and the larger society. These conflicting expectations, rules, and loyalties often compromise the strategies which are available to liberate women of color from violent relationships. This discussion will serve as a foundation for examining the compound effects of oppression which many women of color face even prior to entering the health care system for medical treatment of and protection from domestic violence.

Communities of color in this country have historically been devastated by discriminatory and repressive political, social, and economic policies. It is commonplace to associate high infant mortality, school drop-out rates, criminality, drug abuse, and most other indices of social dysfunction with African-American, Latino, Native-American, and other non-European ethnic groups (Perales and Young 1988). Even among the "model minorities," Asians and Pacific Islanders, groups of new immigrants as well as their assimilated relatives have shown increased rates of HIV and AIDS, mental health problems, and other negative co-factors which are in part attributable to their status as non-majority (nonwhite) people in the United States (Chua-Eoan 1990).

Most everyone, from historians to social scientists to politicians, whether conservative or radical, considers racism to be a significant, if not the primary, cause of this disproportionate level of social deterioration among communities of color (Steinberg 1989). While the dynamics of racism have often been studied from a macro-perspective, comparing the effects of race discrimination on particular ethnic groups vis-à-vis society at large, the differential effects of racism on women versus men of color has not been given due attention. In order to adequately understand any analysis of the combined effects of racism, sexism, and battering, a consideration of gender-based tension within communities of men and women of color, separate from and related to the predominant white society, is required.

There are many stereotypes about women of color which affect not only our understanding of them as women, but particularly our analysis of and sensitivity to them with regard to domestic violence. For example, many portrayals of women of color espouse their inherent strengths as historical, matriarchal heads of households (Rudwick and Rudwick 1971). While this stereotype of women of color as super homemakers, responsible family managers, and unselfish nurturers may be undisputed, such attributions do not mean that all (or most) women of color are therefore empowered and supported in their various family roles or have positions of leadership within their ethnic communities. Many women of color with whom we work state that they face the burden either of having to be overly competent and successful or having to avoid the too-often painful reality of becoming "just another one of those horror stories or pitiful statistics on the front page of the newspaper." For women of color who are experiencing domestic violence, the implicit community and societal expectation to be strong and continue to care for themselves and their families results in their denying not only the actual existence of battering in their lives, but the extent and nature of that abuse (Richie 1992). For example, one Korean woman who was repeatedly punched around her head and face by her husband reported that she used cosmetics extensively each day when she went to Mass with her husband, in order to assure protection of her own, as well as her husband's, dignity among their church and neighborhood friends. When she went to work as a typist in a white business, she was especially careful not to disclose evidence of her abuse, in order to protect both herself and her husband from her co-workers' judgments that "there was something wrong with Korean people."

While public policy makers are concerned about the rapidly escalating crime rate in this country, many leaders in cities predominated by communities of color are becoming increasingly concerned about the profile of those convicted for crimes, i.e., young boys and men of color. The predominance of men of color in correctional facilities (close to 90 percent of the penal population in some cities) has polarized everyone, from scholars to community leaders to policy makers. While most mainstream legislators and public health officials are reluctant to discuss it publicly, there is a rising belief that men of color are inherently problematic and socially deviant. More progressive analysts have ascribed criminal behavior among nonwhite males to historically racist social conditions that are reinforced by criminal, legal, and penal systems which disproportionately arrest and convict men of color at least in part because of their skin color (Kurtz 1990).

There are no equally concerned dialogues about how women of color continue to be victims of crime more often than white women and about the disparate treatment they receive from not only racist, but sexist social systems. An African-American woman who works with battered women as a court advocate states unequivocally that battered women of color are usually treated less respectfully by prosecutors and judges than the white women with whom she works. In addition, when this same court advocate has raised this disparity with her African-American brothers and male friends in her community, she is often derided as being "one of those white women's libbers" who has betrayed "her own" by working on a problem like domestic violence, which will further stigmatize and destroy the men of color who are charged with battering. Unfortunately, this dialectic of the comparable oppression of women and men of color has resulted in a troubling silence about the needs of women of color and led to counterproductive discussions between women and men of color about the meaning and significance of domestic violence, specifically, and sexism in general.

For a battered woman of color who experiences violence at the hands of a man of color from her own ethnic group, a complex and troublesome dynamic is established that is both enhanced and compromised by the woman's relationship to her community. She is battered by another member of her ethnic community, whose culture is vulnerable to historical misunderstanding and extinction by society at large. For the battered woman, this means that she may be discriminated against in her attempt to secure services *while at the same time* feeling protective of her batterer, who might also be unjustly treated by such social institutions as the police and the judicial system. Most battered women of color are acutely aware of how the police routinely brutalize men of color, how hospitals and social services discriminate against men of color, and the ways men of color are more readily labeled deviant than white men. In one Midwestern city, anecdotal reports from court and police monitors have shown that men of color awaiting arraignment for domestic violence charges frequently arrive in court with bruises supposedly inflicted by police officers. One Indian woman stated that when she saw her husband in court the morning after a battering incident, he looked just as bad as she did, with black eyes and bruises about his face. Feeling pity for him, she refused to testify, and upon release he told her of being beaten by police while being transported between the jail and the court house. Although the existence of police brutality is unfortunately not a new phenomenon, it is certainly compromised and complicated in the context of domestic violence, *especially* for men and women of color who are seeking help from this already devastating problem. For battered women of color, seeking help for the abuse they are experiencing always requires a tenuous balance between care for and loyalty to themselves, their batterers, and their communities.

The situation is further complicated by the fact that communities of color have needed to prioritize the pressing social, economic, and health problems which have historically plagued their people and neighborhoods. Because of sexism, the particular concerns of women typically do not emerge at the top of the list. The values of family stability, community self-determination, and protection of one's racial and ethnic culture are often seen as incompatible with addressing the needs of battered women within communities of color. Most of us who have worked in the domestic violence movement are well aware of the gross misconceptions that battering is just a woman's issue or that domestic violence in communities of color is not as serious as other problems. The most dangerous consequence, for battered women of color, however, is that they are often entrapped by these misconceptions and misguided loyalties and thus remain in the confines of violent and abusive households (Richie 1985).

While credit for a broad-based societal response to the problem of violence against women must be given to the feminist movement and its successful grassroots organizing in the mid-1970s, another process of "split loyalties" has emerged, compromising the analysis regarding battered women of color. Those women of color who identify themselves as activists, feminists, and organizers within the battered women's movement often face an additional barrier among their feminist peers when raising issues related to the particular dynamics of domestic violence and race/ethnicity (Hooks 1984). Many white feminists and the organizations they have created become very threatened when women of color, with their concomitant expanded analysis of battering and racism, have moved into leadership roles. Many women of color in the violence against women movement have challenged the long-standing belief of many white feminists that sexism is the primary, if not the only, cause of women's oppression. In a reform movement which has had such a significant impact on the values, behaviors, and subsequent policies regarding women and violence, the reluctance or inability to integrate an understanding of violence against women with other forms of oppression (such as racism, classism, ageism) in addition to sexism has been disappointing (Davis 1985). A more significant concern, though, is the effect of limited analysis on women and children of color who are seeking refuge and safety from both hostile partners and social institutions outside the battered women's movement.

In summary, our understanding of women of color who are battered must be considered against the political, social, and cultural backdrop of their racial and ethnic communities; within the framework of institutional responses that are historically based in racism and other prejudices; and against the background of the feminist agenda, which has been primarily responsible for galvanizing all of the above to address this pervasive social issue. It is in this context that we turn to an examination of the particular influence, concerns, and barriers of the health care system in dealing with battered women of color.

Battered Women of Color: Health Problems and Health Care

Women who are battered are often seriously hurt; their physical and psychological injuries are life-threatening and long-lasting. In one-third of all battering incidents, a weapon is used, and 40 percent result in the need for emergency medical attention (Stark 1977). Research suggests that one-third of all adult female suicide attempts can be associated with battering, and 25 percent of all female homicide victims die at the hands of their husbands or boyfriends (Browne 1987). More women are injured in their homes by their spouses or male partners each year than by accidents or illnesses (FBI 1982).

It is not surprising, therefore, that most battered women report their first attempt to seek help is from a health care institution, even before contacting the police (Stark 1977). This is especially true in communities of color, where police response is likely to be sporadic, at best (Davis 1985). Yet research indicates that of those battered women using the emergency room for acute treatment of injuries related to an abusive incident, only one in ten was identified as battered (McLeer and Amwar 1989). Similar findings have been cited for women using ambulatory care settings. A random sample of women seeking health maintenance visits at neighborhood health clinics revealed that 33 percent were battered women and less than 10 percent received safety information or counseling for domestic violence (Richie 1985). The following story of Yolanda (a pseudonym) illustrates the role of health facilities in the lives of battered women.

> Yolanda is a forty-six-year old who receives primary health care from a neighborhood health clinic. She uses the services of the walk-in clinic two or more times each month, complaining of discomfort, sleeplessness and fatigue. Yolanda never mentions that her boyfriend abuses her, but her clinic visits correspond directly with the pattern of his alcohol binges. The staff of the clinic know about her boyfriend's mistreatment, because he sometimes comes to the clinic drunk and will threaten her if she does not leave with him.

For Yolanda, the clinic symbolizes a safe, public place of refuge. From her experience, she knows it is legitimate to seek assistance when one is sick, and she trusts health authorities to take care of her needs. Health providers lose an important opportunity for intervention when they do not offer assistance to Yolanda, especially since they have clear evidence that her boyfriend is violent toward her. She, in turn, feels that the violence must be hidden and that it is a source of shame, since her health care providers do not acknowledge it or offer to help.

For many battered women of color, the unresponsiveness of most health care institutions is symbolic of the overall reality of social disenfranchisement and deterioration in poor, nonwhite communities across the United States. While lack of quality, affordable housing is a major problem for many people of color, the majority of the homeless are women of color and their children (Perales and Young 1988). The drug epidemic, particularly crack and heroin use, has had a significant impact on violence against women. There is growing anecdotal evidence to suggest that battered women are often forced to use drugs as part of the pattern of their abuse, yet there is a serious lack of treatment programs for women, particularly poor women with children (Chavkin 1990). The spread of HIV and AIDS among many women of color has been compounded by the HIV infection rate among children of HIV-positive mothers. Many women with HIV report that negotiating for safer sex or clean needles is difficult when they are controlled by violent, coercive partners.

With regard to women and the social problems of drugs, homelessness, and AIDS, most public health officials have been quick to label women as the criminals, rather than the victims of a society that is disintegrating before our very eyes. When we add to the above the battering, rape, and psychological abuse of those same women who are homeless, drug addicted, and HIV-positive, it is clear that the health care system can be either a vehicle for assistance or a significant barrier for women who are seeking protection from a myriad of health and social problems.

The experience of Ana illustrates the interrelatedness that can occur between domestic violence, drug use, HIV infection, and the chronic and acute need for health care. Ana's husband was an injection drug user who had battered her severely throughout their ten-year marriage. He had been very ill for a period of months and had tested seropositive for HIV. Ana was already pregnant when her husband was tested, but he insisted that she carry through with the pregnancy. She was battered twice in the four months since she had gotten pregnant, and after one incident she was unable to get out of bed for two days. Her husband Daniel reportedly was concerned about the baby and took her to the emergency room of their local hospital. During the triage interview, the ER (Emergency Room) nurse noticed the tension between Ana and Daniel but was uncomfortable addressing it. The nurse later reported that she did not want to offend them by suggesting that they appeared to be having "marriage problems" because they were Hispanic, and she understood that Hispanics were embarrassed about discussing such matters with health professionals. After being admitted for observation, Ana began to complain of increased pains in her abdomen. After five days in the hospital, Ana hemorrhaged and lost her baby. At that time, she discovered that she had been tested for HIV and was seropositive. She returned home to a distraught and angry husband, who blamed the baby's death on her. She was beaten again and returned to the ER once more.

Ana's case illustrates one of the most troubling examples of the interface between health care and violence against women. With the longstanding lack of adequate and accessible prenatal care for poor women of color, pregnant women of color who are battered are especially vulnerable. Research indicates that 20 percent of all women who are battered experience the first incident during pregnancy (McFarlane 1989). The situation for pregnant battered women is further complicated by the troubling legal trend to hold women accountable for any damage inflicted upon a fetus in utero. If a pregnant woman is battered and the fetus is harmed, she may be criminally liable for not leaving the abusive relationship. Not surprisingly, in most recent "fetal death" cases across the country, the women who are most severely punished are women of color (Pollitt 1990).

As the health care system has labored under increased social and economical stress, specialized programs for women and for certain communities have also been curtailed. For battered women of color this trend has specific and dangerous affects. With a steady increase in immigrants from Central America, South America, and the Caribbean, battered women who do not have legal status in this country are destined to remain invisible and underserved. Because of their undocumented status and other significant barriers, (such as language and cultural differences), many battered women of color are denied assistance by the same organizations established to protect them, e.g., public welfare, legal advocacy, and health clinics (Kanuha 1987). One battered women's program specifically targeted to serve Caribbean women and their children reports that battered women who must use hospital services for their injuries often have to borrow Medicaid cards from other women in order to conceal their undocumented status. Staff from this same program describe the difficulty that one undocumented woman had even getting out of the house, much less to the hospital, as her batterer was rightfully suspicious that reports of his criminal behavior would also jeopardize *his* illegal status.

Most hospital-based crisis intervention programs do not have multi-lingual or multi-cultural staff who are trained in and sensitive to the special issues of women of color. For example, reliance on translators to communicate with non-English speaking women effectively compromises the confidentiality and protection of battered women who are immigrants, from small ethnic communities, or who must use their own family members as translators to describe painful and private incidents of violence in the home. There are numerous stories of women of color receiving insensitive treatment by health care staff who attribute domestic violence to stereotypes such as "I've heard you Latins have hot tempers" or "Asian women are so passive, it really explains why they get beaten by their husbands."

Finally, if a battered woman of color is also a lesbian, differently abled, or from any other group that is already stigmatized, her access to quality care from health providers may be further compromised. One battered lesbian who was an African American described a physician who was continually incredulous about her claims that a "pretty girl like her" would be beaten by her female lover. In fact, she stopped going to the hospital for emergency attention, even though she had no other health insurance, because she was angry at such homophobic treatment and therefore became increasingly reluctant to use the services of that hospital.

As long as health care institutions continue to be the primary, and usually first, access points for battered women of color, we must require them to institute ongoing training, education, and specialized programs, and to hire culturally knowledgeable staff to address the particular needs of this special group of women.

The Response of Women of Color

Despite the philosophical and political contradictions and the practical barriers described in the previous sections, women of color have actively and creatively challenged the discriminatory, institutional practices of health care and crisis intervention services. Against extremely difficult economic, cultural, and political odds, battered women of color and their advocates have initiated a broad-based response to violence against women in communities of color. Aspects of this response will be summarized in the remainder of the chapter.

One of the most significant developments in response to domestic violence in communities of color has been the creation of grassroots crisis intervention services by and for women of color. The majority of these programs have been organized autonomously from white women, privileging the analysis and experience of women of color by assuming the cultural, historical, and linguistic norms of Asian/Pacific Islander, Latin, African-American, Native-American and other nonwhite cultures. Typically located in neighborhoods and communities of color, these programs have a strong emphasis on community organization and public education. While many of these programs struggle for financial support and recognition from mainstream public health agencies and feminist organizations, they endure in great part because they are grounded in a community-based approach to problem solving.

The Violence Intervention Program for Latina women and their children in the community of East Harlem and the Asian Womens' Center in Chinatown are good examples of community-based programs in New York City. Refugee Women In Development (REFWID), in Washington, D. C., has a domestic violence component, as does Arco Iris, a retreat center for Native-American women and other women of color who have experienced violence in Arkansas. In Minnesota, women of color have created a statewide battered women's coalition called Black, Indian, Hispanic and Asian Women In Action (BIHA). In California, California Women Of Color Against Domestic Violence organizes and publishes a newsletter, "Out Loud," and women of color from seven southern states have created The Southeast Women Of Color Task Force Against Domestic Violence. Nationally, the members of the Women Of Color Task Force of the National Coalition Against Domestic Violence have provided national leadership training and technical assistance on the issues of battering and women of color, and their task force has served as a model for the development of programs for battered women of color across the country.

In addition to providing crisis intervention and emergency shelter services to battered women, these community-based programs and statewide coalitions for women of color are involved in raising the issue of battering within other contexts of social justice efforts. Representatives of grassroots battered women's programs are often in leadership roles on such issues as reproductive freedom, immigration policy, lesbian rights, criminal justice reform, homelessness, AIDS policy, and other issues that affect women of color. The National Black Women's Health Project in Atlanta is a good example of this.

Finally, in the past several years there has been a proliferation of literature on violence against women by scholars and activists who are women of color. Seal Press's New Leaf Series published Evelyn C. White's *Chain, Chain Change: For Black Women Dealing With Physical And Emotional Abuse* and Myrna Zambrano's *Mejor Sola Que Mal Acompanada.*

Another good example of analysis by and for battered women of color is a publication by the Center For Domestic And Sexual Violence in Seattle, *The Speaking Profits Us: Violence Against Women Of Color*, a collection of papers edited by Mary Violet Burns. Kitchen Table, Women of Color Press in Albany, New York, has been a leader in publishing writing by women of color, addressing the issue of violence against women in the Freedom Organizing pamphlet series and in many other works (Smith 1985).

By providing direct crisis intervention services, educating communities of color, advocating on broader feminist and social justice issues and publishing culturally relevant resources, Asian/Pacific Islanders, Latinas, Native-Americans, African Americans, Caribbeans, and other women of color have demonstrated a strong commitment to addressing violence against women. Our contributions have significantly enhanced both the conventional research on battered women and the progressive work of the battered women's movement, challenging the accepted analysis that violence against women has equivalent effects on all women. We must continue to develop community-based programs that are culturally relevant and responsive to the complexity of experiences faced by women of color, including inadequate health care, unemployment, homelessness, a failing educational system, and violence. Equally important, we must continue to work within our own cultures to challenge those traditions, assumptions, and values that reinforce male domination and ignore women's needs. In so doing, the struggle to end violence against women of color will include individual liberation as well as social reform. For us, the most compelling motivation for continuing this effort comes from the courage, commitment, and endurance that battered women of color have shown in their personal and collective struggles. On a daily basis they persist in defying the limits that violence, sexism, and racism impose on their lives. Our response must be to let their stories challenge and inspire us—women of color, battered women, white women, and men alike—to work actively to end individual and institutional violence against women.

Note

The women described in this essay are referred to anonymously or by pseudonyms to protect their safety and privacy. Their stories are both composites and individual accounts of women with whom the authors have worked.

Works Cited

Browne, A. 1987. *When Battered Women Kill.* New York: Free Press.

Cazenave, N., and M. Straus. 1979. "Race, Class Network Embeddedness and Family Violence: A Search For Potent Support Systems." *Journal of Comparative Family Studies* 10:281–299.

Chavkin, W. 1990. "Drug Addiction and Pregnancy: Policy Crossroads." *American Journal of Public Health* 80 (4):483–87.

Chua-Eoan, H. 1990. "Strangers in Paradise." *Time* (April). 135:32–35.

Davis, A. 1985. *Violence against Women and the Ongoing Challenge to Racism.* Latham, N. Y.: Kitchen Table Press.

Federal Bureau of Investigation. 1982. *Uniform Crime Reports.* Washington, D. C.: Department of Justice.

Flitcraft, A. 1977. "Battered Women: An Emergency Room Epidemiology with Description of a Clinical Syndrome and Critique of Present Therapeutics." Doctoral Thesis, Yale University School Of Medicine. New Haven: Yale University.

Hooks, B. 1984. *Feminist Theory: From Margin to Center.* Boston: South End Press.

Kanuha, V. 1987. "Sexual Assault in Southeast Asian Communities: Issues in Intervention. *Response* 10:3–4.

Kurtz, H. 1990. "Jail City: Behind Bars with New York's 20,000 Inmates." *New York Magazine.* April 23, 1990.

Lewin, E., and F. Olesen, eds. 1985. *Women, Health and Healing: Towards a New Perspective.* New York: Travistock Publications.

McFarlane, J. 1989. "Battering During Pregnancy: Tip of an Iceberg Revealed." *Women And Health* 15 (3):69–84.

McLeer, S., and R. Amwar. 1989. "A Study of Battered Women Presenting in an Emergency Department." *American Journal of Public Health.* 79 (1):65–66.

Perales, C., and L. Young, eds. 1988. *Too Little Too Late: Dealing with the Health Needs of Women in Poverty.* New York: Harrington Press.

Pollitt, K. 1990. "A New Assault on Feminism." *Nation.* 250:409–11.

Richie, B. 1985. "Battered Black Women: A Challenge for the Black Community." *Black Scholar,* 16:40–44.

Richie, B. 1992. "An Exploratory Study of the Link between Gender Identity Development, Violence Against Women, and Crime among African-American Battered Women." Ph.D. diss., The Graduate School and University Center, City University of New York.

Rios, E. 1985. "Double Jeopardy: Cultural and Systemic Barriers Faced by the Latina Battered Woman." Unpublished paper presented at the New York Women against Rape Conference, New York.

Rudwick, B., A. Meier, and E. Rudwick, eds. 1971. *Black Matriarchy: Myth or Reality.* Belmont, Calif.: Wadsworth Press.

Schechter, S. 1985. *Women and Male Violence.* Boston: South End Press.

Smith, B., ed. 1985. *Home Girls: A Black Feminist Anthology.* Latham, N. Y.: Kitchen Table Press.

Stark, E., A. Flintcraft and W. Frazier. 1977. "Medicine and Patriarchal Violence: The Social Construction of a 'Private Event.'" *International Journal of Health Services.* 9 (3): 461–94.

Steinberg, S. 1989. *The Ethnic Myth: Race, Ethnicity, and Class in America.* Boston: Beacon Press.

White, E. 1985. *Chain, Chain Change: For Black Women Dealing with Physical and Emotional Abuse.* Seattle: Seal Press.

Zambrano, M. 1985. *Mejor Sola Que Mal Acompanada: Para la Mujer Golpeada/ For the Latina in an Abusive Relationship.* Seattle: Seal Press.

Barriers to Birth Control Use among Hispanic Teenagers: Providers' Perspectives

KATHERINE FENNELLY

Introduction

Unmarried Hispanic adolescents in the United States are at higher risk for early childbearing than white teenagers, despite their lower rates of premarital sexual activity. Differences in contraceptive use account for this apparent contradiction. A number of studies have shown that Hispanic adolescents are less likely than white or African-American young women to use birth control, whether the measure is current use of contraception (Becerra and Fielder 1985), use at the time of first intercourse (Mosher and Bachrach 1987; Torres and Singh 1986), use of a method before an unintended pregnancy (Henshaw and Silverman 1988), or attendance at family planning clinics (Mosher and Horn 1987). Even when Hispanic teenagers come to clinics, they are more likely than other teens to present for a pregnancy test (Mosher and Horn 1987) and less likely to adopt a birth control method at the first clinic visit (Torres and Singh 1986). These findings suggest the need for research which elucidates possible social, cultural, or institutional obstacles to the use of birth control methods and services on the part of Hispanic youth.

Methods

The purpose of the present study was to identify specific barriers to contraceptive use and family planning clinic utilization among sexually

300

active Hispanic adolescents in New York City. To do this we subcontracted with a survey research organization to have a cadre of trained interviewers conduct face-to-face interviews with persons who work closely with Hispanic teenagers in a variety of settings. The interviews were designed to elicit information about barriers to birth control and clinic use among these teens, as well as the motivating factors that lead some to use contraception and clinic services. Personal interviews were conducted with 205 "youth-serving providers" in Manhattan. The provider interviews were one phase in a study which included focus group interviews with teenagers about the same issues. Those findings have been reported elsewhere (Schwartz and Fennelly 1986; Fennelly 1984).

Our sampling strategy was designed to yield a diverse group of providers who work with Hispanic youth in a wide variety of programs and services. It was thus important to include both reproductive health programs and non-health youth programs. Providers from programs in the former category might be expected to have had a greater opportunity to discuss sexuality and birth control with their clients and, therefore, to be more expert in the subject matter of the interview. On the other hand, clients in reproductive health programs are more likely to be teenagers who have *overcome* barriers to the use of birth control or to the use of services. Therefore, in order to understand what barriers keep teenagers away, it is equally important to interview providers in non-health-related programs.

Eligible programs for the provider sample included any service or program for normal adolescents which served a clientele that was at least one-third Hispanic. The types of programs sampled were as follows:

Reproductive Health Programs:
Family planning/birth control clinics
Abortion clinics
Prenatal care and gynecological services
Private physicians (gynecologists, obstetricians, pediatricians, general practitioners)
Combination family planning/abortion/gynecological prenatal care services

Non-Health Youth Programs:
Public high schools
Parochial high schools
Youth organizations/recreational programs
Multi-service organizations
Hispanic organizations and services
Job/career/vocational programs

The master list of services and organizations from which the samples were drawn was compiled using several social service and community program directories, listings of clinics and churches from the telephone directory, a list of Catholic churches and schools from the Archdiocese of New York, names of physicians from the New York State Medical Society, and listings of public schools from the New York City Board of Education. Of the 785 programs in this master list, 200 were randomly selected for inclusion in the sample: half from the reproductive health category, and half from non-health programs.

One relevant question is the extent to which research findings regarding predominantly Dominican and Puerto Rican teenagers in New York can be generalized to Hispanic youth of other origins and in various parts of the United States. While many persons talk of a common Hispanic culture, in fact, there are dramatic differences among Hispanic immigrant groups in the United States. For example, the fertility of Cuban adult women and adolescents is remarkably low compared to that of other Hispanic groups, or even non-Hispanics. Other marked differences exist among Hispanic groups with regard to racial origin, socioeconomic status, religiosity, and health status. Certainly it would be desirable to replicate a study of barriers to contraceptive use among providers and adolescents in other parts of the country to compare and contrast the conclusions drawn. In the absence of such comparative data, however, this pilot study concerning predominantly Puerto Rican and Dominican youth does serve as an important starting point for an understanding of barriers which may originate in the shared language, religion, and colonial heritage of various Hispanic groups.

Results

Interviews were completed with 205 youth-serving providers. The largest proportion of respondents were counselors in various kinds of programs, followed by guidance counselors, doctors, and teachers. The physicians included general practitioners, gynecologists, and pediatricians who accepted teenage clients; each of these physicians had a practice which was at least one-third Hispanic. Over one-third of the providers were themselves Hispanic, although this was not a criterion for the selection of respondents. Our screening question sought to identify the person or persons in a program who worked "on a regular basis with Hispanic teenagers." Providers varied in the amount of time they spent working directly with teenagers. This may reflect more or less specialized job functions in agencies of varying size. Our sample included an equal mix of small, moderately sized, and large programs, judged on the basis of the number of teenagers served.

Barriers to the Use of Birth Control

When we asked for the "main" reason why sexually active Hispanic teenagers might not use birth control, the largest proportion of providers

(35 percent) mentioned lack of information. This includes general lack of knowledge about sex, anatomy, and the likelihood of pregnancy, as well as ignorance concerning where to go to get birth control, what methods are available, and how they work. Providers frequently mentioned that these matters are not broached in traditional Hispanic families. As one respondent explained: "In the Hispanic population the mothers do not discuss sexual topics with their daughters. They don't talk about development and the possibility of getting pregnant or gynecological matters—hygiene and things like that. They'll gossip about sex, but they won't really talk about it."

The suggestion that ignorance about sexuality is an important barrier to contraceptive use parallels the findings of other studies of U. S. African-American and white teenagers and may be characteristic of youth in general. On the other hand, some respondents felt that sexual naivete and lack of experience in negotiating the institutions of a new culture were especially important barriers for Hispanic teenagers. In the words of another provider:

> [The main barrier is] a lack of knowledge of the services and where they can obtain them. . . . Especially with the Dominican patients, because of their newness in the country. Girls who have been in the country for a long time or have gone through the school system would probably see their hygiene teacher, or have a special class in sex education, or talk to their gym teachers or other people in the school. But the others who are newly arrived don't have those opportunities. And many who have just come from the Dominican Republic don't realize that they can protect themselves.

Cultural and Familial Factors

The second most frequently mentioned category of barriers was what we called "Cultural or Familial Factors." This includes general religious and cultural proscriptions against sex and birth control, parental strictness and chaperoning customs, and family communication about sex.

Many of the responses in this category reflect what has been called the cult of virginity. As one provider describes it: "Hispanic girls are really sheltered in the home—it just would be unheard of to go to a family planning clinic. The daughter remaining a virgin until she's married is very important in Hispanic culture." If virginity is of paramount importance to many Hispanic parents, it is also of concern to their daughters, but frequently not sufficiently to keep them from becoming sexually active.

> Even though the attitude in the U. S. has changed towards virginity and premarital sex, I think that if Latin teenagers were asked if they were going to participate they would probably tend to respond 'no' because they're still somewhat concerned about maintaining virginity. I certainly don't think that they follow through with that. When the situation presents itself, they go ahead and engage in premarital sex, but it's not necessarily done openly,

and cannot be talked about as openly. Hispanic girls that are raised in the U. S. are a step away from that, except if their parents were raised in the Dominican Republic or Puerto Rico.

Somewhat paradoxically, although sexual activity may be proscribed, for some young women there are also pressures to bear a child. One provider commented that the girls she works with do not object to the idea of becoming pregnant. In fact, they seem to welcome the idea. "I think they are proud to have a baby. Often the girls tell me their boyfriend would like to have a baby. I guess it's proof of masculinity or femininity. Also, it's an environment in which it is socially acceptable to have a child if you're not married." Other providers suggest that pregnancy is not only tolerated, it is indirectly encouraged and highly valued in many Hispanic families. "The Hispanic family quite often makes it easy for the girl to become pregnant and have the birth. They'll support the daughter and the mother will take care of the grandchild. There seems to be less stigma to having an (out-of-wedlock) baby than there would be in another cultural group."

Almost a fifth of the providers mentioned a "main" reason for non-use of birth control which we categorized as a "Psychological Factor." A common one is the idea that teenagers don't plan for sex: it just occurs spontaneously. This frequently mentioned barrier is given several different interpretations. Some providers suggest that many teenagers don't plan because they don't really care about the consequences. "I'm not so sure that sex among the younger kids is with forethought. I think it's that they get high and do it. There seems to be a party attitude, laissez-faire, come what may, what happens happens. And I don't even really see that much remorse." Others imply that teenagers enjoy the risk-taking involved in unprotected intercourse. "They know it all. They know they are not going to get pregnant. They still think they can beat the little sperm. I think that's part of their own rebellion—to take chances." A different interpretation is the notion that teenagers don't anticipate sex because they cannot face up to the fact that they are sexually active. "Teenagers deny that they are having sex. Once you go to a clinic, it is very symbolic, especially for the ones who haven't been sexually active for that long. Using birth control means admitting that you are having sex and dealing with it." Other, somewhat less complex, responses in the "Psychological Factors" category include the notion that teenagers are lazy. This inertia, however, may be the result of a lack of self confidence common to many young people. A plausible series of events and fears keeping teenagers from using birth control are described by one particularly perceptive provider:

It's just *hard* to get on a train or a bus. Well, all these crazy thoughts are going through your head. You are getting dressed to go to the clinic for the first time and you're worried about what they might tell you, what you might have, whether you might be pregnant—even if you know you are not pregnant, they might find something wrong with you. That'll scare anybody. And all those thoughts go on in your head, and you're worried, and your boyfriend might not want to come with you to the clinic, and you would have to go there by yourself. And you might be more scared than anything else in the world, and you might just back out.

Each of the remaining categories of barriers mentioned during the provider interviews accounted for 8 percent or less of the "main" barriers to the use of birth control. These include barriers related to confidentiality; the image, use or side effects of particular methods; the desire for pregnancy; embarrassment over discussing or procuring contraceptives; pressure from males or peers not to use birth control; and clinic or logistical barriers. Nevertheless, their importance should not be discounted, since at least one-fifth of the providers spontaneously mentioned each category of barriers at some point during the interview. Of these, the clinic and logistical barriers are of particular interest because of their relevance to policy. They are discussed in detail in the following section.

Barriers to the Use of Family Planning Clinics

We were interested in ascertaining whether there might be barriers to the use of clinic services which would deter young people who might otherwise want to use contraception. In the opinion of the providers, the fear that parents would find out about a clinic visit was the greatest barrier to service utilization.

> The minute teenagers walk into a clinic they're saying they're sexually active or interested in sex—if it's a family planning clinic. If it is a general clinic where there are a lot of different services, they're not embarrassed because they're not making a statement about their sexuality, they're just going to the doctor. The worry that someone you may know will see you at the family planning clinic is *major*. It's the fear of someone outside of the family finding out and going back and telling. It's like "I could never live it down—my mother thinks that I'm an angel and I'll be making her ashamed of me."

Some of the other clinic and logistical barriers may also overlap with the issue of confidentiality. For example, 26 percent of the providers mentioned cost or perceived expense of the clinic visit as a deterrent. In many cases, if the family is covered by Medicaid, the teenager must ask his or her parent for permission to use the card. This poses a problem: "They are afraid it will be reported. They have to figure out a way to ask their mothers for the Medicaid card, and then they have to come up with a reason they want it. They have to account for the time away from home." It is important to note that the cost of services and Medicaid reimbursement requirements pose economic as well as logistical barriers to service. If a young woman decides to seek contraceptive services without the knowledge of her parents, her own ability to pay, rather than her parents' insurance status, facilitates or inhibits a clinic visit. Furthermore, even if services are offered free to minors, some adolescents may still be kept away by the erroneous belief that they will be required to pay or to present their parents' insurance cards.

Distance from the clinics is another logistical barrier with implications for confidentiality. A few providers suggested that proximity to the home was an advantage, but many more suggested that it poses a barrier, because of the possibility of being recognized at the clinic and becoming the subject of *bochinche* or gossip.

> We have a clinic in our neighborhood and most of the people who work in the clinic are from the neighborhood. Therefore, any discretion ends as soon as they go into the clinic. A girl can go into the clinic for just having "problems." Automatically people are saying she's involved or she's pregnant or she's doing something wrong, and the girls don't like it.

As another respondent put it, "virgins don't need to come to a clinic." Even if the adolescent is not seen by an acquaintance in the clinic, she fears that the clinic will inform her parents of the visit. Several providers mentioned that publicity concerning proposed federal regulations to require parental consent had confused many teenagers into believing that this is the law. A young person may also fear that parents will be notified of the visit later vis-a-vis follow-up calls, laboratory results, or requests for payment or Medicaid information. These findings give credence to the fear of many family planning program administrators that mandating parental involvement or consent would lead to an increase in unintended pregnancies among Hispanic teenagers.

For teenagers who have difficulty speaking English, the lack of bilingual clinic staff may also pose a very tangible barrier to the receipt of services. Sometimes this is connected to concerns about cultural insensitivity or racism. As one provider put it: "There are people who don't speak Spanish in many health care systems. There are people who don't understand the culture, and there are people who might have a non-accepting attitude about the moral values of these youngsters."

Motives for Clinic Visits

To approach the issues at hand from a different perspective, we asked providers what motivates some Hispanic teenagers to utilize birth control clinics. The most frequently mentioned motivating factor was support or permission from a teenager's family. Some providers suggested that clinic users differ from non-users in terms of such personal characteristics as achievement orientation or perspective toward assimilation.

> Those are the teens that have specific plans for the future . . . academic or a job. The ones I see who display an interest in birth control usually speak more English and feel more a part of this society as a whole. If a girl is planning to finish high school or get into a career for herself, she'll mention that as a reason why she's not ready to get pregnant. Sometimes it would be a decision that she and her boyfriend have mutually talked about.

Other providers mentioned that teens are often influenced to use birth control by teachers, counselors or other professionals, or girlfriends who encourage them to go to a clinic to get a contraceptive method. A smaller number cited fear of pregnancy or the experience of a pregnancy as motivating factors. "In some instances [what brings them to a clinic] is the first pregnancy at a young age. The shock of being pregnant, having an abortion." Twenty percent of the providers mentioned lack of knowledge regarding clinics and clinic procedures as obstacles for Hispanic young people.

> They don't think of clinics as preventive services. They think of them as a service you go to when you're sick. You don't go to a clinic when you're feeling fine, and so the association with the clinic is not necessarily a positive one. I think you need information before you go to the clinic. See, somebody has to say what the clinic is there for, what's going to happen when you go there.

Another provider suggests that the distrust of clinics in general is rooted in cultural practices: "In most Hispanic families there's a practice of home remedies. Mom would have a remedy for this, a remedy for that. Going to a clinic on the other hand, represents the unknown."

Suspicion of clinics and procedures also overlaps with the obstacles of fear and embarrassment. Young people don't know what will happen during a visit and may be embarrassed to ask. Some of this is fear of the unknown, and some is fear of specific procedures.

> They don't understand what is going to happen. They are afraid of being asked to get undressed and having an internal exam for the first time. They may not be fully prepared for that, they may be very fearful. They have probably been raised with the idea that you are supposed to cover yourself and the whole idea of virginity, and might have a great deal of reluctance to strip or explain what's been going on with their bodies to unknown adult professionals. They have heard stories—from their older sisters, their cousins about the examination and they fear they're going to be injured. They're frightened of the pelvic examination, the blood work: to actually come in the clinic and to have a physical and have blood taken out of their arm. They're frightened of a man examining them.

Barriers to Male Use of Birth Control

Many barriers to the use of birth control are relevant only for females. For that reason, we asked the providers to identify what prevents Hispanic teenage boys from using birth control or wanting their girlfriends to use it. One-fourth of the providers mentioned *machismo* or a macho image as a deterrent to the use of contraception. They feel that it is unmanly to use birth control and that it is the girls' responsibility, since she is the one who gets pregnant. To a certain extent this attitude may be exhibited to cover lack of experience or embarrassment. "The boys just don't feel comfortable, so they leave it to the girls. They assume that the girls know."

> There is a lot of nervousness around sex and that leads to a failure to bring up the topic. For example, the male is afraid to ask the woman if she has protection or to offer to use protection, and she, likewise, doesn't want to mess up the situation. Frequently it's not brought up because it seems as if it might compromise the relationship or the emotion of the moment.

Other providers suggest a more callous attitude on the part of many males.

> The main thing is that they don't get pregnant. And to them it is nothing more than having intercourse and letting the girl worry about the rest. As far as they are concerned, they are satisfied, and there is no more worry for them.
>
> The boys that I've worked with are very young. The oldest are fifteen or sixteen. They seem to have a very macho sense of themselves. Their definitions of roles are very traditional, and they feel that any birth control would be the girls' responsibility.

Negative feelings about condoms also reduce the willingness of adolescent males to assume responsibility for birth control. According to the providers, young Hispanic males don't like to buy condoms and they don't like to use them. They are embarrassed to be seen purchasing condoms and are concerned that condoms may decrease both the spontaneity of sex and their own enjoyment of the act. Some young men also are unsure about how to interrupt love-making long enough to put on a condom without appearing awkward or inexperienced.

Discussion

It is tempting to draw conclusions about the extent to which important barriers identified in this survey are peculiar to Hispanic adolescents or common to teenagers of all ethnic groups. Since the study was a descriptive one, and the providers and teenagers were exclusively discussing barriers for Hispanics, we have only speculated about differences by comparing findings with studies of barriers among non-Hispanic teenagers. We also asked the providers to comment on whether some barriers were especially relevant for

Hispanic teenagers. Sixteen percent of the providers felt that adolescents face common barriers regardless of ethnicity. Some of these persons disliked the implications that there may be different barriers for different ethnic groups. However, the remaining 84 percent felt that special barriers did exist for Hispanic teenagers.

Lack of information about sexual matters appears to be a major barrier to both contraceptive and clinic use among Hispanic teenagers in New York City. The providers suggest that lack of knowledge poses the greatest barrier for young, inexperienced teenagers and for recent immigrants who have not had sex education in school. Of course, this is not a uniquely Hispanic barrier to birth control use, as demonstrated by the finding from other research that a majority of African-American and white teens in the United States cannot identify the time of greatest risk of pregnancy during the menstrual cycle (Zelnik and Kantner 1980).

Related to lack of knowledge is fear of the unknown, particularly as it relates to clinic procedures. Hispanic girls may be particularly reluctant to have pelvic examinations or to be examined by male providers. Coupled with normal adolescent feelings of embarrassment and anxiety over clinic visits are the culturally determined inhibitions regarding internal examinations and open discussions of physiology or sexuality.

Fear of clinic procedures may also be the result of prior negative experiences in the health care system, or it may stem from reports from friends or family members of degrading or impersonal treatment. Attention to these concerns is of paramount importance in family planning programs. Providers need to take a hard look at their failure to attract many sexually active Hispanic teenagers to clinics before the first unwanted pregnancy. Given the lack of bilingual and bicultural staff and educational materials in many institutions, it is not surprising that Hispanic youth stay away. Bringing them in will require the development of "culturally appropriate" services: i.e., those which are in actuality and are perceived to be accessible, confidential, non-judgmental, and affordable, as well as frequented by other Hispanic youth and staffed with Hispanic personnel.

Confidentiality is an important issue in the provision of services to all teenagers. For example, Zabin and Clark (1983) have shown that the perception that a clinic doesn't inform parents is the most important reason for teenagers' choice of a family planning facility. In a separate article, the same authors (1981) demonstrate that the fear that parents will find out about the visit is an important deterrent to earlier visits for almost one-third of teenage clients.

Fear of parental reactions may be of particular importance to Hispanic youth, judging from the results of the provider interviews. The worries that someone they know will see them in a family planning clinic and that personnel in the clinic would tell parents they had been there might better be termed convictions than fears. Providers describe the majority of teenagers as certain that their parents will find out if they go to a birth control clinic. For this reason, many teenagers perceive a visit to a specialized reproductive health clinic as tantamount to public admission that they are having sex. In a local community clinic, the fear that someone they know or who knows their parents will see them there seems very realistic.

Although most adolescents have conflicts and differences of opinions with their parents, many Hispanic families have the additional strain of opposing cultural values. Parents who were raised outside of the mainland United States may adhere to standards of propriety which their U. S.-acculturated children find difficult to accept. Conflicts over chaperoning, restrictions on the social activities of adolescent girls, and parental concern with appearances and what people will think were mentioned by many of the providers. These conflicts take place in the context of a culture which encourages shared commentary on the activities of friends and neighbors. Parents are often particularly concerned about their daughter's reputation if she is seen in the company of boys while unchaperoned by adults or other relatives. In the face of these expectations and restrictions, Hispanic adolescent girls are often terrified that their parents will discover they are sexually active. Ironically, use of birth control is viewed as a more immediate threat to this secret than is the risk of pregnancy.

Another barrier comes from the fact that Hispanic girls typically date boys who are several years older than they. The boys' relative maturity, coupled with a marked double standard, results in strong male influence concerning the use or non-use of contraception. Many of these males reject birth control because it is "not natural," inhibits spontaneity, or because they want to father a child. More frequently the boys are unconcerned with the subject so long as it doesn't interfere with their enjoyment; birth control is considered completely the girls' responsibility.

One barrier to the use of birth control which is notable for its relative absence in interviews with providers is religious or Catholic Church opposition. Although the majority of Hispanic youth are Catholic, religious values were almost always mentioned as relevant to the parents rather than their children. Of those providers who mentioned religion as a barrier to method use, the response was almost always within the context of the parents' religious values. The childrens' values and actions may be very different.

> Ah, church opposition for birth control. I don't think there are many teen-agers that are interested in God. When they come from families that are very church going, that are God-fearing people, they don't take that into consideration. They may have some guilt feelings because of the idea that nice girls don't have sex, but still and all, I don't think the church plays a major role in their feelings about birth control.

Finally, it is important to consider possible biases on the part of the persons interviewed and the policy implications of study findings. Many of the barriers identified by the providers parallel those described by teenagers in an earlier phase of this study (Schwartz and Fennelly 1986; Fennelly 1984). Some of the key informants were health care providers, and as such they may have been blind to service barriers created by their institutions or themselves. The best examples of this can be seen in the comments supporting the idea of fear of clinic services. The providers most often attributed fear of procedures to lack of information, but it may also be the result of prior negative experiences in the health care system. Attention to these concerns is of paramount importance in family planning programs. Providers need to take a hard look at their failure to attract many sexually active Hispanic teenagers to clinics before the first pregnancy. Given the lack of bilingual and bicultural staff and educational materials in many institutions, it is not surprising that Hispanic youth stay away. Bringing them in will require the development of "culturally appropriate" services: those that both are, and are perceived to be, accessible, confidential, non-judgmental, and affordable, staffed with Hispanic personnel, and frequented by other Hispanic youth.

Note

This research was supported by a grant from the W. T. Grant Foundation.

Works Cited

Becerra, R., and E. Fielder. 1985. "Adolescent Attitudes and Behavior." *Institute for Social Science Research Quarterly* 1:4–7.

Fennelly, Katherine. June 1984. Final Report to the W. T. Grant Foundation "A Study of Barriers to Birth Control among Black and Hispanic Teenagers." Columbia University.

Henshaw, Stanley K., and Jane Silverman. 1988. "The Characteristics and Prior Contraceptive Use of U. S. Abortion Patients." *Family Planning Perspectives* 20(4):158–68.

Mosher, William D., and Christine A. Bachrach. 1987. "First Premarital Contraceptive Use: United States 1960–1982." *Studies in Family Planning* 18(2):83–95.

Mosher, William D., and Marjorie C. Horn. 1987. "First Family Planning Visits by Young Women." *Family Planning Perspectives* 20(1):33–40.

Schwartz, Dana, and Katherine Darabi Fennelly. 1986. "Motivations for Adolescents' First Visit to a Family Planning Clinic." *Adolescence* 21(83):535–46.

Torres, A., and S. Singh. 1986. "Contraceptive Practice among Hispanic Adolescents." *Family Planning Perspectives* 18:193.

Zabin, L. S., and S. D. Clark. 1981. "Why the Delay: A Study of Teenage Family Planning Clinic Patients." *Family Planning Perspectives* 13(5):209–17.

———. 1983. "Institutional Factors Affecting Teenagers' Choice and Reasons for Delay in Attending a Family Planning Clinic." *Family Planning Perspectives* 15(1):25–29.

Zelnik, M., and Kantner, J. 1980. "Sexual Activity, Contraceptive Use and Pregnancy among Metropolitan-Area Teenagers." *Family Planning Perspectives* 12:230–37.

Living with the Threat of AIDS: Perceptions of Health and Risk among African-American Women IV Drug Users

DIANE K. LEWIS

Introduction

There have been few studies of African-American women intravenous (IV) drug-users' life experiences and self-perceptions (see Miller 1986; Rosenbaum 1981),[1] and virtually no published research on the impact of the AIDS epidemic on their outlook and behavior. The few ethnographic studies that do exist were conducted before the widespread adoption of cocaine in African-American IV drug-using communities. Moreover, none of the studies considers implications of the women's own understandings for treatment and prevention. This paper reports preliminary findings from an on-going life history study of African-American women heroin and cocaine injectors who are at risk for AIDS through needle sharing and unprotected sex.[2] The purpose of this report is to present the women's attitudes and behavior regarding drugs, health, and risk and to suggest how their experiences might be utilized to design more effective drug treatment and AIDS prevention programs. To better understand the issues involved, particularly why so little is known about African-American women IV drug users, it is necessary to review briefly the lack of knowledge about minority and women IV drug users, in general.

IV Drug Use, Minorities, and Women

There has been little attempt to do research on and prevent drug abuse in African-American and other minority communities, despite the fact

312

that minorities have long been overrepresented among IV drug users (Tucker 1985) and are now disproportionately reflected in IV drug-use-related AIDS cases (Centers for Disease Control 1990). For example, in 1980, African Americans were reportedly 12 percent, and Hispanics 6 percent, of the population, but they were 28 percent and 12 percent, respectively, of those admitted to drug treatment programs nationwide (Tucker 1985). African Americans now constitute almost half and Hispanics almost 30 percent of all heterosexual AIDS cases linked directly to IV drug use (Centers for Disease Control 1990). Surveys of IV drug users in treatment programs similarly suggest that African Americans and Hispanics are significantly more likely than whites to be infected by the AIDS virus (Hahn et al. 1989; Lange et al. 1988).[3] Moreover, for every addict in treatment, there are an estimated seven not in treatment (Mondanaro 1987; Hahn et al. 1989), a ratio that may be even higher for African American and other minority IV drug users, who often do not enroll in treatment programs where information about AIDS and other disease prevention is disseminated (Lewis and Watters 1989; Burks and Johnson 1978). In most parts of the country drug treatment and prevention programs are often administered and staffed by whites. Where minority-centered programs are available, they tend to be underfunded and understaffed (Tucker 1985; Espada 1979).

A similar situation exists with respect to female IV drug users, who are also, by and large, ignored by researchers (Cohen et al. 1989; Bell 1989), even though one-quarter to one-third of all regular drug injectors are women (Hahn et al. 1989; Cohen et al. 1989) and over half of all female AIDS cases are acquired through IV drug use (Centers for Disease Control 1990). Moreover, there is evidence that the AIDS virus is spreading rapidly among female as well as male IV drug users, with the number of HIV-infected female addicts estimated at between 57,000 and 75,000 persons.[4] The few available studies on women drug users indicate important differences between female and male IV drug users in terms of life experiences, attitudes, and self-perceptions; however, few programs are designed to meet the needs of these women (Cohen et al. 1989; Mondanaro 1987), who bear the additional burden of greater stigma and disapproval than men for their drug-using lifestyles.

African-American Women, IV Drug Use, and AIDS

The inattention to minority and women IV drug users and the consequent lack of effective treatment and education programs has had a devastating effect on African American and other minority women who inject drugs. African-American women IV drug users comprise almost three-fifths (58 percent) of all female addicts with AIDS and may number between 33,000 and 43,000 of those who are infected with the AIDS virus.[5] Furthermore, in New York City, AIDS is the leading cause of death for all women aged twenty-five to thirty-four (Bell, 1989). Nationwide, over half of the women with AIDS in this age group are African American (Centers for Disease Control 1990). These figures underscore the consequences of neglect for African-American women at risk for AIDS, the overwhelming majority of whom are IV drug users.

Past neglect is also reflected in pediatric AIDS cases. Fifty-two percent of all children with AIDS are African American and 61 percent of African American pediatric AIDS cases are linked to mothers who either injected drugs or had sex with an IV drug user (Centers for Disease Control 1990). In San Francisco the number of pediatric AIDS cases is still small; however, there, too, the majority of AIDS cases among African-American children are IV drug related. While 75 percent of all white children with AIDS in San Francisco between 1981 and 1990 were infected through blood transfusions, 89 percent of all African-American children with AIDS acquired the virus from an infected mother (City and County of San Francisco, Department of Public Health 1990).

Methods and Background Information

This paper reports on the lives of a group of twenty-three African-American women IV drug users who are part of a study, in progress, investigating the life histories of thirty black and thirty white women drug injectors in San Francisco. Before recruitment to the life history study, the women were participants in a larger, on-going, HIV seroprevalence survey of IV drug users, where they were given an HIV antibody test and interviewed using a structured questionnaire. Women who agree to participate in the life history study undergo a qualitative, in-depth interview, lasting from one-and-a-half to four hours, during which they are asked about their childhood experiences, past and present drug use patterns, sexual attitudes and activities, perceptions of risk, and reasons for compliance/non-compliance with AIDS prevention efforts. The intent of the life history interview is to elicit the women's own understandings of their lives.

The twenty-three African-American women whose life stories have already been collected came from a variety of backgrounds. One-third of their families were supported by welfare or illegal means and the remainder by parents with middle-class or stable working-class jobs. While some women did not graduate from high school, most had either a high school diploma or the GED. One women was a college graduate. The women ranged in age from twenty-seven to forty-six years, with a median age of thirty-four years. Although initial drug use began for many in their early teens, the median age when drugs were first injected was nineteen years. While the women came from diverse backgrounds, common themes are identifiable in their life stories; these focus around recruitment into and dynamics of drug use, the role of fellow addicts and family members in patterns of addiction and risk-taking, and the women's attitudes toward health and risk. A brief review of these common experiences will contextualize the three case studies to be presented below.

Virtually all the women, regardless of their family's socioeconomic status, grew up in predominantly African-American neighborhoods where drug use was pervasive; the women's use of drugs was but one dimension of their relationship with a family member, a boyfriend, or schoolmate(s). While the majority of the residents in these neighborhoods, including immediate family members, were adamantly opposed to drugs, most of the women in this study were drawn into IV drug-using social networks via people they trusted, and initially they viewed the activity as an exciting, "in" thing to do.

For most of the women, drug injecting began with heroin. At the time of the interview, about half still preferred to shoot either heroin or a mixture of heroin and cocaine (speedball). However, the drug of choice was cocaine for one-fourth of the women, and a substantial minority (17 percent) had recently given up shooting altogether in favor of smoking crack-cocaine.[6] Over two-thirds of the women (68 percent) said they had used crack to some extent in the previous year. Injection frequency varied, for both heroin injectors and cocaine injectors, from several times daily to once or twice a month. A number of the women used alcohol or crack-cocaine to supplement their shots. Compared to the white women in the study, a high proportion of the African American women had never been in treatment; over one-third said they had never enrolled in a drug rehabilitation program.

As long-time addicts, many women faced, on a daily basis, the possibility and sometimes reality of withdrawal symptoms and other IV drug-related illnesses. Nevertheless, the overwhelming majority perceived their health to be as good or better than that of others they knew. Virtually all these women were involved in high-risk needle and sexual behavior. Their relationships with men, as well as with other women IV drug users, often played a critical role in their risk-taking behaviors. The women's ties with men ranged from long-time, stable bonds to fragile, transitory ones, and they were characterized by affection and support as well as abuse and exploitation. Ties with women friends also varied, figuring importantly in the lives of a number of the women. While the women's relationships with boyfriends/husbands and girlfriends varied, almost all said they were close to their families and that family ties were important to them. Each woman had at least one family member she felt she could rely on for help if she needed it.

The foregoing themes are illustrated in the following case studies, excerpted from the life history research described above. The case study excerpts present the women's remembrances of significant events in their lives and focus on IV drug-use-related activities and attitudes that put them at high risk for AIDS.

Case Studies

CASE 1. MAVIS[7]

Mavis is an attractive, neatly dressed woman with fresh needle tracks on her neck. She had injected herself with heroin shortly before the interview and sat throughout most of it with her eyes closed, "cruisin'," as she called it. Nevertheless, she was able to give a detailed, articulate account of her life, demonstrating a vivid, near photographic memory of events from her past.

Born thirty-five years ago, Mavis was raised by her parents in a housing project in a low-income, predominantly African-American neighborhood in San Francisco. Her father held two steady jobs to support his family, one in civil service. Her mother was a homemaker. Mavis had a sister seven years older and two brothers closer to her own age. Neither parent drank or took drugs. Her father was the disciplinarian of the family, raising his children the "strict, old fashioned way." She had always felt distant from her father, but was very close to her mother.

When Mavis was eleven, she discovered that her sister, unknown to the rest of the family, smoked marijuana (weed) and injected amphetamine (speed). Her sister gave her weed to insure her silence. During this period, Mavis had a girlfriend, a year older, who resided with relatives in the project. The girlfriend's mother was a heroin dealer who lived nearby and paid the two girls to clean her apartment every week. She provided weed but refused to give them heroin. When Mavis was twelve, her girlfriend suggested they combine resources and buy their own bag of heroin. As Mavis noted, "It seems like everybody in the projects, they was selling something...[also] I used to make this loop [on the way home from school]...and the people would be out there [near the drug store] selling heroin." After the girls bought a bag from one of the street dealers, they found an older male acquaintance who agreed to inject them for a small sum.

Although that first hit of heroin made Mavis violently ill for several days, each time that she threw up the high felt better. Shortly afterwards, she and her girlfriend were walking home from school when they found a large bag of heroin apparently lost on the street. The girls took their find to Mavis's sister, who agreed to inject them if they shared it with her. After finishing that supply, and before they were fully hooked, the two girls next discovered a hidden cache of heroin while cleaning the apartment of the girlfriend's mother. They stole a quantity and again shared it with Mavis's sister. After almost three weeks of daily injecting and a week before she turned thirteen, Mavis was addicted to heroin.

Mavis discovered that her twenty-year-old sister, who obtained drugs primarily through her sexual liaison with a dealer, also turned tricks to support her habit. Her sister instructed Mavis on how to "date" to support her own habit. Mavis's parents were unaware of her activities until she turned fourteen, when she was first arrested for soliciting. After two more arrests, her parents sent her to live with a relative out of state to avoid juvenile detention. A year and a half later, at age sixteen, Mavis returned to San Francisco and promptly started injecting heroin again. She attended high school until the twelfth grade but did not graduate.

Mavis continued dating to support her habit until she was nineteen, when one of her dates asked her to live with him. An alcoholic who did not inject drugs and who had a good job, he kept her off the streets by supplying her with the money to support her habit. Although he was good to her, she grew tired of him and left him when she was twenty-three, shortly after their child was born. For the next few months, she dated to support her habit until she was hospitalized and almost died after injecting heroin cut with strychnine she had bought on the street. After her release from the hospital, one of her dates asked her to move with him to a different state. She agreed, realizing it was too dangerous for her to continue to inject drugs in San Francisco. The two obtained good jobs in the new locale, and Mavis stopped injecting for four years. She eventually married this man and had another child. Her husband, however, was also an alcoholic and extremely jealous. The last two years of their marriage were marred by continuous fighting over his accusations of infidelities. Mavis left him when she was twenty-seven, after learning she was pregnant for the third time. After delivering her child, she moved back to San Francisco and began injecting heroin again. There she met her current boyfriend, another heroin injector, and has been living with him for the past eight years. Recently her boyfriend was hospitalized with a recurring health problem and was forced to stop shooting heroin. He has been on methadone maintenance for the past six months. Unemployed, he receives disability aid (SSI).

Mavis supports herself and her two younger children on welfare payments. Her oldest child, now a teenager, is being raised by her parents, who moved out of the state when her father retired. Mavis supplements her income and supports her drug use primarily through money she receives from five older men, "regulars" she has "dated" for many years. In addition, she has a reciprocal arrangement with an addict girlfriend she shoots heroin with every day. They pool their money to support their habits: if one does not have enough for heroin, the other one usually does.

Mavis recently reduced her heroin usage from four shots daily to between one and three. She rarely injects speedballs and has never smoked crack, explaining her aversion to cocaine by noting she has a heart murmur and has to be careful. Three or four years ago she started drinking alcohol and now drinks a can of beer daily. During her twenty-three years as a heroin addict, Mavis remembers only two periods when she sought help for her addiction: the year she was twenty-nine and went through a series of twenty-one-day methadone detoxification programs, and the past few months, during which she has made additional attempts at detoxification. Since detoxification is not working, she is waiting for a MediCal slot so she can enroll in methadone maintenance.[8]

Mavis had been exposed to considerable risk through her past needle use and her continuing sexual activities. In earlier years she and her childhood girlfriend often frequented "shooting galleries," where older addicts injected them with used, uncleaned needles. Even after Mavis learned to inject herself, at age seventeen, she continued to share needles. In the early 1980s, when she first heard about AIDS, she stopped sharing needles. She recently learned that her childhood girlfriend had AIDS, but she noted they have not been close friends for many years. As she has gotten older, Mavis has reduced the number of men she dates. Nevertheless, she estimates she had sex with at least one hundred different men over the previous five years and admits that her clients do not always wear condoms. Her boyfriend never wears condoms, but she feels certain he has never had sexual contact with anyone carrying the AIDS virus. Despite her heart murmur and her heavy addiction, Mavis feels her health is better than that of most people she knows.

Mavis currently lives with her children and her boyfriend in the home of non-drug-using friends of her parents. She has a fairly stable life centered on her children, from whom she derives great enjoyment. She is actively involved in their lives, taking them on frequent outings and field trips. She also telephones her mother weekly and refers to her as "my best friend." She has no doubt her mother would quickly offer help if she needed it.

CASE 2. ROSEMARY

Rosemary is a slender woman who appears younger than her thirty-two years. She came to the interview looking distracted and wary. She was one of the few women who did not seem to enjoy talking about her life.

The oldest girl of five children, Rosemary was born on the East Coast and moved to the housing projects in San Francisco with her mother and grandmother when she was small. She was raised until age nine by her mother, with whom she never got along. Her mother, who drank too much, never married and supported the family through welfare payments. According to Rosemary, her mother favored the other children and gave her undeserved corporal punishment. In retaliation, Rosemary disobeyed and was always in trouble. When she was nine she got drunk on liquor left over from one of her mother's parties and was severely beaten. Her mother threatened to send her to Juvenile Hall, but her grandmother intervened and took Rosemary to live with her. She has a very close relationship with her grandmother, whom she calls her mother.

At age thirteen, Rosemary began to smoke weed with her friends. Three years later she met the man, a few years older than she, who later became her husband. At seventeen, she had the first of five children by him, and when she was twenty-three they were legally married. Rosemary went to the twelfth grade, but did not graduate from high school. When she was eighteen, her boyfriend's older sister introduced both of them to heroin. "I wanted to find out what it was about, and I went right along wid 'em." Rosemary and her husband have been regular heroin injectors since that time. When Rosemary was thirty, the authorities took her children away, after her sister reported she was a drug addict and said she was neglecting them. Three of the children are with her sister and two are with her sister-in-law, the former addict who introduced them to heroin but is now drug-free. It hurts Rosemary to see her children with others, but she is grateful they are with her own people, and she can see them whenever she wants to.

Rosemary learned to inject herself with heroin when she was nineteen, and now hits herself three times a day, or as often as she can. Two years ago she started crack and smokes, on an average, every other day. She also drinks alcohol daily and is fond of inexpensive wine.

Since Rosemary lost her children, she receives disability aid (SSI) as a drug addict. Her husband receives indigent aid (General Assistance or G. A.). Rosemary derives additional income from panhandling. She has never turned tricks or held a regular job. The couple supports their heroin habits through the husband's robberies and their welfare checks. Rosemary obtains crack from girlfriends, who give her a share of their supply in exchange for the use of her pipe and a place to smoke.

Rosemary and her husband resolved to stop IV drug use when their kids were taken. For the first time in twelve years of heroin use, they entered a methadone maintenance program. During the two years they were on methadone to control their heroin addiction, they began to smoke crack. About six or seven months ago they stopped methadone and started injecting heroin again. Heroin use not only led to the loss of their children; it had a direct impact on their daily interactions. Rosemary and her husband used to fight violently over the division of the drug. In her view, he often tried to shortchange her, and she refused to tolerate it. The fights stopped when they were on methadone and now occur infrequently.

Rosemary's major risk for AIDS stems from her husband, whose heroin habit is heavier than hers. In addition to daily shots with her, he goes out and shoots with others. She does not know how many more times he injects every day or who he shares needles with. She shares only with him and admits they just started cleaning needles with bleach or alcohol several months ago, after learning about AIDS in the methadone maintenance program. Her husband never uses condoms, nor does she feel it is necessary, since she has a monogamous relationship with him.

Rosemary has had abscesses from IV infections a few years ago. She also suffers from anemia, which probably stems from her IV drug use (Mondanaro 1987). Nevertheless she considers herself to be very healthy and feels her health is better than that of other women she knows.

The lifestyle of Rosemary and her husband is focused almost exclusively on "chasing drugs." She is the only one of her siblings involved with IV drugs and considers herself to be the black sheep of the family. Although she realizes she can have her children whenever she quits drugs, she claims she does not want them back until she and her husband can afford to move from the crime-ridden housing project where they currently live. Despite their lifestyle, she continues to have a very warm relationship with her grandmother and feels she can depend on her whenever she is in difficulty.

CASE 3. CORA

Cora is a well-groomed, good-looking woman who also appears younger than her thirty-nine years. A direct, matter-of-fact person, she was very alert and appeared to enjoy the interview.

The oldest of seven children, Cora grew up in the housing projects in San Francisco until age thirteen, when her parents separated. Her father was a laborer unable to find steady work, and her mother was a homemaker. Neither of her parents used illegal drugs; however, her father was an alcoholic. After the separation, her mother supported the family on welfare and moved them to a housing project in Los Angeles. Shortly after their arrival there, Cora was raped on her way home from a babysitting job.

When she was fifteen, Cora started smoking weed and experimenting with pills, and at sixteen she spent the summer visiting relatives in San Francisco. There she hung out with a "fast" crowd, and at the end of the summer refused to return to Los Angeles. Not wanting Cora away from her, her mother decided to move the rest of the family back to San Francisco; her boyfriend came with them. Cora learned that her mother's boyfriend, unknown to her mother, injected speed, when she unexpectedly encountered him at a mutual friend's house. She had taken too many pills and was unable to go home, and he suggested injecting her with speed to mask the effect of the pills. She liked the high and began using speed off and on for the next year. She avoided her mother's boyfriend after he introduced her to drug injecting, but she always had friends willing to supply her with the drug whenever she wanted it.

Cora was married twice. At age seventeen, she married for the first time, and she had a child when she was eighteen. Her husband disapproved of injecting drugs and got her off speed. However, he was an aspiring pimp and became abusive when she refused to go on the street. After several severe beatings, she left him and got a divorce. At twenty-one, she married a military man, but stayed with him only a year because he was too strict with her child. She never bothered to formally divorce him. Cora did not use drugs at all between ages seventeen and twenty-five, the eight-year period of her two marriages; however, she did start drinking. When she was twenty-five, she met a fast crowd again and started snorting cocaine. She and a girlfriend used to inject cocaine privately, on the sly. At age twenty-six she lived with a heroin injector and her daily cocaine injections increased. A year later, after he was jailed, Cora met her current boyfriend, a cocaine injector, and has had a steady, monogamous relationship with him for the past twelve years.

Until recently, Cora injected cocaine an average of twice a week. At times she might inject up to five times a day and then stop for a week or so. When she was thirty-seven, Cora and her boyfriend began smoking crack. Although she would rather inject cocaine than smoke it, it is increasingly difficult to find decent powder, while crack is readily available. Cora now smokes crack almost every day and injects an average of every other month. Cora also drinks two bottles of wine a day and uses alcohol, in part, to cushion her "comedown" from crack. Although she admits she drinks "too heavily," she does not feel she has an alcohol problem.

A high school graduate, Cora is one of the few women in the study who has held a series of legal jobs. Despite her first husband's insistence, she never turned tricks to support her drug use, although when she was younger she occasionally boosted (shoplifted). Her current boyfriend has been her main source of support through a long-time job as a gardener, a job he lost almost two years ago (in part because of his involvement with crack). Cora also had jobs caring for the elderly, but has not worked for the past four years, claiming she gets too upset when her clients die. Since her boyfriend lost his job, they have an unstable living situation, moving in and out of a series of temporary hotel rooms paid for by the city. They each receive indigent aid (G. A.) and supplement it by collecting cans to sell. They rely on his mother for occasional financial help. Cora estimates they spend 75 percent of their limited income on drugs.

Cora has never been in a treatment program and believes she can stop using drugs if she wants to. However, the week before the interview, she had been high four days straight from injecting and smoking cocaine. She says, "I can control it, I do believe. Until I get to using it, you know." Although some of Cora's siblings were drug users, two of them, a brother and sister, managed to stop and now have good, well-paying jobs.

Cora appears to be involved in fewer risky activities than many of the other women in the study. While she has never learned to inject herself and shares needles with her boyfriend, from the beginning of their relationship she has insisted they sterilize their needles after using them. She and her boyfriend are very discreet about their injecting, and most of their acquaintances are not aware they shoot drugs. Her boyfriend never uses condoms. Cora does not feel it is necessary, because he is almost never out of her sight.

When she was twenty, Cora had cancer of the uterus, which resulted in a hysterectomy. Other than that she reports no specific health problems and appears to be quite healthy. Her perception of her own health, however, is that it is merely "fair."

Cora is starting to get bored with cocaine, especially with smoking it. "It's not enjoyable as it use to be. I find myself getting better blast just by drinking." Her goal is to eventually get a job and have her own place with her boyfriend. She feels her mother and her siblings would help her if she needed it and that she can also rely for immediate assistance on her boyfriend's mother, with whom she has a good relationship.

Discussion

These case studies suggest that lack of appropriate services as well as behavioral and attitudinal factors may help account for why many of these women are reluctant to enroll in drug treatment programs. One factor relates to pattern of drug use. A growing proportion of the African-American women currently inject or smoke cocaine exclusively, and no existing treatment for cocaine injection is as effective as methadone maintenance is for heroin users (Chaisson et al. 1989). There is also a belief shared by a number of cocaine injectors that cocaine is not as addictive as heroin. It may take longer, therefore, for these women to acknowledge that help is needed. Thus Cora and other cocaine users may not have attempted treatment in part because they do not consider themselves truly addicted.

Yet even African-American women who are heroin addicts, such as Mavis and Rosemary, have only rare encounters with the treatment system. In San Francisco, where drug treatment programs for low-income persons tend to be multicultural and community based, applicants often must wait several months for services (City and County of San Francisco, Department of Public Health 1990). The lengthy waiting period may discourage many women from applying.[9] In addition, attitudes about health may reinforce their avoidance. Despite their addiction, the majority of these women perceive themselves to be in good or very good health. For women like Mavis and Rosemary, relative to women addicts they know, this may indeed be the case. (Cora, who considers herself in fair health and whose drug injecting is hidden, may use non-injecting women as her reference group). That the women IV drug users in this study were sufficiently concerned about their health to get tested for the AIDS virus probably indicates they are more health-conscious than other addicts who did not get tested. If, as seems likely, one prerequisite to enrollment in drug treatment is a feeling of ill health, then the self-perception of good health on the part of such a high proportion of the women may help explain why so many never enter treatment. Furthermore, many heroin users who had unsuccessfully tried detoxification programs balked at the treatment considered most effective, methadone maintenance, in part because of beliefs that methadone is highly addictive and that it is more dangerous to their health than heroin (Hunt et al. 1986). In their view, except for the fact that methadone is legal and subsidized, addiction to methadone is not much of an improvement over addiction to heroin. These viewpoints indicate a need for the development of drug-free treatment programs that are effective for both cocaine and heroin users (Gawin and Kleber 1984). Clear-cut messages are also needed that health problems stemming from chronic IV drug use— such as immune system depression, malnutrition, diabetes, and gynecological and dental problems (Mondanaro 1987)—can often be long-term and hidden. These messages could be modeled on educational campaigns proposed to control hypertension in the African-American community (National Black Health Providers Task Force 1980), a number of which have been successful in convincing hypertensives of the necessity of treatment even when they lacked symptoms of disease (Kong 1989).

The women's stories illustrate other themes from the study that need to be considered in formulating appropriate treatment and AIDS prevention strategies. All of the women continue to be involved in high-risk sexual behavior: the majority have sexual relations with IV drug users and/or other men whose sexual histories are largely unknown to them. None of the women reported that their sexual partners consistently wear condoms. Many say their primary sexual partner never wears one. Thus the fact that the virus is spread through dirty needles has caused virtually all of the women to take recent steps to protect themselves either by no longer sharing or by cleaning their needles with bleach or alcohol, but the fact that the AIDS virus is also spread through unprotected sexual intercourse has not evoked a similar preventive response. For some women, non-compliance with safe-sex guidelines may stem from their partners' refusal to wear condoms, despite their own wishes. However, many African-American women IV drug users seem as strongly opposed to the use of condoms as their sexual partners. All three women in the case studies appear to determine the timing and frequency of sexual relations with their partners. For example, Rosemary notes that she and her husband have sex about once a week, but "then sometimes I don't want to be doing it then. We don't do it unless I want to." Similarly, Cora, noting that she and her boyfriend have sex about once a month, said, "I mean, it bothers him but it doesn't bother me at all." It is therefore urgent that the need for sexual risk reduction be more effectively conveyed to these women as well as to their sexual partners. This information might be most persuasively presented by African-American men and women IV drug users and former users who have themselves successfully adopted safe-sex behaviors. Such sexual risk reduction efforts could be modeled on the AIDS prevention programs that former IV drug users are spearheading among IV drug users in New York City (Friedman et al. 1987).

In discussing their lives, the women revealed the extent to which alcohol is integrated with IV drug use. Over one-third (38 percent) of the women said they drink alcohol in addition to injecting drugs. Like Cora, some drink wine or beer to moderate an otherwise unpleasant "comedown" from crack and to alleviate the craving for more. Others use alcohol when they reduce or stop injecting heroin or cocaine. For example, Mavis started drinking as she began reducing her dosage of heroin. Cora began drinking when she stopped using drugs altogether for an eight-year period and now affirms she would rather get high on alcohol than on crack. Rosemary currently drinks alcohol as often as she shoots heroin. Thus treatment programs that help women stop injecting drugs need to incorporate techniques to prevent subsequent dependency on alcohol.

Like almost all of the women, the three women in the case studies grew up in neighborhoods where drug use was widespread and where injecting heroin formed another bond in an existing, emotionally charged relationship: for Mavis with her admired older sister, and for Rosemary with her future husband. Even Cora was first injected by her mother's boyfriend, someone she initially trusted. These experiences suggest that just as people close to African-American women addicts were instrumental in their entrance into drug use, people with personal ties might be most effective in helping them get out of it. However, most drug treatment programs tend to be somewhat impersonal and to rely solely on professional staff, an approach that may reach white IV drug users but that may be culturally inappropriate for many African American and other minority IV drug users (Lewis 1990). Since all of the African-American women IV drug users in the study derive considerable emotional support from one or more relatives (a pattern not found among the white women), it seems fitting that appropriate family members be incorporated as part of the treatment strategy. This could be particularly apt when the relative has herself or himself successfully stopped using drugs, such as Rosemary's sister-in-law or Cora's brother and sister. To succeed, preventive programs must also focus on the women's immediate living situation. It is instructive, for example, that Mavis's recent willingness to cease heroin injecting occurred when her boyfriend was forced to do so. It is unlikely that either Cora or Rosemary will enter, much less succeed, in treatment as long as they live with men who continue to use.

Finally, the study shows how ingeniously the women network to support one another in obtaining and using drugs, as shown by Mavis's arrangements with her daily shooting partner and Rosemary's exchanges with her crack associates. These patterns suggest that the same networking skills could be exploited by the women to support one another in risk reduction and in creating feasible alternatives to IV drug use. Thus women injectors with similar experiences, backgrounds, and goals need to be encouraged to work together to share resources and develop their own strategies to help one another reduce risk and, ultimately, stop dependency on drugs.

Conclusion

This research suggests that many African-American women IV drug users have general notions about the importance of AIDS prevention measures. However, most do not seem sufficiently aware of the concrete reality of their own risk. They are in urgent need of culturally relevant information about the extent of the risks they face, followed by drug treatment programs, available on demand, that will help them stop their drug dependency and acquire the resolve they need to change their lives. The women's own understanding and self-perceptions provide important clues regarding strategies and techniques that should be considered in designing and planning culturally specific risk reduction efforts.

Obviously any attempt to help African-American and other minority women and men with problems of drug addiction will be merely palliative until the underlying conditions of drug use in minority communities are eliminated (Tucker 1985; Espada 1979). Although a discussion of these conditions is beyond the scope of this paper, the effects of racism, inadequate education, and unemployment are evident in the neighborhoods where most of these women grew up. In addition to eradication of the legacy of racial injustice, there is an immediate need to redirect national concern from punishment to the prevention and treatment of drug addiction in minority communities. It is unconscionable that our society is allowing the lives of so many people of color to be lost to drugs and AIDS. The need to fight this conspiracy of neglect must be brought to the attention of the nation (Espada 1979).

Notes

1. Miller's (1986) study of street women discussed the lives of underclass African-American women, but dealt primarily with criminal activities rather than drug use. Rosenbaum's (1981) study of one hundred female heroin users included the life experiences of thirty-eight African-American women; however, her focus was the common experience of heroin use, and ethnic differences were not discussed.
2. The AIDS virus is transmitted through the exchange of bodily fluids. It can be acquired via contaminated needles, unprotected sexual intercourse, and through perinatal transmission from mother to child. Preventive measures include sterilizing needles before use and using condoms during sexual intercourse.
3. A person who is infected with the AIDS virus can look and feel healthy. Full-blown AIDS can occur after a period of time in those infected with the virus.

326 | Diane K. Lewis

4. This figure is based on the estimate by Hahn et al. (1989) that there are 226,000 IV drug users infected with the AIDS virus. The assumption is that infection rates for males and females are similar (Hahn et al., 1989).
5. This figure is derived by multiplying the estimated number of infected female IV drug users by 58 percent (58% X 57,000 to 58% X 75,000).
6. Crack is a rock-like derivative of cocaine from which the hydrochloride has been removed.
7. All names used are pseudonymous.
8. Drug detoxification programs are short-term, usually twenty-eight days, and may be drug-free or methadone-based. Maintenance programs are long-term and require supervised daily doses of oral methadone.
9. In 1988, during a six-month period, a total of 3,798 people were waiting for drug treatment services in San Francisco. Federal funds awarded in 1989 reportedly reduced the waiting period for all substance abuse programs to an average of 3.7 weeks (6.6 weeks for methadone maintenance) (City and County of San Francisco, Department of Public Health 1990).

Acknowledgments

I am indebted to John K. Watters, Ph.D., whose collaboration made this research possible. I am also grateful to Askia Muhammud, Patricia Case, M.Ph., and Jennifer Lorvick, who helped recruit women to the study; to Ellen Opie, M.Ph., and Christy Ponticelli, M.A., for research assistance; and to Dena Taylor, M.S.W., for comments on an earlier draft. I especially thank the women who shared their lives with me.

This research is supported by a grant from the State of California on the recommendation of the Universitywide Task Force on AIDS and by funds allocated from the University of California, Santa Cruz.

Works Cited

Bell, Nora Kizer. 1989. "AIDS and Women: Remaining Ethical Issues." *AIDS Education and Prevention* 1:22–30.

Burks, Ethel B., and Tyron S. Johnson. 1978. "The Black Drug Abuser: The Lack of Utilization of Treatment Services." In Arnold J. Schecter, ed. *Drug Dependence and Alcoholism* Vol. 2: *Social and Behavior Issues.* New York: Plenum Press.

Centers for Disease Control. 1990. HIV/AIDS Surveillance Report. February:1–18.

Chaisson, Richard E., Peter Bacchetti, Dennis Osmond, Barbara Brodie, Merle A. Sande, and Andrew R. Moss. 1989. "Cocaine Use and HIV Infection in Intravenous Drug Users in San Francisco." *Journal of the American Medical Association* 261:561–65.

City and County of San Francisco, Department of Public Health. 1990. "Strategic Plan for Mental Health, Substance Abuse and Forensic Services." San Francisco: Division of Mental Health, Substance Abuse & Forensic Services.

Cohen, Judith B., Laurie B. Hauer, and Constance B. Wofsy. 1989. "Women and IV Drugs: Parenteral and Heterosexual Transmission of Human Immunodeficiency Virus." *The Journal of Drug Issues* 19:39–56.

Department of Public Health, City and County of San Francisco. 1990. "Strategic Plan for Mental Health, Substance Abuse and Forensic Services: Preliminary Version for Submission to the San Francisco Board of Supervisors."

Espada, Frank. 1979. "The Drug Abuse Industry and the 'Minority' Communities: Time for Change." In R. L. Dupont, A. Goldstein, and J. O'Donnell, eds. *Handbook on Drug Abuse*. Washington, D. C.: U. S. Government Printing Office.

Friedman, Samuel R., Don C. Des Jarlais, Jo L. Sotheran, Jonathan Garber, Henry Cohen, and Donald Smith. 1987. "AIDS and Self-Organization among Intravenous Drug Users." *International Journal of Addictions* 22:201–19.

Gawin, F. H., and H. D. Kleber. 1984. "Cocaine Abuse Treatment: Open Pilot Trial with Despiramine and Lithium Carbonate." *Archives of General Psychiatry* 41:903–09.

Hahn, Robert A., Ida M. Onorato, T. Stephen Jones, and John Dougherty. 1989. "Prevalence of HIV Infection among Intravenous Drug Users in the United States. *Journal of the American Medical Association* 261:2677–84.

Hunt, D. E., D. S. Lipton, D. S. Goldsmith, and D. L. Strug. 1986. " 'It Takes Your Heart': The Image of Methadone Maintenance in the Addict World and Its Effects on Recruitment into Treatment." *International Journal of Addictions* 20:1751–71.

Kong, B. W. 1989. "Community Programs to Increase Hypertension Control." *Journal of the National Medical Association* 81 (Suppl):13–16.

Lange, W. Robert, Frederick R. Snyder, David Lozovsky, Vivek Kaistha, Mary A. Kaczaniuk, Jerome H. Jaffe, and the ARC Epidemiology Collaborating Group. 1988. "Geographic Distribution of Human Immunodeficiency Virus Markers in Parenteral Drug Abusers." *American Journal of Public Health* 78:443–46.

Lewis, Diane K. 1990. "Life Histories of Female IV Drug Users: A Progress Report." Paper presented to the Scientific Meeting of the Universitywide Task Force on AIDS. San Diego, Calif.

———, and John K. Watters. 1989. "Human Immunodeficiency Virus Seroprevalence in Female Intravenous Drug Abusers: The Puzzle of Black Women's Risk." *Social Science and Medicine* 29:1071–76.

Miller, Eleanor M. 1986. *Street Woman*. Philadelphia: Temple University Press.

Mondanaro, Josette. 1987. "Strategies for AIDS Prevention: Motivating Health Behavior in Drug Dependent Women." *Journal of Psychoactive Drugs* 19:143–49.

National Black Health Providers Task Force on High Blood Pressure Education and Control. 1980. "Final Report of the National Black Health Providers Task Force on High Blood Pressure Education and Control." Bethesda, Md.: U. S. Dept. of Health and Human Services, Public Health Service, National Institutes of Health.

Rosenbaum, Marsha. 1981. *Women on Heroin*. New Brunswick, N. J.: Rutgers University Press.

San Francisco Department of Public Health. 1990. "AIDS Monthly Surveillance Report." San Francisco: AIDS Office-Surveillance Branch.

Selik, Richard M., Kenneth G. Castro, and Marguerite Pappaioanou. 1988. "Racial/ Ethnic Differences in the Risk of AIDS in the United States." *American Journal of Public Health* 78:1539–45.

Tucker, M. Belinda. 1985. "U. S. Ethnic Minorities and Drug Abuse: An Assessment of the Science and Practice." *International Journal of Addictions* 20:1021–47.

Poverty, Drug Use, and AIDS: Converging Issues in the Life Stories of Women in Harlem[1]

MICHAEL C. CLATTS

Introduction

In some societies, sickness and death are routinely attributed to the malevolence of sorcery and are often blamed on rivals in competing tribes. Such events are understood as an attack on the integrity of the community itself, and survivors believe themselves to be morally obligated to seek revenge for their fellows and retribution from their enemies, often through counter-sorcery or ritualized warfare (Glick 1967, 54). These customs reflect a conceptualization of disease in which the misfortunes of illness are believed to be closely bound to the social circumstances in which an afflicted individual lives. In Western medical practice, by contrast, descriptions of the causes of illness and death have generally focused upon the identification and control of specific biological agents. Here the medical practitioner rather than the village sorcerer is looked to for treatment and relief.

Yet concepts of disease and death in Western societies are often no less bound to prevailing social and cultural beliefs. Within recent history, no where is this more clearly demonstrated than in the current medical, religious, and political discourses on Acquired Immune Deficiency Syndrome (AIDS). Primarily associated with sexual transmission in homosexual acts and with the sharing of "dirty" needles during intravenous drug use, AIDS has rapidly become linked with entrenched metaphorical complexes. These involve fundamental cultural fears and fantasies, beliefs and moral ideologies, concerning not simply disease, but the nature of virtue and vice as well.

Some of the "risk groups" initially identified with AIDS (e.g., homosexuals) have at least partially succeeded in altering the way in which they are represented in relation to the disease; they are also reported to have made substantial changes in their risk behavior (Siegel et al. 1988). However, those whose risk is associated with the use of illegal narcotics (a "high risk group" composed largely of minority men and women living in impoverished communities) often do not possess comparable access to the social, economic, and political sources of power. They have had little opportunity to affect the way in which they are represented in relation to this disease. Moreover, individuals in diverse social and economic circumstances relate differently to the risk behaviors implicated in infection with Human Immuno-Deficiency Virus (HIV) and, similarly, are constrained in different ways in their ability to alter the behaviors which place them at risk for HIV infection. Many minority women, for example, have reported that safe-sex guidelines conflict with their reproductive roles and ambitions (Worth 1988).[2]

This essay focuses on women in Harlem, a community in the upper part of Manhattan in New York City. A recent study of mortality patterns there indicated that cirrhosis, drug dependency, and alcohol use are among the leading factors contributing to "excess mortality" rates. These rates exceed those of such Third World nations as Bangladesh (McCord and Freeman 1990; see also Selwyn et al. 1989). The same study noted that since 1980, the number of deaths of persons between twenty-five and forty-four years of age in Harlem had increased by more than 30 percent and that AIDS has become the leading cause of death in that age group.

In the course of an AIDS intervention program in Harlem, nine hundred intravenous drug users (IVDU's) and their sexual partners were contacted. Data indicates that *knowledge* about risk from sharing drug injection equipment and from unprotected sex is widespread in the community, but that several high-risk behaviors continue to occur with alarming frequency. Nearly 70 percent reported using IV heroin, and/or 70 percent IV cocaine, and approximately 75 percent reported using crack. Nearly 40 percent of the women had exchanged sex for money, and nearly 65 percent had exchanged sex for drugs. This data is consistent with nationwide studies of female spouses of IV drug users, over 40 percent of whom support their own drug habits, as well as that of their spouses, through the sex-for-drugs exchange (Sowder and Weissman 1989).

Much of our everyday understanding of these statistics, however, derives from the stark images of contaminated needles and dusty crack vials appearing on the front pages of our newspapers. We know relatively little about the meaning which these substances have in the everyday lives of users, and we know even less about the way in which their use is related to the prevailing social and economic institutions in these communities. In the absence of voices from these communities, we have been left with inadequate and often inaccurate representations of the drug user as a social failure. This image has often functioned as a larger metaphor for notions of race, class, and gender.[3]

To redress the inadequacy of these representations, this essay profiles three women from Harlem. Life histories were obtained through open-ended ethnographic interviews conducted by the author. They provide the basis for a reassessment of the discourse on AIDS, particularly as it relates to risk behavior among minority women. The primary significance of the narratives is not whether the women have AIDS. The focus is on demonstrating the interrelationship between behaviors which place these women at risk and the social and economic roles they occupy.

Case Studies

SALLY

"It's really scary out there!"

Sally is a thirty-nine year old woman who moved to Harlem in her early twenties. She recounts a turbulent childhood—the death of her mother when she was ten, her father's re-marriage and his subsequent death, perennial shifts in and out of foster care when her father was unable to find work or pay the rent. One of her earliest and most vivid childhood memories involves repeated sexual assaults by one of her cousins. She says she worries now about what he is doing to his own daughter. Her adult life has been no less traumatic. Several relationships have failed, and she has been beaten and abandoned, sometimes relying on prostitution and drug-peddling to make her way.

She first "skin popped" when she was nineteen.[4] Her boyfriend was a dealer, and she wanted to "feel included in what everyone else was in to." Over the years she tried almost every drug on the streets (uppers, downers, pot, alcohol, LSD, cocaine, crack), but she says that "heroin is still king." When asked about her experience with heroin, however, she says that "psychologically it makes you feel inferior, you tend to dog yourself." She rolls up her sleeve and her pant leg, revealing long stretches of scar tissue from numerous abscesses. She tells about her collapsed veins and the times she shot dope cut with meat tenderizer and cocaine possibly laced with mercury. She describes addiction in terms of fears of withdrawal, but also in terms of how it has affected her perception of herself. She says she no longer feels like she can "fit socially into the world of people that are straight, with clean clothes . . . it changes your self, your body stinks and is corroded."

She has been a Catholic, a Methodist, a Protestant, and now a Buddhist. She attributes her strong sense of spirituality to her father's Native-

American heritage, which he imparted to her. Consistent with this, she notes that her parents died on the same day ten years apart, a fact that she believes has cosmic significance. In another instance she recalls the day when two pigeons appeared at her window; she knew someone close to her had died, and later she learned a cousin had died of AIDS that morning.

Sally talked for over three hours, incredulous that someone was really interested in her story. She described her nights on "the stroll," of "mixing and selling drugs," of hours she lingered in "shooting galleries" and crack houses. There she sold sex for "fifty cents" or "just one hit on the crack pipe." Her descriptions parallel observations of institutional incarceration, in which "the territories of the inmate's self—his body, his thoughts, actions, possessions, are all violated" (Goffman 1961, 23). She "only shoots up at home now." Consequently she believes that she is no longer at risk for AIDS, noting also that she has "a place to stay and clothes, and I keep myself clean." Yet she worries about the kids who have taken her place on the stroll. She knows that they will be beaten and exploited. Like herself, they are tired, hungry, and sick. She fears that many will "disappear and that no one will even know it."

The latter prognosis is described in the context of anxieties which she has about herself, one of which is about AIDS. She says that she has not been tested, but thinks about AIDS constantly. The interview itself has provided an opportunity to look back to her work on the streets and the dangers of street prostitution and to reassess their meaning and purpose. Initially she struck a reminiscent pose, much like a retiree might review an illustrious career. As we moved through the years of violence and death, however, she recalled having lost contact with most of her family. Her parents, her siblings, her children, and most of her friends "have come and gone." Suddenly she sees a reflection of herself in the glassy eyes of the girls who have taken her place on the stroll. There is a sudden flash of panic in her eyes, as if she has been startled by her own anonymity.

BEATRICE

"... that's what drugs are for, to fill the empty spaces"

Beatrice, wary of the interview, broke the "conversational ice" by mockingly describing her breasts. When the joke elicited a laugh, she relaxed a little. She'd had personal experience with oral history, noting that "every family is like a folk song, it reminds us of who we are." "Some of us are Elks, some evangelists, or Masons, or tea readers, or dream interpreters," and, she said, "everyone is born with a gift." I was immediately struck by her vivid sense of history, by the connectedness she sees in the world, and the incongruity between this and what I already knew about the circumstances of her daily life.

Beatrice, a black woman born in a coastal town in South Carolina in 1953, says hers was "a beautiful family." They enjoyed "wide open spaces, and open signs of expression and affection." She grew wistful as she recounted stories supporting this image: grandmother bringing grandfather his favorite cookies while they sat in their rocking chairs on the front porch, and how she wondered how often they had sex to produce eleven children. Her family has always been involved in what she calls "chemical dependency." Her grandfather owned various stores in their home town that fronted the illegal corn liquor black market. Similarly, her father and uncles "wrote numbers" and later organized a cocaine network between New York and the South.

Beatrice started using drugs when she was fourteen. Her sister's crib death the year before caused her mother to have a nervous breakdown, and she began using her mother's valium. "My girl friends and me tried them, and then we graduated to marijuana, and acid, and then liquid methadone." "We used to get them [acid] on these little pieces of paper with cartoons on them and the character indicated how high the high was, you got goofy off of Goofy." She went to college for a year and studied psychology because she was "interested in what people were thinking." This brief time in college was the only period in her life when she did not use drugs, she explains, "'cause I had something to fill my mind."

Her father died soon after the family moved from South Carolina to New York. She took care of her mother, who never recovered from her nervous breakdown. She offers few details about the next several years. Apparently she became increasingly involved in street prostitution, but she reports that she has "moved off the stroll now, by the power of God, and the word of God." Although she elaborates little on her formal religious beliefs, much of her conversation is punctuated with references to God. She also frequently alludes to a spiritual transformation associated with drug use. She describes a kind of out-of-body experience in which drugs allow her to escape from her body, to look down upon herself and "to see what it is I have to do." The things she describes in this vein, however, all center around the "things" she has to do in order to survive economically, particularly through prostitution. Sadly it is these same "things," and the risk for AIDS resulting from them, which in fact critically threaten her survival.

She schedules each of her regular johns at a specific day and time. They come and tell her, "Hey Baby, I got four bottles [crack], do you want to get busy?" Many bring her cash to buy drugs for them, since she knows where to get "the best deal." "We get high on the drugs they've paid for," she tells me very matter of factly, and "they pay separately for anything else" [sex]. She adamantly claims never to trade sex for drugs; she always insists on being paid in cash. This makes her feel "more wanted" and regulates her spending and consumption of crack. Many of her men are older. "They went through school and made their Mama proud." "They have raised children, had their jobs, bought and sold their houses," and "now they're all alone." "They live in one room with their hotplates and memories." Beatrice reflects,

> Now they want to put together photo albums of all of us crack girls. Most of them come to my house to spend time with me. They speak to my Mama and bring her a little something that they've boosted [stolen] as a token of thanks for her hospitality, and then we go to my room and everyone knows not to bother us. Sometimes I go to their place, and they have my money all set out for me in a nice little candy dish.

She believes her work is therapeutic for the johns. She boasts about a famous photographer who came to see her after he was paralysed with a stroke. She smiles wryly, "he ain't paralysed no more."

Beatrice knows she is at high risk for AIDS. She says that she does not have penetrating sex any more because she wouldn't know how to tell her sexual partners if she got AIDS. She grows suddenly fidgety and for the first time in the interview avoids eye contact. She is obviously anxious about the subject. She demonstrates her knowledge about AIDS and her belief that she is in control of the johns, but she does not want to dwell on any details. I ask her if she has been tested, but she deflects my question as if she hasn't heard it. I try another tack, asking if she knows how to prevent becoming infected. She responds, "you know I can prolong HIV from turning to AIDS if I drop my sex to a point . . . you know I swear to God that I have it in me now, and I am scared to death, but I can slow it down." "I don't want to know yet." She directs the discussion to the girls she knows who are still "out on the streets" (prostituting), of the risks they are taking and the danger they are in. She has shifted the focus from herself, but in so doing has also revealed the boundary she imagines to exist between herself and the disease. It is as if the disease only exists on the streets. She believes she is safe in her own apartment, behind closed doors with her family, in a place where she is in control.

Power and control issues surrounding sex surface frequently in the interview. She indicated that she knows "how to come across sensual enough so that it doesn't matter if my skin color is light enough, or my hair is long enough." "At the moment of your orgasm I know you, and I control you," she explains. One john, she recalls, "had the nerve to ask me afterwards if I had an orgasm." She told him flatly, "I gets mines from counting those greens" [money].

Sex is always associated with the use of drugs, particularly crack. She recounts an anti-cocaine commercial that she saw on television.

> They show you this pretty little nose, and a radio goes by and sniff—it turns to cocaine; a car goes by and sniff—it turns to cocaine; a yacht goes by and sniff—it turns to cocaine; then a trip to Paris goes by and sniff—it

turns to cocaine. You know when I saw that I said they're full of shit. I can't go to Crazy Eddy's every ten minutes with three dollars and get a radio, and I can't go to Chrysler and get a car without a down payment, and if I go to a travel agency to book a trip to Paris I have to have a credit card and a good job. But I can go to that crack man every ten minutes and at the end of the day he'll even throw me a bottle free. Where else can I go to get something like that?

She concluded, "most of the things I want are impossible to get without a higher state of being," again alluding to a spiritual transformation achieved by the use of crack.

Crack has "a dark side," Beatrice admits. In an animated voice she describes a series of "lies which a little voice inside your head whispers, coaxing you to take another hit."

You're not tired. You can walk those twenty blocks to get another fifty cents that will buy you another hit. You're not hungry. You don't need to spend that three dollars on food. What you do to get the money, it doesn't matter. Step over that shit, step over that piss, give that man a quick one. It doesn't matter. It's okay if that baby is crying or hungry. That watch he gave you for Christmas, you can get a jumbo bottle for that and then you'll be smoking lovely.

She says the "facts change and the lies tune into your eyes." "Cocaine causes you to see everything and everyone in terms of the *quantity* of rock [crack] that you can get."

Lois

"At the end of the rainbow"

Lois, a thirty-two year old woman, has lively and searching eyes, a sure and engaging smile, but a frail and emaciated body. She walks slowly, using a cane, and even in conversation she stops to catch her breath. Lois was born in southern New Jersey, to a woman who was unmarried and unable to care for her. She was raised by her maternal grandmother, a strongly religious person with a generous and fair spirit. Lois succeeded in elementary and high school. She first used drugs when she began working toward a career in business.

She began "partying" in the clubs in Atlantic City and Philadelphia, and later in New York. "It was a weekend thing," she recalls, "snort cocaine, shoot heroin, take pills, and get wasted." She recalls that "it was okay," for the drugs helped relieve pressures she felt "to succeed as a black woman trying to make it in the white man's world." When her lover died in a car accident, Lois began doing "speedballs" on a daily basis, shooting cocaine and heroin together. Eventually she had "a breakdown." She underwent residential treatment for drug abuse, but soon after returning to work she got pneumonia.

In the last two years she has been unable to work, and she has been hospitalized repeatedly with various AIDS-related opportunistic infections. She is frequently incontinent, must wear a diaper, and has difficulty eating because of swelling in her mouth and throat from oral candida (thrush). Like many in this community suffering from AIDS, she articulates that her principal fears lie in the imagined consequences of "people knowing," rather than in the actual illness or the ultimate threat of death. After several years of illness, her chief concern is still "other people's finding out." Transfixed in some kind of nightmare, she imagines being disowned by her family, disdained by her neighbors, and discriminated against by her landlord.

Lois initially described herself as "in remission," but her arms and legs and face are marked with the red blotches characteristic of Kaposi's Sarcoma. Amid silent tears, she whispers that she feels "near the end of her rainbow." Earlier the interview was filled with resonant laughter over the ironies of human life, the friends she had known and the times they had enjoyed together. As we moved through the years, however, the tone changed, revealing her exhaustion from years of chronic illness, fear, and abandonment. For a moment she was overcome by the darkening horizon she glimpsed, and she quietly grasped my hand as we sat in a shared silence. Yet she was anxious to tell her story and relieved by the chance to do so. She was angry at God, who was supposed to be looking out for her, and, as if describing a bad dream, recounted thoughts of jumping off the roof of her building. She vacillated between despair and the hope that a cure will be found. But she was also convinced that she would never be able to afford it—the cost of food and rent had already overwhelmed her. She thanked me repeatedly for *not* asking what she says everyone asks her: "how do you feel?"

Implications for Health and Illness

The scope of this paper does not permit a complete exegesis of these ethnographic narratives. The material does, however, have a direct bearing upon our understanding of drug use and other risk behaviors among minority women. The life history materials substantiate the evidence reported in a number of quantitative studies which indicates that chronic drug use among women, particularly of cocaine and coca-based products such as crack, is highly correlated with behaviors implicated in the spread of a number of sexually transmitted diseases, including HIV infection. In order to adequately understand the motivations which underpin the use of narcotic substances, however, and the relationship to other risk behaviors such as unprotected sex, we must examine the experiential functions which the use of these drugs accomplish.

It is noteworthy that within our own social history, the drugs which have most often been the objects of social control are precisely those which are associated with releasing inhibitions—those, such as crack, that are perceived as providing the user an experience which in some way stands outside the confines of social realities (i.e., roles and statuses) designated as legitimate, somehow inherently "right." Often it is precisely the immorality associated with failure to maintain these socially proscribed inhibitions that is central to the way in which drug addiction as an "illness"—or indeed any of the "illnesses" which have come to be conceptualized as indicative of an individual's own *failure*—is itself characterized (Agar 1985; Clatts and Mutchler 1989; Foucault 1980; Sontag 1978).

Each of these women chronicles a lifetime of experiences in which she was discriminated against because of the color of her skin and the accent in her speech. All continue to suffer from chronic economic impoverishment, necessitating participation in particular sexual roles which they find both demeaning and exploitative. Both Sally and Beatrice detailed much self-doubt and self-incrimination about their participation in street prostitution. Significantly, within this context it is noteworthy that all described their experience of crack and cocaine in terms of feeling powerful and in control in relation to men. One of the ways in which this power was manifested was through the open expression of anger against men, in effect to turn their anger outward against the world, rather than inward against themselves. Even though it is the object of formal sanction, anger among men is generally interpreted as somehow consistent with maleness. By contrast, females—black and Hispanic women, in particular—rarely have a comparable forum in which to "act up." Women are expected to "hold the family together," to be the "peacemakers" and disregard their own feelings and frustrations.

The life story narratives suggest that the frequent assumption that it is the drugs themselves which cause users to have destructive feelings is problematic. The causes of the emotions these women reported are clearly external to the women themselves. They are better understood as the consequence of the social and economic roles the women occupied as a function of their poverty. Thus it is not that drugs like crack cause such feelings as anger, but rather that they provide an experience in which users (and apparently minority women in particular) are able to express emotions which otherwise remain socially proscribed and therefore silenced. One of the implications of this functional relationship is that the formulation of effective therapeutic approaches to drug dependency among women is likely to be contingent upon alternative modalities in which to explore such emotions and their causes.[5] Moreover, sustaining independence from drugs like crack will be similarly contingent upon minority women being afforded alternative economic choices to that of street prostitution.

Conclusion

In "Tally's Corner," an ethnographic study of men who congregated on a ghetto streetcorner, E. Liebow (1967) pointed out that in contrast to the prevailing representation of these men as lacking ambition and an orientation to the future, more properly speaking they were oriented "to different futures." To a large extent the employment choices these men made were defined by the structure of economic opportunity available to them. The system provided inadequate remuneration for their work and afforded them few opportunities for mobility. A similar conclusion can be drawn about the risk behaviors of the women whose lives have been chronicled here.

In formulating programs which seek to intervene in behaviors compromising health (i.e., "risk behaviors") and in attempting to evaluate compliance with such programs, we ought to be mindful that choices are imbedded within a host of perceived opportunities and constraints whose meaning and interrelationship are bound by an emergent system of social relations.[6] Thus communities like Harlem which have been hardest hit by AIDS are also fraught with acute levels of economic displacement (Davis and Schoen 1978; Hamid 1989; Kitagawa and Hauser 1973). Here a dearth of affordable housing has left many to sleep in the streets or seek shelter and comfort in one of the many burned-out and abandoned buildings which serve as "shooting galleries" or "crack houses." Similarly, decades of inadequate employment and educational opportunities in the community have bequeathed to yet another generation of women a single "marketable" resource—their bodies.

A host of AIDS educational efforts in New York City seek to provide drug users with information about ways to reduce risk for HIV infection (Friedman et al. 1986). Participants in the Harlem project from which the research presented here is derived have expressed an eagerness to learn about AIDS (Deren 1989). However, as a growing body of literature shows, behavioral change is not determined solely by knowledge of the mechanisms of HIV infection (Kelen et al. 1989; Morgan et al. 1989; Ragni and Nimorwicz 1989). The experiences of prejudice, exploitation, and economic immobility documented here betray the inadequacy of mechanistic models of disease control and atomistic approaches to disease prevention. These life stories demonstrate that educational programs are unlikely to succeed if the individuals targeted for these efforts continue to lack opportunities for equitable employment and decent housing. AIDS is only one of the dangers confronting poor minority women in Harlem, but for many it is proving to be the last.

Notes

1. Unless otherwise noted, both the quantitative and ethnographic data presented in this paper are from studies conducted by the Harlem AIDS Project and supported by Grant DA05746 from the National Institute on Drug Abuse. The project is

administered by Narcotic and Drug Research, Inc., and S. Deren serves as the Principal Investigator. The ethnographic research was conducted by the author and is presented with the consent of the subjects involved, whose names have been changed to protect their privacy. Views expressed in this paper are solely those of the author and do not necessarily represent those of NIDA or NDRI. In addition to thanking the women participating in the study, I would like to acknowledge the assistance of R. Davis, J. Sotheran, E. Springer, and both editors of this collection in the preparation of this paper.

2. Similarly, homeless youth involved in the sex industry consistently report difficulty in engaging in safe-sex practices (e.g., the use of condoms), because they are economically dependent upon an economy controlled by "johns" who refuse to do so or who will pay more for not doing so (Clatts 1990).

3. For more detailed discussion, see Clatts and Mutchler (1989).

4. "Skin-Popping" involves injecting narcotic substances—such as heroin or heroin mixed with cocaine—into the skin surface rather than into veins ("mainlining"); it is often described as the way in which experimentation with IV drugs begins.

5. Anger in particular is an emotion which social service providers, including those responsible for drug treatment, are often ill-equipped to manage. Individuals participating in such programs are expected not to exhibit anger outside specifically circumscribed contexts, and they are formally and informally sanctioned when they do so. The client role is defined by an expectation of behavioral deference and demeanor toward the practitioner. At least on an interpersonal level, compliance is often signified in clients' expressions of gratitude and satisfaction, and anger is represented as indicative of both a lack of compliance and individual failure (Clatts and Mutchler 1989; Goffman 1961).

6. Lewis (1966) created considerable controversy when he proposed the concept of a "culture of poverty," by which he argued that the poor are systematically enculturated into this role (Valentine 1969). The scope of this paper does not permit an adequate treatment of this debate. In arguing that some methodological attention be paid to the larger social and economic environment in which risk behavior occurs, I intend no causal inference about them. The latter is properly understood as an empirical question, and it is not within the confines of this paper.

Works Cited

Agar, M. 1985. "Folks and Professionals: Different Models for the Interpretation of Drug Use." *International Journal of the Addictions* 20 (1): 173–82.

Clatts, M. 1990. "The Clinical Dynamics of the Crack Menace: An Ethnographic Perspective." Paper presented at the Sixth Annual Family Therapy Network Conference, Washington, D. C.

———, and K. Mutchler. 1989. "AIDS and the Dangerous Other: Metaphors of Sex and Deviance in the Representation of a Disease." *Medical Anthropology* 10: 105–14.

Davis, K., and C. Schoen. 1978. *Health and the War on Poverty: A Ten Year Appraisal.* Washington D. C.: Brookings Institution.

Deren, S. 1989. "The Harlem AIDS Project: Description and Preliminary Findings."
Paper presented at the First Annual National AIDS Demonstration and Research
Conference, Rockville, Maryland, October 1989.

Foucault, M. 1980. *The History of Sexuality*, Vol. 1. Chicago: University of Chicago
Press.

Friedman, S., D. Des Jarlais, and J. Sothern. 1986. "AIDS Health Education for
Intravenous Drug Users." *Health Education Quarterly* 13 (4): 383–93.

Glick, L. 1967. "Medicine as an Ethnographic Category: The Gimi of the New Guinea
Highlands." *Ethnology* 6 (1): 31–56.

Goffman, E. 1961. *Asylums: Essays on the Social Situations of Mental Patients and
Other Inmates*. Garden City, N. Y.: Anchor Books.

Hamid, A. 1989. "The Political Economy of Drugs." Paper presented at the Fall
Session of the New York State Psychological Association, September 27, 1989.

Kelen, G., T. DiGiovani, L. Bisson, D. Kalainov, K. Sivertson, and T. Quinn. 1989.
"Human Immunodeficiency Virus in Emergency Department Patients." *Journal of
the American Medical Association* 262 (4): 516–22.

Kitagawa, E., and P. Hauser. 1973. *Differential Mortality in the United States: A Study
in Socio-Economic Epidemiology*. Cambridge: Harvard University Press.

Lewis, O. 1966. "The Culture of Poverty." *Scientific American* 215 (4): 19–25.

Liebow, E. 1967. *Tally's Corner: A Study of Negro Streetcorner Men*. Boston: Little,
Brown.

McCord, C., and H. Freeman. 1990. "Excess Mortality in Harlem." *New England
Journal of Medicine* 322 (3): 173–77.

Morgan, T. R., M. Plant, and D. Sales. 1989. "Risk of AIDS among Workers in
the 'Sex Industry': Some Initial Results from a Scottish Study." *British Medical
Journal* 299: 148–49.

Ragni, M.V., and P. Nimorwicz. 1989. "Human Immuno-Deficiency Virus Transmission and Hemophilia." *Archives of Internal Medicine* 149 (6):1379.

Selwyn P., D. Hartel, W. Wasserman, and E. Drucker. 1989. "Impact of AIDS
Epidemic on Morbidity and Mortality among Intravenous Drug Users in a New
York City Methadone Maintenance Program." *American Journal of Public Health*
79 (10): 1358–62.

Siegel, K., L. Bauman, G. Christ, and S. Krown. 1988. "Patterns of Change in Sexual
Behavior among Gay Men in New York City." *Archives of Sexual Behavior* 17
(6): 481–97.

Sontag, S. 1978. *Illness as a Metaphor*. New York: Strauss and Giroux.

Sowder, B., and G. Weissman. 1989. "NADR Project Revealing New Data on High-
Risk Behavior among Women." *Network* 1 (2).

Valentine, C. 1969. *Culture and Poverty: Critique and Counter-Proposals*. Chicago:
University of Chicago Press.

Worth, D. 1990. "Minority Women and AIDS: Culture, Race, and Gender." In D.
Felman, ed., *Culture and Aids*. New York: Praeger Publishers.

Latinas and HIV Infection/AIDS: Reflections on Impacts, Dilemmas, and Struggles

GLORIA J. ROMERO, LOURDES ARGUELLES, AND ANNE M. RIVERO

Introduction

Latinos and African Americans represent about 40 percent of Acquired Immune Deficiency Syndrome (AIDS) cases in the United States (Centers for Disease Control 1992). Twenty-nine percent of these cases are among African Americans and 16 percent are among Latinos. Relative to their proportion of the total population, African Americans and Latinos have an incidence of AIDS two or three times higher than homosexual/bisexual white males and over twenty times higher than white heterosexual males (Mays and Cochran 1988).

Women comprise about 11 percent of AIDS cases nationally. African American and Latina women constitute approximately 74 percent of all female cases of AIDS in the nation. The high incidence of AIDS among African Americans and Latinos influences the very survival of these communities. Indeed, 80 percent of all AIDS pediatric cases are Latino and African-American babies.

Such statistics require that HIV/AIDS prevention education and treatment approaches that are sensitive to culture, class, sexual orientation, and gender be developed and implemented on an ongoing basis in our communities. Yet development and implementation of these approaches have been delayed partially by the dearth of information about HIV infection and AIDS among people of color in the United States and about women of color in particular. Such research has focused on white homosexual and bisexual men.

340

Consequently, research illuminating the reasons for these women's vulnerability to becoming infected has been delayed. More important, there has been an almost total absence of information about Latino and African-American sexual practices and other high-HIV-risk behaviors. Additionally, there is a significant lack of information on effective educational strategies and clinical treatment for use among heterogeneous segments of both communities.

An end result is that prevention programs, typically designed and implemented by white, male researchers, have been insensitive to the complex ways in which race, class, gender, sexual orientation, and national origin mediate health in this society. They fail to consider Latinas' behaviors and attitudes and how they affect the success of AIDS prevention campaigns. We contend such actions are not only unethical but are doomed to failure.

We will offer a set of fundamental considerations necessary to understanding the nature and dynamics of HIV infection and AIDS among Latinas—primarily those of Mexican origin residing in Los Angeles County. Some of these observations, previously discussed in the AIDS literature (Amaro 1988; Mays and Cochran 1988), are supplemented by community practitioners' observations in AIDS education, research, and clinical work with Latinas. This "underground" knowledge is primarily communicated through community-based conferences, in-service training, and sharing of personal experiences among AIDS practitioners and activists. It seldom finds its way onto the pages of academic or popular discourse journals.

Additionally, we will draw from empirical data banks we have compiled over the years. These include: in-depth interviews with Latino community practitioners and Latinas whose lives have been directly and indirectly influenced by the HIV epidemic (Arguelles and Rivero 1988); focus groups with Latina amnesty applicants (Arguelles 1990); evaluations of AIDS prevention education classes with Latina immigrants (Arguelles and Pino 1988); interviews from a recently completed telephone survey of 998 African Americans and Latinos in Los Angeles County (Romero and Arguelles 1990; Garcia et al. 1990); and interviews with white, Latina, and African-American female sex partners of IV drug users (Rivero and Arguelles 1989).

Finally, we will draw from our own experiences with Latina friends and allies who have become HIV-infected and/or died from AIDS. Combining research with practice, and reflecting on everyday life in Latino communities, we propose a prototype for grasping the multiplicity of issues involved in understanding Latinas and AIDS and for formulating AIDS education and treatment strategies for Latinas.

Latinas and the Latino Community

The statistical category "Latino" obscures and conceals the political and cultural implications of different and contradictory social histories within

Latino/Latina populations. "Latina" is an umbrella term including Chicana, Mexican, Cuban, Puerto Rican, and Central and South American women. Thus, using "Latina" in AIDS-related education, prevention, and outreach programs is problematic. The generalization persists, despite the diverse neo-colonial history, ethnic mix, gender socialization, and immigration status of these women. Understanding their diversity is critical in developing and providing education and clinical services, for these differences influence an individual's perceived personal power and her ability to effect changes in her own life.

In Los Angeles the majority of Latinas are of Mexican ancestry. Yet there is an increasing influx of Central and South American Latinas and a steady immigration from the Caribbean. These women constitute a significant and growing sector of the labor force in Los Angeles County. Their economic and social existence is characterized by ethnic, class, and gender-based exploitation and oppression, both in this country and in their countries of origin (Arguelles and Romero, in press). They have suffered excess morbidity and mortality prior to the advent of the HIV epidemic (Trevino and Moss 1984).

Latinas differ not only on the basis of national origin and unique social histories. Other variables which differentiate between and within groups include: linguistic capability, urban versus rural background, education, socioeconomic and employment status, life-cycle stage, and degree of "acculturation" into the socio-cultural mainstream. Typically, AIDS practitioners conceptualize "the Latino community" as merely the geographical place of residence of large numbers of Latinos. However, location is just one factor in Latinos' community identification; the concept of community must be expanded. "Belonging" is internalized and individualized, and it is rooted in such variables as: language (Spanish), place of parental or ancestral origin, adherence to cultural traditions, or identification with the Latino reference group in the face of competing identity ideologies.

These identity factors are of particular importance in AIDS-related work. Though Latino barrios have existed throughout history, an increasing number of Los Angeles Latinos who identify as part of the Latino community are being dispersed and intermingled with other populations due to massive economic restructuring (Soja 1989). Social and cultural links with traditional family and church institutions are lost as Latinos struggle to adapt to a rapidly changing urban morphology.

Latina Sexuality

What little research on HIV prevention exists fails to take into account the social and sexual contexts of Latinas. For example, most education programs focus on "safer sex" messages. Yet in reality very little is known about Latina sexuality. There is no Kinsey Report on Latina (or Latino) sexuality or popular culture studies (e.g., Hite, *Playboy*, or *Redbook* reports, and so on) (Romero 1989; 1990). In fact, only recently has Latina sexuality become a salient issue in the academic world. With different purposes in mind, entrepreneurs, health planners, and educators alike incessantly penetrate larger and larger areas of the private lives of these women in search of information on their sexual behavior. For capitalists this information is key in securing new advertising markets. The production and socialization of desire is fundamental to their selling strategies. Therefore they need knowledge of sexual ideologies and practices (Romero and Arguelles 1990).

What do we know about Latina sexuality? Academic works on "la mujer" have described her in many aspects but ignored her sexual ideologies and practices. This is true among mainstream Anglo researchers, as well as Latino/a scholars (e.g., Mirande and Enriquez 1979; Mora and del Castillo 1980; Sanchez and Martinez Cruz 1977). In twenty years of the National Association of Chicano Studies (NACS) meetings, only three panels raised the issue of sexuality. Two have been offered since 1988. Interestingly, *Chicana Voices*, the publication produced from the 1984 conference proceedings devoted to "la mujer," excludes any attention to sexuality. There have been no shortages of racist stereotypes about Latino and Latina sexuality (Padilla and O'Grady 1987; Romero and Arguelles 1990). When Latino sexuality has been considered, the Latina has been ignored (Romero and Arguelles 1990).

Latina sexuality—in all its diversity—must be perceived within its socio-historical context. And understanding the Mexican-American woman's knowledge, attitudes, and beliefs about AIDS must include knowledge of the cultural belief systems produced by the conquest of Mexico by Spain, the resultant *encomienda* system, and the colonial Catholic Church. As A. Nieto-Gomez (1976) argues, the social-psychological roles of *La Hembra*, the Woman, and *El Hombre*, the Man, are the products of circumstances spanning centuries of conquest. The resultant creation of a people suffering sweeping class, race, and gender stratification cannot be ignored in AIDS education work.

Latina sexuality is also presumed to be consistently heterosexual. Interestingly, the workshop on Latina lesbians at the 1990 NACS conference produced the first major challenge to both men and heterosexual Chicanas with regard to this fallacy. Certainly, research has well documented the diversity and variability in women's sexual behaviors and identities across the life cycle (Golden 1987). Though lesbianism is understood to exist in virtually every society, it seems to be less formalized and less visible than male homosexuality. Furthermore, despite significant constraints on the activities of women, the expression of lesbianism has been documented cross-culturally (Anzaldua 1987; Blackwood 1984; Lugones 1990; Perez 1990; Ramos 1987).

Latino culture is no exception, and Latina lesbians face distinct cultural pressures and difficulties (Espin 1984).

Risk Perception

Despite the multiple discourses and an exponential increase in HIV-prevention education, efforts with ethnic minority peoples, researchers, and AIDS community workers continue to document a high incidence of low perception of personal risk of infection in the Latino population at large. This is particularly true among Latinas (Arguelles and Rivero 1988). In addition to sociocultural differences in conceptualizing illness and understanding vulnerability to infection vis-à-vis a chain of transmission through seemingly healthy individuals, a variety of other factors contribute to their sense of low personal risk. They continue to view HIV infection as a white, gay male disease (Mays and Cochran 1988). This is reinforced by the mainstream media, whose programming features white male educators addressing a white, gay male audience. The Latino media, in its HIV-related programming, has compounded the problem by avoiding the issue of bisexuality in the community—this pattern represents a major infection route for Latina women.

Data from the Romero and Arguelles (1990) telephone interviews with 250 Latinas residing in Los Angeles county indicate that whereas 73 percent of respondents believe that everyone is at risk for getting AIDS, they tend to feel somewhat personally invulnerable. Fifty-three percent of the women responded that they are not worried about getting AIDS, while 79 percent responded that they will be able to protect themselves from being exposed to the virus. Seventy-eight percent of the women responded, "I consider my own AIDS risk to be very low." Furthermore, 77 percent responded, "I'm sure that none of my present or former sex partners have AIDS."

Latinas' false sense of security is compounded by several factors. These include: a focus on intravenous drug use as the risk factor and a pervasive denial of the existence and practice of homosexual/bisexual behavior. HIV infection is also thought to be rare among Latinos because most of them are unaware of having had personal contact with an HIV-infected person. Demonstrably, data from our telephone survey indicate that 61 percent of Latinas report not knowing anyone who had yet tested positive for HIV infection. Eighty-nine percent responded not knowing anyone with AIDS. This may well represent both a low percentage of Latinos who have been tested and a high level of denial.

Our (1990) data also reveal that danger of infection lacks the saliency and urgency of other stressful daily issues, risks, and immediate survival-related problems faced by these already highly stressed women. Thus the risks are not accorded a high ranking in their personal hierarchy of problems.

However, 71 percent of the Latinas agreed with the statement, "AIDS is a major threat in the Latino community."

At-risk Latinas

Despite their perceptions of relatively lower vulnerability to HIV infection, the epidemic has begun to have significant impact on Latinas' everyday lives—as wives, partners, mothers, and workers. AIDS service providers in the Los Angeles area recognize that in addition to the "high profile" risk factors (IV drug use, multiple sex partners, and so on), there are other rarely discussed transmission considerations. These include needle sharing for injecting vitamins and medications and for ear piercing, both common practices. Other high-risk behaviors include anal intercourse and/or sex with homosexual/bisexual men, usually by those naive to their partners' various sexual behaviors.

Risk Differences Among Latinas

As noted, it is a mistake to presume universal heterosexuality among Latinas. Although lesbians in general are at much lower risk of HIV infection than heterosexual women (Marmour et al. 1986), many Latina lesbians are likely to be at high risk because of societal and cultural pressures to maintain a facade of heterosexual identity and/or their desire to have children. This frequently results in alliances and sexual involvements with gay and/or bisexual men. Some lesbians may also be at high risk of infection because of involvement in sex work (prostitution) and IV needle-sharing practices.

Another stigmatized group is Latina sex workers, many of whom are IV drug users. They may service many men in rapid succession to survive and support their drug use. Informants to our research as well as others (Magana 1989) concur that these women are often in poor health, lack basic HIV information, and are unable to use condoms with their clients (largely undocumented Latino men) for fear of being rejected. Unprotected sex with large numbers of partners, coupled with IV drug use (including needle sharing), places these Latinas at even higher risk.

Non-drug-using sexual partners of male IV drug users are a large, hidden group of women at risk. Los Angeles Latinas in this population are characterized by service providers and researchers as one of the most psychologically dependent and resource-poor groups in the community. Many of these women are homebound and closely controlled by their partners. They frequently do not suspect their partners are IV drug users. Latinas are more prone to stay with their men—out of a sense of duty and of fate (*destino*)—despite negative life conditions than are black or white non-drug-using female partners. Frequently, undocumented immigration status, coupled with years of informal-economy patterns of work can be insurmountable barriers to their independence. In turn, Latino male IV drug users, unlike many of their African-American and white counterparts, may try to keep the family together by working or hustling money for its upkeep (Rivero and Arguelles 1989). Such relationship patterns put Latina sex partners of IV drug users at high risk of infection.

Women partners of bisexual Latino men constitute a large, invisible, group. These women, socialized into perceiving sexual orientation as a strict sexual dichotomy between heterosexual or homosexual, are naive to the dynamics and prevalence of bisexuality among Latino males (Rogers and Williams 1987). A Latina's ability to accept the idea that her partner engages in homosexual relations is hampered by a belief that only "feminine" males can be sexually involved with other males. Preliminary observations from AIDS community workers suggests that many female partners of bisexual Latinos engage in anal intercourse, a practice known to carry high risk for transmitting the HIV virus (Arguelles and Rivero 1990). Careful exploration and verification of this practice is necessary, however, since confusion about both genital physiology and vocabulary may result in unclear differentiation between anal intercourse and rear-entry vaginal intercourse. The words "anus" or "rectum" are often unfamiliar. Women frequently use the phrase "sex from behind" to describe their sexual practices. Clinicians and health educators highlight the need to clarify such terminology for purposes of HIV/AIDS-prevention education. For example, M. Davila (1989) observed the high incidence of women reporting their (presumed heterosexual) partners' insistence on anal intercourse. They explained it as the man's preferred sexual activity, thus refuting the commonly suggested notion of anal intercourse among Latinos as a means of contraception and/or preservation of virginity.

Infected Latinas

There is little in the AIDS literature about the consequences of HIV infection and AIDS among Latinas. Commonly, HIV-infected Latinas have suffered advanced progression of illness before diagnosis. Hence they experience a shorter than average time of survival after diagnosis. Delay in diagnosis may be partially attributed to attending to the needs of others before their own. Moreover, they may fail to recognize and respond to symptoms of deteriorating health. Our telephone survey indicates that 43 percent of the women responded that they did not know of any symptomatology associated with AIDS. Frequently, appropriate medical care may be inaccessible and/or unaffordable. Another serious concern is that accelerated progression of the illness is likely to be exacerbated by such co-factors as poor nutrition, other preexisting health problems, pregnancy, and chronic stress (Livingston 1988; Romero et al. 1988).

Ironically, one avenue for obtaining an earlier diagnosis is through the "amnesty" program enacted by Congress as part of comprehensive immigration reform in 1986. Undocumented Latina women (or couples), primarily Mexican, wishing to apply for citizenship and/or legal residence under the "amnesty" provision of the Immigration Reform and Control Act of 1986 must submit to mandatory HIV testing to comply with Immigration and Naturalization Service (INS) regulations. Yet many of these women are not helped by this information, but instead they are further confused. They do not understand the often contradictory information about AIDS itself, what a seropositive outcome means, or what legal consequences (including involuntary deportation) may follow. Immigrants' rights activists who monitor AIDS find it difficult to interpret these complex regulations. Additionally, they are uncertain what advice to give to those who may test HIV positive on the basis of as yet untested legal challenges. Therefore Latina amnesty applicants who are HIV positive not only fear uncertainty regarding their poor health and life expectancy, but about their immigration and legalization status as well.

Once diagnosed, Latinas suffer the cruel consequences surrounding AIDS. They often find themselves abandoned by their husbands/partners (who are most often the source of their infection), cast out from their families, and severed from their extended family support system. For example, an eighteen-year-old HIV-infected teenager we will call Emilia took an HIV test as part of her application for citizenship with the amnesty program. When she learned of her diagnosis she told her mother. She did not fully comprehend what a positive test result meant. Emilia painfully recalled: "the first thing my mother wanted to know was, 'how many guys have you been sleeping around with?' " Her mother's suspicion of her "promiscuity" distanced them from one another. Others rationalize rejection or avoidance by those around them as a response motivated by fear of contagion. For many who have tested positive, increasing isolation becomes a way of life at a time when support is most needed.

The infected Latina's failing health usually renders her unable to continue with employment. As is the case for other infected women of color, this results in increased economic deprivation for her and her family (Gross 1987). She worries that her increasing inability to be a proper homemaker will cause disintegration of her household and loss of her children.

Also ever present is the tragic reality that her small children may be infected. However, Los Angeles has not yet seen the avalanche of pediatric cases that is overwhelming Northeastern cities. The HIV-ill Latina mother, weak, facing her own illness and loss, must still manage care for a sick child who needs frequent hospitalizations, expensive medications, and complicated home care. They may both be unwelcome among family, friends, and neighbors due to the fear of AIDS. If her life is to end before her child's, she may not have any of the traditional resources (extended family and friends) to assume the care of her child after her death. She may face the pain of envisioning her child's abbreviated future in the hands of strangers. Amalia, an immigrant woman from Mexico who also learned of her HIV infection via the amnesty program, has developed AIDS symptoms and has seen her spouse die. Her two-and-a-half-year-old daughter, however, has not yet tested positive. Amalia grieves over the loss of her husband, her own infection, and the threat to her daughter's health. She is preoccupied with who will care for her child when she becomes unable to do so. Her worry is exacerbated by the fact that she has no immediate family in the United States.

Latinas with Infected Adult Family Members

Latina women are more likely to be faced with the issue of AIDS-infected adult or adolescent sons or daughters (most likely gay or bisexual sons) than with contracting AIDS themselves. Given the primacy of motherhood in Latino cultures, this is a devastating scenario. Controversy exists in the literature regarding the cultural importance and demands of motherhood for Latinas. Typically it is seen as the central value and achievement in a woman's life. This view is particularly prevalent among low-income, often immigrant Latinas. In a series of focus groups conducted recently with female amnesty applicants, this view was very strong. The saliency of motherhood in Latina women's lives strongly confirms that the birth of a child signals the beginning of an endless chain of obligations. Women are socialized to understand that they are accountable for all aspects of their children's well-being, including their development, behavior, personality, success/failure, and social acceptability.

When a son or daughter becomes ill with AIDS, his/her mother is almost always the first, and often the only, person s/he tells. Such a revelation is usually postponed as long as possible. Consequently the mother often suffers extreme grief and surprise when confronted with the child's severe illness and impending death. There may also be the shock of having to confront their child's gay or bisexual lifestyle. If the illness is related to IV drug use rather than sexual practices, there is less stigma. But the illness itself is so stigmatized and arouses so much suspicion that the family usually feels deeply threatened. Once her son or daughter has confided in her, the mother attempts to mediate between her ill offspring and other family members. The success of her efforts may determine whether her child is accepted, supported, or banished. Over time, the mother will also assume the burden of caring for her child as the illness progresses. This often requires either resorting to informal-economy employment to raise extra funds or missing work because of caretaking demands, thus adding monetary worries to the already overwhelming situation.

During these extremely stressful times, the Latina mother is vulnerable to guilt and blame, both imposed internally upon herself and applied by others. She searches her history as a mother to understand where she "went wrong" in rearing a gay/bisexual son or a sexually active or drug-using daughter. In some cases she ends up the family scapegoat, bearing as much blame and rejection as her child. To spare her family shame she must often withdraw from traditional social supports and bear the burdens alone.

Like mothers of gay sons, Latina wives/partners of infected bisexual men often face the dual trauma of their loved one's life-threatening illness and the shock of discovering their mate's affectional/sexual behaviors. Intertwined with grief, fear, and loss is the struggle with anger, betrayal, resentment, and self-blame. Stigma, again, plays its destructive role, often closing the doors to traditional support systems. These women have little choice but to remain with and care for their sick partners, for they would face even more severe shame and stigma were they to leave them. Economic loss is often extreme as the male partner becomes unable to work. The woman forfeits stable employment as her time and energy are increasingly needed for the care of her deteriorating mate. Realistic anxieties develop over her own future health and that of her young children or of a fetus carried in her womb. For some women those anxieties turn to despair as their fears are realized in their own (or their children's) HIV diagnosis.

Concealment from some family members is common. In a recent videotaped interview Ricardo, a Latino with AIDS, poignantly describes his peers' concealment of their illness from their families. Often when families do know the truth, they say their HIV-infected family member has "cancer" or another illness which is more socially acceptable. Public statements are rarely made for fear of bringing shame and pain to the family (Arguelles and Rivero 1990).

Implications for Praxis

What should be done in response to the increasing incidence of HIV infection among Latinos and Latinas? As outlined previously (Arguelles and Rivero 1988), the time has come for health workers and AIDS practitioners to formulate specific answers to this fundamental question. We must recognize closeted male bisexuality as a major vector for HIV infection to Latinas. Latinas must be cognizant of the high incidence of bisexuality among Latinos. The pattern of hiding and denying is in accordance with the cultural and societal norm of rampant homophobia among Latinos: this needs deconstructing.

Women must understand significant cultural co-factors which compound the risk of infection. Emotional, sexual, and economic abuse by males results in their being forced or cajoled into participating in the highest risk practice, anal sex (Hearst and Hulley 1988). Those who attempt to say "no" to unprotected, high-risk sexual practices may open themselves to a high risk of violence. More than simple facts, they must be given skills, strategies, and attitudinal options to better assist them in preventing and/or coping with HIV infection. They need to develop a working knowledge and open, relaxed understanding of female (and male) sexual anatomy and physiology. Additionally, assistance is necessary in developing better, more empowered communication skills with male partners. Support and encouragement for initiating and asserting changed sexual behavior must come from a culturally sensitive appreciation that threatening the male's sense of power and superiority may result in physical harm or destruction of the relationship—oftentimes, a relationship that a woman maintains out of the need for economic and social survival.

Such assertiveness training cannot be conducted in terms of a white, heterosexual, middle-class framework that presumes relationships are formed on a "friendship" model where open communication is advocated. As V. M. Mays and S. D. Cochran observe (1988), economically and politically disenfranchised women of color may not have "friendship-based" relationships. Additionally, the assumption that all Latinas are heterosexual is unwarranted as a basis for HIV/AIDS prevention and education. Until more research is done on women of color, it may, in fact, not even be practical to speak of adopting "safer sex" practices when *safe relationships* may not exist. Thus any campaign targeting disease prevention and health promotion needs to address the layers of oppression and exploitation faced by Latinas in this society.

Though these are more women-centered approaches, work with the male partners is also necessary if any real change is to come. Interventions encouraging these men toward greater self-acceptance and higher overall self-image are needed. These can be coupled with strategies encouraging more openness and honesty within their intimate relationships. History can be advantageously evoked here: reference to the acceptance and respect of homosexuality, bisexuality, and gender mixing in indigenous and traditional cultures and communities (Williams 1986) provides a positive framework.

Latinas who confront HIV infection and the contradictions it elicits deserve emotional support (via individual or group counseling) and assistance in obtaining needed resources. Bringing these women together in peer support groups and service/outreach networks (such as Mothers of AIDS Patients in Los Angeles) facilitates mutual support and collective empowerment. It is also concordant with Latinas' cultural tradition of reciprocal help and protection in times of struggle.

Works Cited

Amaro, H. 1988. "Considerations for Prevention of HIV Infection among Hispanic Women." *Psychology of Women Quarterly* 12: 429–43.

Anzaldua, G. 1987. *Borderlands/La Frontiers: The New Mestiza*. San Francisco: Spinsters/Aunt Lute.

Arguelles, L. 1990. Focus groups with Latina amnesty applicants. Unpublished data.

———, and N. Pino. 1988. "Flor de Vida: AIDS Prevention Education for Latina Women." Unpublished mimeographed manuscript.

———, and A. M. Rivero. 1988. "HIV Infection/AIDS and Latinas in Los Angeles County: Considerations for Prevention Treatment and Research Practice." *California Sociologist* 11: 69–89.

———. 1990. Latinas and AIDS: a study. Unpublished data.

Arguelles, L., and G. J. Romero. In press. "The Communication Networks of Transnational Mexican Female Labor in Los Angeles: A Critical Investigation with Implications for Policy and Program Formulation." In A. Mattelart, ed., *Communication and Class Struggle*. Paris: General Press.

Blackwood, E. 1984. "Breaking the Mirror: The Construction of Lesbianism and the Anthropological Discourse on Homosexuality." In E. Blackwood, ed., *The Many Faces of Behavior*. New York: Harrington Park Press.

Center for Disease Control. 1992. *HIV/AIDS Surveillance Report*. 1 (July): 1–18.

Davila, M. 1989. Personal communication to the authors.

Espin, O. 1984. "Cultural and Historical Influences on Sexuality in Hispanic/Latina Women." In C. S. Vance, ed., *Pleasure and Danger: Explorations and Challenges*. Boston: Routledge and Kegan Paul.

Garcia, H., L. Arguelles, G. J. Romero, G. Cadena, and A. M. Rivero. April 1990. "Distrust of AIDS Public Information: A Study of Latino and African-American Attitudes." Paper presented at the annual meeting of the National Association of Chicano Studies, University of New Mexico.

Golden, C. 1987. Diversity and Variability in Women's Sexual Identities. In Boston Lesbian Psychologies Collective, eds., *Lesbian Psychologies: Exploration and Challenges*. Champaign: University of Illinois Press.

Gross, J. 1987. Bleak Lives: Women Carrying AIDS. *New York Times*, August 27, A-1.

Hearst, N., and S. B. Hulley. 1988. "Preventing the Heterosexual Spread of AIDS: Are We Giving Our Patients the Best Advice?" *Journal of the American Medical Association* 80: 49–59.

Livingston, I. L. 1988. "Co-Factors, Host Susceptibility and AIDS: An Argument for Stress." *Journal of the National Medical Association* 80: 49–59.

Lugones, M. 1990. "Playfulness, 'World'-Travelling and Loving Perception." In G. Anzaldua, ed. *Making Face, Making Soul*. San Francisco: Aunt Lute.

Magana, R. 1989. Personal communication to the authors.

Marmour, M., L. R. Weiss, M. Lyden, S. H. Weiss, W. C. Saxinger, and T. J. Spira. 1986. "Possible Female to Female Transmission of Human Immunodeficiency Virus." *Annals of Internal Medicine* 64: 969.

Mays, V. M. and S. D. Cochran. 1988. "Issues in the Perception and Risk Reduction Activities by Black and Hispanic/Latina Women." *American Psychologist* 43: 949–57.

Mirande, A., and E. Enriquez. 1979. *La Chicana: The Mexican-American Woman*. Chicago: University of Chicago Press.

Mora, M., and A. R. del Castillo. 1980. *Mexican Women in the United States: Struggles*

Past and Present. Los Angeles: Occasional Paper No. 2, UCLA Chicano Studies Research Center.

Nieto-Gomez, A. 1976. Heritage of La Hembra. In S. Cox, ed., *Female Psychology: The Emerging Self.* Chicago: Science Research Associates.

Padilla, E. R. and K. E. O'Grady. 1987. "Sexuality Among Mexican Americans: A Case of Sexual Stereotyping." *Journal of Personality and Social Psychology* 2: 5–10.

Perez, E. April 1990. "A Chicana Lesbian Feminist Plenary." Annual meeting of the National Association of Chicano Studies, University of New Mexico.

Ramos, J. 1987. Ed., *Companeras: Latina Lesbians.* New York: Latina Lesbian History Project.

Rivero, A. M., and L. Arguelles. 1989. Female sex partners of IV drug users in Long Beach and surrounding areas: a needs assessment study. Unpublished data.

Rogers, M. F. and W. Williams. Spring 1987. "AIDS in Blacks and Hispanics: Implications for Prevention." *Issues in Science and Technology*, 91.

Romero, G. J. August 1989. "Latina Sexuality." Paper presented at the National Conference on HIV Infection and AIDS Among Racial and Ethnic Populations, Washington, D.C.

———. February 1990. "The Politics of Latina Sexuality." Paper presented at the Latinas and AIDS: Nuestra Conference, Los Angeles.

———, and L. Arguelles. July 1990. "La Malinche, la Virgen, y Sonia Braga: A Critical Assessment of Latina Sexuality." Paper presented at the IV International Conference on Hispanic Cultures, University of Mainz, Germersheim, Federal Republic of Germany.

———. 1990. Technical Report on Knowledge, Attitudes and Beliefs about AIDS. Prepared for Avance Human Services, Los Angeles, Calif.

Romero, G. J., F. G. Castro, and R. Cervantes. 1988. "Latinas without Work: Family, Occupational, and Economic Stress Following Unemployment." *Psychology of Women Quarterly* 12: 281–87.

Sanchez R., and R. Martinez Cruz. 1977. *Essays on la Mujer.* Los Angeles: UCLA Chicano Studies Research Center.

Soja, E. W. 1989. *Postmodern Geographies: The Reassertion of Space in Critical Social Theory.* London: Verso Press.

Trevino, F. M. and A. J. Moss. 1984. "Health Indicators for Hispanic, Black, and White Americans." *Vital Health and Statistics* 10: 148, DHHS Pub. No. (PHS) 84-1576.

Williams, W. 1986. *The Spirit and the Flesh: Sexual Diversity in American Indian Culture.* Boston: Beacon Press.

The Use of Women's Culture in AIDS Outreach

MARY ROMERO

Introduction

Epidemiological studies have segmented populations at high risk for contacting Human Immunodeficiency Virus (HIV) infection (Allen and Curran 1988; Brown and Primm 1988; Fineberg 1988; Heyward and Curran 1988). Although more than 90 percent of Acquired Immune Deficiency Syndrome (AIDS) cases in the United States are male, several recent studies have detailed the spread of the disease among women (Guinan and Hardy 1987a, 1987b; Haverkos and Edelman 1988; Schneider 1989). They have also noted that heterosexual male cases and female cases are disproportionately represented in minority communities. In 1986, 70 percent of infected women were Latinas or African Americans (Guinan and Hardy 1987a).

Until recently preventive measures against the AIDS virus were aimed primarily at gay males and male intravenous (IV) drug users. However, there is a small but growing literature dealing with the prevention of AIDS in women. Some of this literature comes from the popular press and has been published in *Self*, *Playgirl*, *Vogue*, and the like. Unfortunately, this literature is unlikely to reach those most at risk—poor women of color. Several investigators have emphasized the necessity of understanding issues of status, power, and cultural background in tailoring educational messages to women at risk (Flaskerud 1988; MacCormack 1988; Mitchell 1988; Weissman 1988; Staver 1987; Shaw and Paleo 1986; Shaw 1988).

353

Most of the literature focuses on defining female at-risk populations, delimiting specific risk behaviors, identifying appropriate educational messages, and discussing factors which might inhibit the adoption of risk reduction procedures. Two populations have received specific attention: female intravenous drug users (IVDUs) (Cohen, Haver, and Wofsy 1989; Schneider 1988) and prostitutes (Cohen, Alexander, and Wofsy 1988; Rosenberg and Weiner 1988; Seidlin et al. 1988; Shaw 1988).

It was not until recently that another female at-risk population, the sexual partners of male IV drug users, began to be studied. Previously there have been no studies of projects specifically designed to introduce behavioral changes among poor women of color at risk for HIV infection. Beginning in 1988, the National Institute of Drug Abuse (NIDA) required the demonstration outreach and education program workers that it funded to include female sexual partners of IV drug users. Unable to rely on existing models, program workers faced new challenges in creating outreach techniques to reach this previously ignored population. A sexual partners unit called "SOULS" was created as part of a Northwestern City Program. The following paper reports preliminary findings of an ethnographic and participant observation study aimed at identifying and describing specific components of the SOULS' outreach.

Background

The National Institute on Drug Abuse (NIDA) was created by the United States Congress in 1971 to prevent heroin abuse. As AIDS appeared among intravenous-drug-using populations, the agency gained a new concern. In 1987 the National AIDS Demonstration Research (NADR) and the AIDS Targeted Outreach Model (ATOM) were created. Twenty-seven cities received NADR funding to develop models for providing education about safe sex and the transmission of the HIV virus via contaminated injection equipment. Directed primarily by drug researchers (including ethnographers, sociologists, epidemiologists, and psychologists), NADR projects developed a street-based ethnography and outreach approach—the reach and teach bleach model—to combat AIDS among IV drug users. Using models generated from the NADR projects, the ATOM projects provided education and distributed condoms and bleach to IV drug users. Although both NADR and ATOM projects sought to hire persons from the indigenous communities they served, almost all professional staff and administrators were white males. Regardless of educational experience, Latinos and African Americans tended to be concentrated in positions aimed at outreach rather than research.

The emphasis on changing male drug-use practices and sexual behavior is in part a historical artifact. When AIDS began to threaten drug users, it was predominately white male drug ethnographers and Latino and African-

American male street gang workers who first offered a practical technology for reaching what was thought by some to be an unreachable population. Using ethnographic data primarily collected by Latino and African-American male outreach workers, researchers described IV drug practices and social networks of inner-city IV drug users and developed outreach and educational programs based on the findings. Ethnographers from several cities more or less simultaneously developed a "bleach protocol" as a result of examining needle-sharing routines (Watters 1987; Margolis and Broadhead 1989). It was within this male-dominated setting that programs to educate female sexual partners were introduced. The street approach has been demonstrably successful in convincing male IV drug users to use bleach to clean their injection equipment. But this style of outreach is essentially gender specific, geared toward the lifestyle of males who congregate on the street corners rather than females who are less likely to participate in street culture. Analysis of the development of specific programs aimed at serving women reveals how entrenched male culture has been in the battle against AIDS.

Even though the original NADR/ATOM program included women IV drug users and prostitutes, it soon became apparent that women were not being well served. Rather than develop specific models and programs for women, NIDA targeted the wives and female lovers of IV drug users as the unserved population. Consequently, in 1988 NIDA awarded specific grants to NOVA Research Company to develop programs for outreach and prevention to the "sexual partners" of IV drug users. The grants funded programs to provide services to women as "sexual partners" of male IV drug users. From its inception, the program was geared at reaching women; however, NIDA's definition of the target population as non-using sexual partners of male drug users did not include IV drug users and prostitutes. Furthermore, the assumption was that programs aimed at IV drug users were not gender specific and served both men and women. Although NIDA's social construction of a new social group, the "sexual partners" of IV drug users, did not challenge the outreach and prevention model based on male drug use, the new program did create an opportunity for exploring new alternatives to AIDS outreach.

The Female Sexual Partners Unit of the Northwestern City's Consortium to Combat AIDS was initiated in February 1988—at a time when the rate of sero-conversion for sexual partners of IV drug users was estimated to exceed the rate of new infection among IV drug users. Although the general wisdom among program directors had been that the traditional outreach and education aimed at male IV drug users was inappropriate for women, a model of prevention had not yet been developed. Various methods being tested in outreach and education included: empowerment, negotiation skills and safer-sex-skills training, holistic approaches, self-help groups, and professionally led support groups. My initial interest in the SOULS' outreach was to examine their development of an innovative approach that is based on a practical understanding of *women's culture.*

SOULS and the Initial Stages

The unit consisted of a full-time program coordinator with a master's degree in social work, a consultant, and four Community Health Outreach Workers (CHOWs), referred to as the "SOULS." Although in this city the largest numbers of needle users are white males, presumably with female partners, the white male project directors identified the at-risk population of female sexual partners of IV drug users as largely made up of low-income African Americans and Latinas. Consequently, the CHOWs recruited to be SOULS were African-American and Latina women who had personal histories working or living in the communities they served. The original team of SOULS consisted of three African-American women and one Latina woman, ranging in age from mid-twenties to mid-fifties. The team included both lesbians and heterosexuals. All the SOULS had completed some college courses, and one had started graduate work.

Unlike other units in the Northwestern City Consortium, the sexual partners' unit attempted to work closely together, utilizing a team approach in their activities. Most of the other Community Health Outreach Workers (CHOWs) employed by the Northwestern City Consortium were assigned a particular area and worked individually in their outreach efforts. Furthermore, the SOULS were the only all-woman unit in the agency; however, several of the other units were staffed only by men. All other units of the Northwestern City Consortium were headed by a male coordinator, and the units were assigned specific neighborhoods of the city. The significance of these differences became more evident as I conducted my research.

Several phases occurred in the development of an adequate model to reach the wives and women lovers of IV drug users. All new CHOWs, including the SOULS, were required to attend a ten-day, comprehensive training program. Although the training included discussions about women and drugs, the program was overwhelmingly aimed at work with male IV drug users. The basic outreach procedure consisted of working the streets—that is, locating areas where IV drug users congregate, giving out one-ounce bottles of bleach and condoms, developing rapport with street corner groups, and using that rapport to explain AIDS risk factors and how to prevent transmission of the virus.

Proposals for shaping outreach to sexual partners reveal how entrenched male culture was among the various program administrators working with IV drug users. Proposals were predicated on assumptions about the sexual partners of male IV drug users. Suggested techniques included hanging out at street corners talking to women about safe sex, *paying* male drug users to bring in their sexual partners to fill out questionnaires, and soliciting the sexual partners of drug users currently in recovery programs. Other than vague concepts like carrying outreach activities into laundromats, the training offered few techniques to reach the wives and female lovers of IV drug users.

Following the training, the SOULS began to explore specific methods for locating the targeted population and began to develop types of educational programs that might reach women sexually involved with IV drug users. Importantly, the SOULS coordinator began establishing team spirit by incorporating her new-hires directly into program planning. Possessing professional and personal expertise in street and ethnic community outreach, the women of color on the SOULS team looked for ways to translate the basic goals of providing AIDS education and the technology of prevention into specific patterns of outreach to women.

The next phase in the development of an outreach model occurred in a two-week-in-service workshop, during which researchers from Northwestern City working in the area of AIDS and women, particularly prostitutes, met to share findings and discuss current programs. The SOULS followed up by visiting agencies in the city and surrounding communities to collect detailed information on the operational techniques of other programs. Two of the most advanced programs that shared intervention techniques and offered to assist in the SOULS activities were programs serving the prostitute community in Northwestern City.

Phase three consisted of ethnographic mapping of the target population. The goal of the ethnography was to locate women and identify their various ages, ethnic groups, and activities. By analyzing various characteristics of the target population of women, outreach workers determined the best way to access the population. The SOULS explored the areas where IV drug users lived. They talked to people on the streets, in the hotels and public housing projects, searching for families, particularly wives and lovers of IV drug users.

Identifying the characteristics of the target population revealed several problems with NIDA's construct of sexual partners of IV drug users as non-drug-using women. First of all, IV drug users were both men and women. Secondly, the sexual partners of IV drug users included men. Thirdly, NIDA's categories of target populations were based on the assumption that the wives or lovers of male IV drug users were not addicts themselves. While male IV drug users "often prefer and have spouses or old ladies who are not addicts," women "had mates who are either addicts or ex-addicts" (Rosen-baum 1981, 1201). The mapping process uncovered a small population of women who were not using drugs and who were the sexual partners of IV drug users. This finding was most likely the function of male IV drug users concealing their drug usage from their wives and lovers. Committed to the creation of a women's unit, the SOULS rejected the inclusion of male sexual partners of IV drug users and broadened their client load to include all women who were *potential* partners of IV drug users, regardless of their own drug use.

Gradually all the units in the Northwestern City Consortium came to define "sexual partners" as women and all women clients as the service domain of the sexual partner's unit. When the target population was broadened to include essentially all poor women in the service area, many of the CHOWs in the other units began referring women clients to the SOULS. By solidifying relationships with other agencies addressing the needs of poor women, the SOULS became known as the women's unit in the Northwestern City Consortium. They began to distribute condoms and bleach and provide education to these outside agencies.

Phase four was direct intervention, or, as one SOUL commented, "taking the office to the street." However, in this case the office was actually taken to single-room occupancy hotels, shelters, public housing projects, laundromats, and anywhere else women could be found.

The path was not easy. The SOULS had to educate both their bosses and their co-workers about how women's lifestyles were different from the IV drug culture of men. The first obstacle the SOULS faced was creating an identity as an administrative unit distinct from the male-dominated parent outreach program serving IV drug users. Innovative outreach methods and requests for autonomy were met with opposition from the all-male administrative staff. The women struggled to establish precedence for participating in untraditional street outreach.

Wives and lovers of IV drug users did not congregate on street corners, and female IV drug users who may hit the streets to "cop" generally did not hang out. Women sexually involved with male IV drug users typically were either employed or spent much of their time in their homes caring for children. Many of the clients were African-American women with two to three children living in a single-room occupancy hotel and on welfare. Because of the structure of government programs such as AFDC and welfare, poor women are made responsible for the home and housing. They take responsibility for the family and coping with the daily problems of the poor—paying the rent, clothing their children, buying food, standing on line for health care: the list goes on.

The SOULS realized they faced two major obstacles in reaching their targeted population:

> (1) they had to gain access to these women and compete for time with pressing family obligations. As one women client put it, "If you want to talk to me about AIDS you better get in line with the rest of the shit!"

> (2) AIDS education had to be packaged to a population whose daily worries might also include homelessness, hunger, illness, and physical abuse.

Developing a Prevention Model
Based on Women's Culture

Using the insight they were developing into the lifestyle of women involved with IV drug users, the SOUL team incorporated a strong sense of women's culture into their outreach. Outreach was shaped around an understanding of the lifestyle and needs of poor women. Building bonds of trust with the women was accomplished by serving as advocates in the process of helping clients gain public assistance. The SOULS listened closely to their needs—such as food, housing, clothing, and health care—and assisted the women in contacting agencies and walking them through the system. In order to create an environment to discuss AIDS, the SOULS had to help out with each woman's present crisis. They conceived strategies that placed AIDS education within a larger context that took into account the more pressing priorities in the women's lives.

One of the SOULS observed that a "home"—or, as she termed it, a "nest,"—was an extremely high priority in these women's lives. If they wanted to reach these women they had to find a way to be invited to their "nest." So the SOULS acquired a room in a hotel where many of their clients resided. They named the space "A Room of Her Own," and they invited women in the hotel to come and visit. They offered coffee and cookies and a place to relax and talk. Having a physical space in the hotel near their target population provided entrée to these women, who are closely tied to home and family. The "home-like" environment created an atmosphere in which women could discuss their intimate relations and explore ways to change their sexual behavior. Women needed more than information about AIDS and access to condoms. They needed the opportunity to discuss ways to introduce condoms into their relationship. Unlike CHOWS distributing condoms to gay or heterosexual male IV drug users on street corners and in parks, the SOULS team had to confront the cultural baggage attached to condom use before many of the women would take the condoms. Creating a space for women to congregate allowed frank discussions about male and female conflict over safe sex. In a female-dominated setting, the SOULS could use women's sexual joking to lessen their clients' inhibitions and to provide detailed information about safe and unsafe sex practices. Because males were not present, cultural constraints that favor women thinking about sex as passive actors were lessened.

Another way in which the SOULS team established contact was to bring the women a "gift." The SOULS built on the CHOW practice of exchanging "gifts" with clients. CHOW gifts included bottles of bleach, Kwell shampoo, condoms, posters, counseling, education, meals, and referrals. In exchange, clients introduced CHOWs to other potential clients, distributed bleach, guarded CHOWs' cars, and provided protection. Although the SOULS considered the "gift" to be related to the courting ritual that men used, the "gift" was actually an extension of the CHOWs' practice of gift-giving, which might best be described by what A. Daniels referred to as "ingratiating oneself" in the field (1983, 197). Montini (1989) suggested that the exchange of gifts served to keep clients and CHOWs equals, taking the "sting" out of the kind of item offered as a gift and transforming the gift into an expression of affection from the CHOWs to the clients.

Gifts could be simple—a friendly smile and a brief explanation: "I'm from Northwestern City Consortium and I'd like to give you a gift to keep you from getting AIDS." A few condoms and some literature might suffice. But SOULS also used gifts to establish a more enduring relationship. A weekly give-away of used clothes attracted women from the neighborhood to "a room of her own." This activity provided needed and much appreciated clothes for the women and their families. Going "shopping" fulfilled family obligations and also provided the women living with men a "legitimate" excuse to spend time away from home. During the holiday season, food baskets were distributed and presents were given to the children. During all these activities AIDS education proceeded informally and condoms and bleach were distributed. Events centered around "women's work" functioned as a way to separate the women from their IV drug partners in order to provide them with information about the risks they confronted.

The IV drug users that these women were sexually involved with did not necessarily approve of the SOULS' work, particularly the distribution of condoms. In a setting where the male IV drug user denies use or is hiding his use from non-using partners, the introduction of the condom often leads to confrontation. While the distribution of condoms to male IV drug users, alcoholics, and homeless men in the park and street corners stroked male egos and was symbolic of manhood, the distribution of condoms among women carried a negative cultural message. Even women prostitutes who faithfully use condoms with all their johns reported not using a condom with their steady partner. Northwestern City Consortium CHOWs also reported several instances in which women were beaten for attempting to introduce condoms into their sexual relationship. For many heterosexual liaisons, particularly between male IV drug users and female non-users, condoms presented a threat to the relationship. The condom may also be construed as an attack on the man's virility, since IV drug users usually have an absence of or decrease in sexual activity (Rosenbaum 1981). Thus outreach to women had to be particularly sensitive to dangers inherent in the educational message itself. Clothing and food drives helped diffuse the situation. Husbands or lovers became less hostile to participation in the SOULS' activities because they were also obtaining clothes or food. Clothes drives offered an unexpected return as well. New clothes made a real difference in the self-image of women who suffered from low self-esteem. The act of obtaining a "new" dress, sweater, shoes, or handbag allowed women to begin to feel good about themselves. The SOULS' strategy was built on the premise that women need to feel good about their personal worth before they can begin to be empowered to practice safe sex with their partners.

"A room of her own" accomplished more than simply reaching the target population. It created a female-dominated space in which an atmosphere of trust was created. Several afternoons a week, the SOULS would open the room and provide an activity, such as the clothing drive or a workshop. Throughout the week, the space was used by individual SOULS to educate, counsel, and service neighborhood women on a one-to-one basis. "A room of her own" celebrated women's culture and, in the process, helped women make changes in their relationships with their sexual partners. The concept of women's culture has recently appeared in studies exploring the coping and resistance strategies used by women in community organizing and in organizing work places outside the home. By creating the "room of her own," the SOULS team reproduced women's culture to create an environment that not only attracted the population they wished to address, but also produced an ideal setting for empowering women to change sexual practices. The SOULS team's approach to reaching the sexual partners of IV drug users was based on "indigenous" knowledge about women's culture and its use to reach a previously invisible and ignored population. At the same time, it offered insight into a concept that transcends this particular application.

Discussion

The original street outreach to IV drug users aimed at a simple modification of the intravenous drug ritual—introducing bleach to clean their works. Outreach to women is overwhelmingly more complicated and problematic than the model developed for male IV drug users. Preventing AIDS among women invokes profound cultural change; deep seated community norms must be overturned. In general, heterosexual females do not control their bodies or their sexuality. Men initiate sex and generally determine the specific activity. In order to prevent AIDS, women must refuse to participate in unsafe sex and must introduce condoms into their relationships. Unlike bleach, condoms carry cultural stigma. Outreach workers have discovered that condoms frequently represent infidelity, and some women have faced physical danger as a consequence of trying to introduce their use in the relationship.

Although outreach specifically targeted to the sexual partners of IV drug users is still being developed, the inclusion of women's culture will be crucial in the prevention of AIDS among all women. The use of women's culture in developing an outreach model is vital. It is necessary to find and develop sources of empowerment to change culture by leaving or changing sexist relationships. However, this process is extremely slow. Meanwhile, the HIV virus continues to spread, particularly among African-American and Latina women. We have to employ traditional aspects of women's culture to reach women. There is also a parallel need to work with men on issues of sexism and to bring home the message that sexism can kill. AIDS outreach to men must similarly engage in changing community norms and confront the sexist attitudes and values that support unsafe sex. Working with men is essential, because heterosexual women are confronted with the daily reality that men often determine how safe sex will be. Work must be done to help ensure that both partners are recognized and respected as active agents in determining decisions about safe sex.

Acknowledgments

I have profited greatly from my discussions with Teresa Montini and Eric Margolis, and I appreciate their criticisms and suggestions. I also express my thanks to Patrick Biernacki for inviting me to do the study on the Sexual Partners Unit.

The names of the program and the city cited in this essay are pseudonymous.

Works Cited

Allen, J. R., and J. W. Curran. 1988. "Prevention of AIDS and HIV Infection: Needs and Priorities for Epidemiologic Research." *American Journal of Public Health* 78:381–6.

Brown, L. S., Jr., and B. J. Primm. 1988. "Intravenous Drug Abuse and AIDS in Minorities." *AIDS Public Policy Journal* 3(2):5–15.

Cohen, J., P. Alexander, and C. Wofsy. 1988. "Prostitutes and AIDS: Public Policy Issues." *AIDS Public Policy Journal* 3(2):16–22.

Cohen, J., L. B. Haver, and C. Wofsy. 1989. "Women and IV Drugs: Parental and Heterosexual Transmission of the HIV Virus." *Journal of Drug Issues* 19(1):39–56.

Daniels, A. 1983. "Self-Deception and Self-Discovery in Fieldwork." *Qualitative Sociology* 6(3):195–214.

Fineberg, H. V. 1988. "The Social Dimensions of AIDS." *Scientific American* October: 128–34.

Flaskerud, J. H. 1988. "Prevention of AIDS in Blacks and Hispanics: Nursing Implications." *Journal of Community Health Nursing* 5:49–58.

Guinan, M. E., and A. Hardy. 1987a. "Epidemiology of AIDS in Women in the United States, 1981 through 1986." *Journal of the American Medical Association* 257:2039–42.

———. 1987b. "Women and AIDS: The Future is Grim." *Journal of the American Medical Women's Association* 42:157–58.

Haverkos, H. W., and R. Edelman. 1988. "The Epidemiology of Acquired Immune Deficiency Syndrome and HIV Infection among Heterosexuals." *Journal of the American Medical Association* 260:1922–29.

Heyward, W. L. and J. W. Curran. 1988. "The Epidemiology of AIDS in the U. S." *Scientific American* October:72–81.

MacCormack, C. P. 1988. "Health and the Social Power of Women." *Social Science and Medicine* 26:677–83.

Margolis, E., and R. Broadhead. 1989. "Street-Based Outreach in Combating AIDS among IV Drug Users: A Case Study of a Model Project." Unpublished manuscript.

Montini, T. 1989. Unpublished field notes and personal communication.

Mitchell, J. L. 1988. "Women, AIDS, and Public Policy." *AIDS Public Policy Journal* 3(2):50–2.

Rosenbaum, M. 1981. "When Drugs Come into the Picture, Love Flies out the Window: Women Addicts' Love Relations." *International Journal of the Addictions* 16(7): 1197–1206.

Rosenberg, M. J., and J. M. Weiner. 1988. "Prostitutes and AIDS: A Health Department Priority?" *American Journal of Public Health* 78:418–23.

Schneider, B. E. 1988. "Gender, Sexuality and AIDS: Social Responses and Consequences." In R. A. Berk, ed., *The Social Consequences of AIDS in the United States*, pp. 1–11. ABT Books.

———. 1989. "Women and AIDS: An International Perspective." *Futures.*

Seidlin, M., K. Krasinski, D. Bebenroth, V. Itri, A. M. Paolino, and F. Valentine. 1988. "Prevalence of HIV Infection in New York Call Girls." *Journal on AIDS* 1:150–54.

Shaw, N., and L. Paleo. 1986. "Women and AIDS." In L. McKusick, ed., *What To Do About AIDS: Physicians and Mental Health Professionals Discuss the Issues*, pp. 142–54. Berkeley: University of California Press.

Shaw, N. S. 1988. "Preventing AIDS among Women: The Role of Community Organizing." *Socialist Review* 18(4):76–92.

Staver, S. 1987. "Minority Women Grappling with Growing AIDS Problem." *American Medical News* November 6: 61.

Watters, J. K. 1987. "Preventing Human Immunodeficiency Virus Contagion among Intravenous Drug Users: The Impact of Street-Based Education on Risk Behavior." Paper presented at the III International Conference on AIDS, Washington, D. C.

Weissman, G. 1988. "Promoting Health Behavior among Women at Risk for AIDS." *NIDA Notes* Winter:7–8.

NOTES ON CONTRIBUTORS

Lourdes Arguelles, Ph.D., is an Associate Professor of Women's Studies and Chicano Studies, and holds the MacArthur Chair in Women's Studies at Pitzer College, Claremont, California. A former director of the AIDS Research and Education Project in Long Beach, California, she is a licensed psychotherapist working through the Pomona Valley Gay and Lesbian Coalition Counseling Services. Dr. Arguelles also teaches at the Claremont Graduate School and at the University of California, Los Angeles. She has published numerous articles on Latinos and Latinas in national and international academic journals.

Caroline Westbrook Arnold, D.Sc., is an Assistant Professor at the University of Massachusetts, Boston, and a Research Associate at the Center for Research on Women at Wellesley College, Wellesley, Massachusetts. A native of Austin, Texas, she was educated in the public schools there, at Mills College, Howard University, and Harvard University School of Public Health.

Brenda Child is a doctoral candidate in American History at the University of Iowa. She is a member of the Red Lake Band of the Chippewa Tribe. Her dissertation is entitled "A Bitter Lesson: Chippewas and the Government Boarding School Experience, 1879–1940." She teaches in the History Department at the University of Wisconsin, Milwaukee.

Michael C. Clatts is a doctoral candidate in the Department of Anthropology at the State University of New York at Stony Brook. His principal area of interest is the study of social change, particularly the formulation of strategies with which to direct it. His doctoral research was sponsored by the Agency for International Development and concerned the role of gender systems in community responses to economic development programs in the Philippines. He began research relating to AIDS in 1982, while working with the National Cancer Institute on the first multi-city epidemiological study of risk factors. For the past several years he has been engaged in street-based ethnographic research relating to AIDS in New York City, and he is currently conducting research in Harlem in conjunction with an AIDS intervention program supported by the National Institute on Drug Abuse.

Priscilla Ferguson Clement is an Associate Professor of History at Pennsylvania State University, Delaware County Campus. A specialist in the field of U. S. social welfare history, she is the author of *Welfare and Poverty in the Nineteenth Century City, Philadelphia 1800 to 1854* (Fairleigh Dickinson University Press, 1985), as well as several articles and book chapters on impoverished children, the aged, and the wandering poor in nineteenth-century America. She is co-editor of two forthcoming volumes on the history of juvenile delinquency in Western nations and is currently working on a study of how impoverished women were cared for in representative American cities from 1800 to the present.

Carol M. Cummings, M.A., A.B.D., is a doctoral candidate in the Department of Psychology at the University of Michigan. Her primary research interests are health and medical psychology; psychosocial factors in health status; blood pressure; immune deficiency; and women's health issues. She is a native of Louisville, Kentucky.

Sheila P. Davis, R.N., M.S.N., is an Assistant Professor at the University of Alabama School of Nursing, University of Alabama at Birmingham. A doctoral candidate in Nursing at Georgia State University, her research interests include bicultural stress among ethnic nurse educators and issues involving cultural diversity. As a master's-prepared cardiovascular nurse specialist, she has engaged in numerous health promotion/disease prevention activities that have targeted ethnic communities. Presently she is completing a study documenting nurses' knowledge regarding dark skin assessment.

Frenzella Elaine De Lancey is an Assistant Professor in the Humanities Department at Drexel University, Philadelphia, where she is currently coordinator of the African American Studies Minor. She is the former recipient of a Ford Foundation Fellowship for Minority Students. Her dissertation, "Intertextuality and Willful Transformation as Narrative Strategies in African-American Women's Writing," which she has recently revised for publication, received honorable mention from the National Council for the Humanities. Her principal area of research at this time is the work of Sonia Sanchez.

Denise Drevdahl, R.N., M.S., is an Assistant Professor in the Department of Nursing, Northern Arizona University, Flagstaff. Her background is in community health, with an emphasis on assessing needs and implementing community-based programs. Her research interests include Native American women's health beliefs, health policy, and development of community-support interest groups promoting health programs for the underserved.

Linda Dumas, R.N., Ph.D., is a nurse sociologist and Assistant Professor in the College of Nursing, University of Massachusetts at Boston. She is in practice with the Boston Visiting Nurses Association as an inner city, home care clinician and has worked with individuals and families in urban communities for twenty years. She continues to focus applied research interests on health program planning for low-income community individuals and families. Her research interests are focused on urban health problems related to poverty, gender, race, and aging.

Katherine Fennelly, Ph.D., is an Associate Professor of Health Education at Pennsylvania State University, where she also holds an appointment at the Population Issues Resource Center and is an affiliate of the Women's Studies Program. Previously an Associate Professor of Clinical Public Health at Columbia University, she has lived and worked in Latin America, first as a CARE representative in Ecuador, and later as a Field Representative for the Latin American Regional Office of the International Planned Parenthood Federation. For the past several years she has conducted research and written extensively on childbearing among Hispanic adolescents in the United States.

Nikky Finney, author of *On Wings Made of Gauze* (New York: William Morrow, 1986), has recently completed another book of poetry, *Rice*, and her first novel, *While Others Played and Chased the Sun*. She is a frequent contributor to *Catalyst* and *Essence* magazines as well as the regional literary journals *Callaloo* and *Southern Black Writer*. She was a Visiting Professor of Creative Writing at the University of Kentucky, Lexington, in 1990, and became an Assistant Professor in the English Department in 1991. She has since returned to the Bay Area in California to write and teach.

Wonda Lee Fontenot, Ph.D., University of California, Berkeley, is Director of Wommanuse Institute for the Study of Arts, Culture, and Ethnicity, Post Office Box 92342, Lafayette, Louisiana, 70509. Her scholarship is concerned with ethno-medicine, specifically the link between culture and physiological factors affecting the well being and health care quality of rural and ethnic populations. She has also studied racial/cultural mixing between African Americans and Native Americans in the United States.

Barbara Frye, R.N., Dr.P.H., is an Associate Professor in International Health at Loma Linda University School of Public Health. Her background is in refugee health, both in the United States and internationally. Her specific area of interest is the health seeking behavior of refugee populations.

Shirley A. Hill is a doctoral candidate in the Department of Sociology, University of Kansas, where she is specializing in the family and medical sociology, with a specific interest in how families cope with chronically ill children.

Cora A. Ingram, R.N., M.S., C.N.S., is an Assistant Professor at the University of Alabama School of Nursing, University of Alabama at Birmingham. She has held numerous positions in both academic and clinical settings, and has presented papers to professional groups on a wide variety of issues. Her teaching and research interests include policy development in schools of nursing, minority health issues, at-risk students, cultural diversity, and family dynamics. Currently she is a doctoral student in the Program in Administration in Higher Education at the University of Alabama at Tuscaloosa.

Teresa C. Jacob, Ph.D., was born in Brazil, where she first began her studies in psychology. In 1978 she moved to the United States and received her Ph.D. in psychology from the University of California, San Diego, in 1985. Her research endeavors focus on women of color and health issues. She presently teaches at Grossmont College and is affiliated with the UCSD School of Medicine as a Research Associate.

Valli Kanuha, M.S.W., has worked in community health settings and the battered women's movement since 1975. She has organized numerous programs for women of color, facilitated support groups for battered lesbians, and served as a consultant, trainer, and volunteer with many battered-women's programs and feminist organizations. She is the author of several articles on violence against women, feminist therapy, and HIV/AIDS and other health issues. She has been the Assistant Director of Education at Gay Men's Health Crisis, a large AIDS organization in New York City, and is currently Deputy Director at the Hetrick-Martin Institute in New York City.

Diane K. Lewis, Ph.D., is a Professor of Anthropology at the University of California, Santa Cruz. During a sabbatical year (1986-1987) she returned to school to study epidemiology and received an M.P.H. Since 1987 she has been a collaborator in the San Francisco-based Urban Health Study, which does outreach, HIV testing, and interviewing about risk behaviors and AIDS awareness among IV drug users, with the goal of monitoring and preventing the spread of the AIDS virus. She has published articles on IV drug users and risk in *Social Science and Medicine* (1989), *American Journal of Public Health* (1990), and *AIDS* (1991). She plans to continue studying the impact of the AIDS epidemic on women of color.

Alice Longman, Ed.D., is a Professor in the College of Nursing at the University of Arizona, where she has taught at the graduate and undergraduate levels for fifteen years. Her clinical research is in the area of oncology nursing.

Gretchen E. Lopez, M.A., A.B.D., is a doctoral candidate in psychology at the University of Michigan. Her research addresses the impact of social contexts on political thinking. Her specific research interests include the development of gender and race consciousness within higher education. She is a native of Buffalo, New York.

Lois Lyles, Ph.D., is an Assistant Professor of English at San Francisco State University. Her areas of specialization are English Renaissance poetry and twentieth-century African-American literature. She writes poetry and fiction.

Joanne B. Mulcahy, Ph.D., is affiliated with the Northwest Writing Institute at Lewis and Clark College, where she teaches interdisciplinary courses on gender, culture, and folklore. She is the former Coordinator of the Oregon Folk Arts and Folklife Program at Lewis and Clark College. Among her areas of specialization are women's life histories, traditional arts and aesthetics, and narrative theory. She is working with Mary Petersen on a longer version of Mary's life history and conducting research on women's stories about sexual violence. She was previously the Program Coordinator for the Kodiak Women's Resource Center, where she was responsible for the arrangement of safe homes for women in danger from domestic violence.

Nolan E. Penn, Ph.D., is currently a Professor in the Department of Psychiatry at the University of California, San Diego, School of Medicine, as well as Associate Chancellor. He received his doctoral degree in psychology from Denver University in Colorado, and completed post-doctoral work in the Department of Psychiatry at the University of Wisconsin, Madison, and at the Harvard Medical School. His longstanding interest in illness prevention and comprehensive health care delivery has motivated his study of issues affecting the early detection and prevention of disease.

Mary Petersen lives part of the year in the village of Akhiok on Kodiak Island, Alaska, and an additional part at a fish camp near the village. She was born near Akhiok and raised according to Alutiiq traditions. Trained as a traditional healer, she recently returned to the village to work as the Community Health Aide. She has also taught the Alutiiq language and traditional Aleut basketmaking in the Anchorage and Kodiak schools.

Beth E. Richie, M.S.W., Ph.D., is an activist in the movement to end violence against women. She is the former co-chair of the Women of Color Task Force Against Domestic Violence and a founding member of the Women of Color Organizing Project, Leadership Institute for Women. Currently she is a faculty member in the Program in Community Health Education at Hunter

College. She earned her doctorate in the Program in Sociology at the City University of New York.

Anne M. Rivero, M.S.W., L.C.S.W., is a Clinical Social Worker with the Day Treatment Program of the Pomona Valley Mental Health Center, Pomona, California, and the Pomona Valley Gay and Lesbian Coalition. Previously a therapist with the Los Angeles County-University of Southern California Mental Health Clinic, she has worked extensively with persons living with AIDS. She has also published and conducted numerous workshops on Latinas and AIDS.

Adrienne M. Robinson, B.A., is a graduate of the University of Michigan Department of Sociology. She is currently a graduate student in Public Policy at the New School for Social Research in New York, where she is specializing in urban renewal and development issues. She is originally from Detroit, Michigan.

Gregoria Rodriguez is the project director of a multidisciplinary study of contributing factors associated with an increase of neural tube defects in Cameron County, Texas. She is a doctoral student in the Sociomedical Sciences Division of the Department of Preventive Medicine and Community Health at the University of Texas Medical Branch, Galveston, Texas. Her interests include minority and Third-World women's health issues, minority and international health policy, and U. S.–Mexico border health.

Gloria J. Romero, Ph.D., is an Associate Professor of Psychology at California State University, Los Angeles. She is the former recipient of both a Ford Foundation Postdoctoral Fellowship for Minority Group Scholars and a Rockefeller Foundation Postdoctoral Fellowship. Her research interests include Latinas and unemployment, Latinas and AIDS, and Latinos and political empowerment. She has published widely on these issues and has spoken about them at local, national, and international conferences. She is actively involved in several Chicano community organizations.

Mary Romero, Ph.D., is an Associate Professor in the Department of Sociology at the University of Oregon, Eugene. She has published numerous articles on Chicana workers, the impact of affirmative action and the appropriation of Chicano culture. She has been extensively involved in the development of curricula for Chicano studies courses in sociology and the integration of women of color into ethnic studies and sociology course curricula.

Michelle Saint-Germain, Ph.D., is an Assistant Professor in the Department of Political Science at the University of Texas at El Paso. She is a former

Research Associate at the Southwest Institute for Research on Women at the University of Arizona. Her research interests include women, politics, and public policy, with specializations in the areas of health, Hispanics, and Central America.

Ama R. Saran, M.S.W., is a mediator, translator, activist, and academic. From 1984 to 1990 she was Core Consultant with the National Black Women's Health Project. By May 1992 she plans to have a Ph.D. in one hand in Africana women's studies, and by June 1992, an M.P.H. in the other in maternal and child health. Current work and future plans center on domestic and international work in health education and promotion on women's health and AIDS.

Leslie E. Spieth, B.A., traveled extensively overseas during her childhood. Her father taught English literature and moved the family from place to place while garnering experiences and observations for his own writing. During this time, Spieth was exposed to a variety of cultures and lifestyles, which led to her interest in studying human behavior and medical systems. She graduated with honors from the University of California, San Diego, and is currently completing a Master's degree in psychology at San Diego State University. She intends to pursue doctoral work in the area of psychological applications to medicine.

Françoise Vergès is from Reunion Island (Indian Ocean) and has participated in the anti-colonialist movement there. After moving to France in 1971, she became involved in the women's liberation movement (through the group Pyschoanalysis and Politics) and, as a journalist for the magazine *Des Femmes en Mouvements*, she wrote extensively on women's movements in the Third World. She is presently a graduate student in the political science Ph.D. program at the University of California, Berkeley, and is currently working on women, creolization, and *metissage*. Her forthcoming publications include "Memories of Origins: Sexual Difference and Feminist Polity," *RAGE* (1991), and, with Kathleen B. Jones, "Toutes avec Tous: Women, Politics and the Paris Commune of 1871," *Women's Studies International Forum* (1991), and "Aux Citoyennes: Women's Politics, Democratic Culture, and the Paris Commune of 1871," *The History of European Ideas* (Summer 1991).

Gloria Waite, Ph.D., is an Assistant Professor at Southeastern Massachusetts University, where she teaches African and African-American history. Her publications include *A History of Traditional Medicine and Health Care in Pre-Colonial East-Central Africa* (1991); "The Politics of Disease: The AIDS Virus and Africa," in *AIDS in Africa: The Social and Policy Impact*, eds.

Norman Miller and Richard Rockwell (1988); "Some Useful Plants in East-Central Africa: A Cross-Cultural Ethnobotanical Survey," in *Monographs in Systematic Botany, Missouri Botanical Garden* (1988); "Public Health in Pre-Colonial East-Central Africa," in *Social Science and Medicine* (1987); "Spirit Possession Dance in East-Central Africa," in *Journal of the Association of Graduate Dance Ethnologists UCLA* (1980); and "The Socio-Political Role of Healing Churches in South Africa," in *Ufahamu* (1976).

ABOUT THE EDITORS

Barbara Bair, Ph.D., is a Fellow of the Virginia Center for the Humanities, Charlottesville, and was for many years an Associate of the James B. Coleman African Studies Center at the University of California, Los Angeles. She has taught interdisciplinary courses in American literature, women and health, and American cultural and social history. She has published in the fields of feminist literary criticism, health care policy, Pan-Africanism, and African-American and women's history. Before pursuing her graduate degrees, she worked as a nursing assistant and home health aide for the Social Services Department of the County of Santa Cruz, California. An expert on the Garvey movement, she is the author of work on women in the movement; the associate editor of volumes six and seven of *The Marcus Garvey and Universal Negro Improvement Association Papers* (University of California Press, 1989, 1990) and of *Marcus Garvey: Life and Lessons* (1987); and a consulting and contributing editor for *Africa for the Africans: The Marcus Garvey and Universal Negro Improvement Association Papers African Series*. She has been the recipient of Mellon and Rockefeller post-doctoral fellowships, the latter in affiliation with the program for the integration of race, class, and gender at the Institute for Research on Women, Rutgers University. She is currently at work on a book on African-American women's activism and the construction of gender.

Susan E. Cayleff, Ph.D., is Professor in the Department of Women's Studies at San Diego State University. She teaches American women's history from a multi-cultural perspective, women and health, women's sexuality, and women and sports. Her research and publication interests include folk healing ways, self-help and patent medicines, women in alternative healing sects, women within biotechnical medicine, and Western conceptions of female physiology. She has published *Wash and Be Healed: The Water-Cure Movement and Women's Health* (Temple University Press, 1987, 1992) as well as numerous articles and reviews on women's history and the history of medicine. Prior to teaching at SDSU, she taught at the University of Texas Medical Branch at Galveston (1983–87). There she taught women's history, the history of medicine, and medical ethics to medical students and clinical faculty. She also developed a clinical teaching affiliation with the Department of Obstetrics and Gynecology and the School of Nursing. She has recently completed *The Golden Cyclone: The Life and Legend of Babe Didrikson Zaharias 1911–1956*, for the University of Illinois Press. Other forthcoming books include *Breaking Trails: An Oral History of Women Athletes in Twentieth-Century America* (Temple University Press) and *Keeping to the Path: A History of Naturopathic Healing and Professionalism in Twentieth Century America.*

SOME FURTHER SOURCES

Approaches within the fields of women's studies have in many ways
paralleled developments in ethnic studies: the two meet in the subject area of
health and women of color. As academic disciplines which—like women's
studies—originated in a sociopolitical movement, African-American Studies
and its counterparts (Native-American, Asian-American, and Chicano studies)
have emphasized the scrutiny of institutions of repression, the politics of
disenfranchisement, and unequal access to rights and opportunities, including
unequal access to medical education and medical care. Researchers have also
sought to regain knowledge about heritage and pay tribute to outstanding
individuals of color. In terms of the study of health care, this has meant
fostering appreciation for self-help movements, philosophies, and traditions
of care within communities of color and heralding the contributions of lay
and professional practitioners of color to medicine and healing. In response
to these kinds of emphases in ethnic studies, scholars in other fields began
to introduce the issues of poverty and ethnicity into work that previously
considered only the experiences of middle-class or working-class whites.

The burgeoning of the field of women's history in the 1970s brought
with it the growth of a sub-specialty in the history of health care, one
which focused on the white female experience. The growth of this subfield
mirrored the range of approaches to women's history itself, which began
with a focus on individual women who succeeded in traditionally "male"
professional fields and on the history of women's exclusion or oppression.
Later interpretations branched out into studies of representative women; their
work culture; their participation in social movements, labor unions, and
professional organizations; and the patterns of their daily lives. Researchers
also began to ask questions about the cultural "difference" between men and
women and about the patterns of social and psychological construction of
traditionally-gendered values and orientations. Only in the past few years
has this social-historical approach been significantly broadened beyond the
study of the experiences of middle-class and working-class white women
to include women of color and cross-cultural comparisons. Similarly, the
subfields of the history and sociology of women and health began in force

in the 1970s with studies of women as practitioners (midwives, healers, nurses, and physicians); their access to or exclusion from educational and professional institutions; their regulation by the medical infrastructure and the legal system; their acceptance or limitation within given circumstances and according to social mores; and the experience of women as patients in a male-dominated health care system. While women's historians have focused on nineteenth-century medicine, feminist social scientists have analyzed contemporary medical institutions.

Examples of work on the African-American experience of health and on African-American women as health practitioners include V. Gamble, "The Negro Hospital Renaissance: The Black Hospital Movement, 1920–1940" (Ph.D. diss., Philadelphia, University of Pennsylvania, 1987); J. W. Robinson, "Black Healers During the Colonial and Early 19th C. America" (Ph.D. diss., Carbondale, Southern Illinois University, 1977); T. Savitt, *Medicine and Slavery: The Diseases and Health Care of Blacks in Antebellum Virginia* (Urbana: University of Illinois Press, 1978); L. Snow, "Popular Medicine in a Black Neighborhood," in E. H. Spicer, ed. *Ethnic Medicine in the Southwest* (Tucson, Ariz.: University of Arizona Press, 1977): 19–25; A. Vrettos, "Curative Domains: Women, Healing and History in Black Women's Narratives," *Women's Studies* 16 (1989): 455–73; and W. Watson and D. Wilkinson, *Black Folk Medicine: The Therapeutic Significance of Faith and Trust* (New Brunswick, N. J.: Transaction Books, 1984). The dynamics of race and class are considered in B. Bullough and V. Bullough, *Poverty, Ethnic Identity and Health Care* (New York: Appleton-Century-Crofts, 1972); E. Martin, "Birth, Resistance, Race, and Class," Ch. 8 in *The Woman in the Body: A Cultural Analysis of Reproduction* (Boston: Beacon Press, 1987); M. S. Simms and J. Malveaux, "Health Issues of Black Women," a section in *Slipping Through the Cracks: The Status of Black Women* (New Brunswick, N. J.: Transaction Books, 1986); and R. Abram, ed. *Send Us a Lady Physician: Women Doctors in America, 1835–1920* (New York: W. W. Norton, 1985), which features a chapter by Darlene Clark Hine on nineteenth-century black women physicians. Hine's *Black Women in White: Racial Conflict and Cooperation in the Nursing Profession, 1890–1950* (Bloomington and Indianapolis: Indiana University Press, 1989) is an excellent new overview of the history of black women in nursing. The central role of slave and free women of color in midwifery and healing has been the focus of a number of studies, including L. Holmes, "Traditional Afro-American Midwives," in P. Eakins, ed. *The American Way of Birth* (Philadelphia: Temple University Press); L. Holmes, "Louvenia Taylor Benjamin, Southern Lay Midwife," *Sage* 1, no. 2 (Fall 1985): 51–54; O. L. Logan, *Motherwit, an Alabama Midwife's Story: Onnie Lee Logan as told to Katherine Clark* (New York: E. P. Dutton, 1989); and S. Robinson, "A Historical Development of Midwifery in the Black Community, 1600–1940," *Journal of Nurse-Midwifery* 29 (1984): 247–50.

While a growing amount of literature has elucidated the patterns of traditional care, the growth of institutions, and the roles of minority practitioners, relatively little published material exists about the experiences of illness of African-American women; even less is published about Latina, Native-American, and Southeast Asian-American women's health. Book-length treatments of women of color and health are especially needed. Until the last few years, this major subject area has been treated primarily as a subset within larger works focusing on white women and health or within those principally concerned with men of color.

Evelyn C. White's *The Black Women's Health Book: Speaking for Ourselves* (Seattle: Seal Press, 1990), now in its third printing, is an excellent example to the contrary. White gathers material from forty-two black women, including Angela Davis, Lucille Clifton, Faye Wattleton, Alice Walker, Barbara Smith, and Zora Neale Hurston, to discuss a range of health issues from survival to cancer to abortion to incest. She also includes a listing of organizations that address black women's health issues (pp. 289–90). Evelynn Hammonds has reviewed White's book in "No Trifling Matter," *The Women's Review of Books*, 7, no. 9 (June 1990): 1.

Angela Davis's "Sick and Tired of Being Sick and Tired: The Politics of Black Women's Health," in *Women, Culture, and Politics* (New York: Random House, 1989), pp. 53–65 and her "Racism, Birth Control, and Reproductive Rights," in *Women, Race, and Class* (New York: Random House, 1983), pp. 202–21, as well as Beverly Smith's "Black Women's Health: Notes for a Course," in *All the Women Are White, All the Blacks Are Men, But Some of Us Are Brave: Black Women's Studies*, ed. Gloria T. Hull, Patricia Bell Scott, and Barbara Smith (Old Westbury, N. Y.: Feminist Press, 1982), pp. 103–14, have become standard assignments in the area of African-American women and health, as have the writings of Audre Lorde. Patricia Bell-Scott and Beverly Guy-Sheftall have devoted a special issue of *Sage: A Scholarly Journal on Black Women* to black women's health (2, no. 2, Fall 1985). Scott and S. R. Murray have also edited a special issue on African-American women for *Psychology of Women Quarterly* 6, no. 3 (Spring 1981). And Byllye Avery has joined E. Hinton-Hoytt, P. E. Drake and J. M. Stewart in editing a special issue on African-American women's health issues for *Spelman Messenger* 100, no. 1 (Spring 1984).

A sampling of the range of studies that consider aspects of the health of African-American, Asian-American, Latina or Native-American women include: C. Carrington, "Depression in Black Women: A Theoretical Appraisal," in L. F. Rodgers-Rose, ed. *The Black Woman* (Beverly Hills, Calif.: Sage, 1980): 265–72; F. G. Castro, P. Furth, and H. Karlow, "The Health Beliefs of Mexican, Mexican-American and Anglo-American Women," *Hispanic Journal of Behavioral Sciences* 6, no. 4 (December 1985): 365–83; M. S. Chavis, "My Life with Sickle Cell Disease: A Conversation with Rita

Edwards," *Sage* 2, no. 2 (Fall 1985): 20–24; A. Clark, ed. *Culture, Childbearing, Health Professionals* (Philadelphia: F. A. Davis Co., 1978), which includes material on Latina and Asian-American women; B. Dillingham, "Indian Women and Indian Health Service Sterilization Practice," *American Indian Journal* 3, no. 1 (1977): 27–28; J. Duncan, "Cambodian Refugee Use of Indigenous and Western Healers to Prevent or Alleviate Mental Illness" (Ph.D. diss., Seattle, University of Washington, 1987); O. Espin, "Spiritual Power and the Mundane World: Hispanic Female Healers in Urban U. S. Communities," *Women's Studies Quarterly* 3 & 4 (1988): 33–47; A. Hernandez, "Chicanas and the Issue of Involuntary Sterilization," *Chicano Law Review* 3, no. 3 (1976): 3–37; J. Jackson, *Aging Black Women: Selected Readings* (Washington, D. C.: College and University Press, 1975); S. Jasso and M. Mazorra, "Following the Harvest: The Health Hazards of Migrant and Seasonal Farmworking Women," and L. Mullings, "Minority Women, Work, and Health," in *Double Exposure: Women's Health Hazards on the Job and at Home*, ed. W. Chavkin (New York: Monthly Review Press, 1984); D. E. Jones, *Sanapia: Comanche Medicine Woman* (Prospect, Ill.: Waveland Press, 1972); M. Kay and M. Yoder, "Hot and Cold in Women's Ethnotherapeutics: The American-Mexican West," *Social Science Medicine* 25, no. 4 (1987): 347–55; F. B. Linderman, *Red Mother: Pretty Shield, Medicine Woman of the Crows* (New York: John Day Co., 1972); J. Macklin, "All the Good and Bad in This World: Women, Traditional Medicine, and Mexican American Culture," and other articles on Latina women's health in M. B. Melville, ed. *Twice a Minority: Mexican American Women* (St. Louis: C. V. Mosby, 1980): 127–48; R. A. Martinez, ed. *Hispanic Culture and Health Care: Fact, Fiction, Folklore* (St. Louis: C. V. Mosby, 1978); R. Modesto and G. Mount, *Not for Innocent Ears: Spiritual Traditions of a Desert Cahuilla Medicine Woman* (Arcata, Calif.: Sweetlight Books, 1980); W. Noble, *African Psychology: Toward Its Reclamation, Reascension, and Revitalization* (Oakland, Calif.: Black Family Institute, 1986); L. Nsiah-Jefferson, "Reproductive Laws, Women of Color, and Low-Income Women," *Women's Rights Law Reporter* 11 (Spring 1989): 14–39; C. Perales and L. Young, eds., *Too Little, Too Late: Dealing with the Health Needs of Women in Poverty* (New York: Harrington Press, 1988); B. Perrone, H. H. Stockel, and V. Krueger, *Medicine Women, Curanderas, and Women Doctors* (Norman and London: University of Oklahoma Press, 1989); D. T. Putney, "Fighting the Scourge: American Indian Morbidity and Federal Policy, 1897–1928" (Ph.D. diss., Milwaukee, Marquette University, 1980); B. Roeder, "Health Care Beliefs and Practices Among Mexican Americans: A Review of the Literature," *Aztlan* 12, nos. 1 & 2 (1982): 223–56; L. Rose, *Disease Beliefs in Mexican-American Communities* (San Francisco: R & E Associates, 1978); M. Sanchez-Ayendez, "Puerto Rican Elderly Women: The Cultural Dimension of Social Support Networks," *Women and Health* 14, no. 3–4 (1988): 239–52; J. Schreiber and J. Homiak, "Mexican-Americans," in A. Harwood, ed. *Ethnicity and Medical Care* (Cambridge: Harvard University Press, 1981); M. C. Sobralske, "Perceptions of Health: Navajo Indians," *Topics in Clinical Nursing* 7 (1985): 32–39; T. M. Theim, "Health Issues Affecting Asian/Pacific American Women," in *Civil Rights Issues of Asian and Pacific Americans* (Washington, D. C., Proceedings of the Conference on Civil Rights Issues of Asian and Pacific Americans, May 1979); U. S. Department of Health and Human Services, *Report of the Secretary's Task Force on Black and Minority Health* (Washington, D. C.: GPO, 1986); R. Wood, "Health Problems Facing American Indian Women," *Conference on the Educational and Occupational Needs of American Indian Women* (Washington, D. C.: National Institute of Education, October 1980); R. E. Zambrana and M. Hurst, "Work and Health Among Puerto Rican Women," *International Journal of Health Services* 12, no. 2 (1984): 261–73; and R. E. Zambrana, ed. *Work, Family and Health: Latina Women in Transition* (Bronx, N. Y.: Hispanic Research Center, Fordham University, 1982).

To date, no cross-cultural multidisciplinary collection exists that gathers together materials about the health of women members of these various "minority" groups into one study, and few focus on methods of staying well and maintaining physical and mental harmony.

There has been a slowly growing number of scholarly articles in the humanities, social sciences, and medical sciences that examine the experience of women of color and illness. The popular press has also begun to cover issues of concern to women of color and to report on the results of new studies. See, for example, "A Few More First Birthdays" [on infant mortality rates], *Time* (22 April 1991): 33; "AIDS Testing Ignores Women," *San Francisco Chronicle*, 19 June 1991; "Chinese Medicine Rights," *Seattle Post-Intelligencer*, 25 November 1990; "Hospital to Adjust Childbirth Services to Ethnic Needs," *San Jose Mercury News*, 12 September 1991; S. Chin, "Asian Health: A Special Prescription," *San Francisco Examiner*, 7 July 1991; P. Cooke, "Blinded by the Pain of the Killing Fields," *San Francisco Chronicle*, 7 July 1991; R. Cowen, "Finding a Transplant Match for Blacks," *Science News* 137 (7 April 1990): 223; M. Douglas, "Health Care for Hispanics Found Lacking," *San Jose Mercury News*, 20 September 1991; H. Freeman and L. Villarosa, "Emergency: The Crisis in Our Health Care," *Essence* (September 1991): 59; C. Gorman, "Why Do Blacks Die Young?" *Time* (16 September 1991): 50–52; K. Huckshorn, "Minority Women Avoid Birth Control," *San Jose Mercury News*, 12 September 1991; J. Kay, "Minorities Bear Brunt of Pollution: Latinos and Blacks Living in State's Dirtiest Neighborhood" and " Minority Groups Taking Stand Against Toxic Sites," *San Francisco Examiner*, 7 April 1991; W. King, "No Insurance, Little Hope," *Seattle Times*, 7 October 1990; C. Johnson, "Blacks and Cancer," *U. S. News and World Report* 109 (22 October 1990): 21; B. Laker, "Seattle:

An Unliveable City for Black Babies" and "Seattle Probably Won't Get Nod: Bush Infant Mortality Plan Will Peg 10 Cities Using Overall Rates," *Seattle Post-Intelligencer*, 8 February 1991; V. W. Pinn-Wiggins, "NMA President Leads National Crusade for Equal Health Care," *Ebony* (April 1990): 58–59; G. Spears, "New Mothers Turn from Breast-feeding," *San Jose Mercury News*, 26 September 1991; R. Ramirez, "Latino Seniors Suffer Behind Barrier," *San Francisco Examiner*, 5 May 1991; L. Saul, "AIDS and Its Toll on Women," *New York Times*, 17 September 1989.

The short literature is so plentiful that bibliographic directories have been produced as readers' guides. Sheryl Ruzek, Patricia Anderson, Adele Clarke, Virginia Olesen, and Kristin Hill have collaborated on an excellent guide to sources on African-American, Native-American, Latina, and Asian-American women and health (including journal articles and educational and audiovisual resources) in *Minority Women, Health and Healing in the U. S.: Selected Bibliography and Resources* (San Francisco: University of San Francisco and Other Sponsors, 1986). The Women, Health, and Healing Program at the University of California, San Francisco, also makes curricular materials on women and health available for order. Other helpful bibliographic sources include Roberto Abello-Argandona, Juan Gomez-Quinones, and Patricia Herrara Duran, eds. *The Chicana: A Comprehensive Bibliographic Study* (Los Angeles: University of California, Chicano Studies Center, n.d.); Elizabeth Higginbotham, *Selected Bibliography of Social Science Readings on Women of Color in the United States* (Memphis: Memphis State University, 1989); the Pan American Health Organization, *Women, Health and Development in the Americas: An Annotated Bibliography* (Washington, D. C.: Pan American Health Organization, 1984); and Andrea Timberlake, Lynn Weber Cannon, Rebecca F. Guy, and Elizabeth Higginbotham, eds. *Women of Color and Southern Women: A Bibliography of Social Science Research, 1975 to 1988* (Memphis: Memphis State University, 1988).

Recent literature on minority health directed for use by physicians includes R. P. Bain, R. S. Greenberg, and J. P. Whitaker, "Racial Differences in the Survival of Women with Breast Cancer," *Journal of Chronic Disease* 39, no. 8 (1986): 631–42; R. Baron, et al., "Sudden Death Among Southeast Asian Refugees: An Unexplained Phenomena," *Journal of the American Medical Association* 250 (2 December 1983): 2947–51; P. Blanchard, et al., "Isoniazid Overdose in Cambodian Population of Olmsted County, Minnesota," *Journal of the American Medical Association* 256 (12 December 1986): 3131–33; R. J. Blendon, L. H. Aiken, H. E. Freeman, and C. R. Corey, "Access to Medical Care for Black and White Americans: A Continuing Concern," T. F. Kirn, "Research Seeks to Reduce Toll of Hypertension, Other Cardiovascular Diseases in Black Population," C. K. Svensson, "Representation of American Blacks in Clinical Trials of New Drugs," M. B. Wenneker and A. M. Epstein, "Racial Inequalities in the Use of

Procedures for Patients with Ischemic Heart Disease in Massachusetts," and R. Wilson, "Glaucoma in Blacks: Where Do We Go From Here?" in *Journal of the American Medical Association* 261 (13 January 1989): 278–81; 195; 263–65; 253–57; 281–82; M. E. Guinan and A. Hardy, "Epidemiology of AIDS in Women in the United States, 1981–1986," and C. B. Wofsky, "Human Immunodeficiency Virus Infection in Women," *Journal of the American Medical Association* 257 (17 April 1987): 2039–42, 2074–76; A. Harwood, "The Hot-Cold Theory of Disease: Implications for Treatment of Puerto Rican Patients," *Journal of the American Medical Association* 216 (1971): 1153–58; T. Jacob, N. Penn, and M. Brown, "Breast Self-Examination: Knowledge, Attitudes, and Performance Among Black Women," *Journal of the National Medical Association* 81, no. 7 (1989): 769–76; W. W. Marsh and K. Hentges, "Mexican Folk Remedies and Conventional Medical Care," *American Family Physician* 37, no. 3 (1988): 257–62; P. R. McGinn, "Report Hits Racial Bias in Health Care," *American Medical News* 32 (15 December 1989): 11; D. K. Rassin, et al., "Incidence of Breastfeeding in Low Socioeconomic Group of Mothers in the United States: Ethnic Patterns," *Pediatrics* 73 (1984): 132–37; S. Rostand, "Diabetic Renal Disease in Blacks: Inevitable or Preventable?" *New England Journal of Medicine* (19 October 1989): 1121–22; and E. Stark, A. Flitcraft, and W. Frazier, "Medicine and Patriarchal Violence: The Social Construction of a Private Event," *International Journal of Health Services* 9, no. 3 (1979): 461–92.

Literature prepared for public health workers includes: "AIDS and Black America: Special Psychosocial Issues," *Public Health Reports* 102 (1987): 224–31; R. Burak, P. Gimotty, W. Stengle, D. Eckert, L. Warbasse, and A. Moncrease, "Detroit's Avoidable Mortality Project: Breast Cancer Control for Inner-City Women," B. Campbell, E. Kimball, S. Helgerson, I. Alexander, and H. Goldberg, "Using 1990 National MCH Objectives to Assess Health Status and Risk in an American Indian Community," V. Hutchins and C. Walch, "Meeting Minority Health Needs Through Special MCH Projects," A. Lanier, L. Bulkow, and B. Ireland, "Cancer in Alaskan Indians, Eskimos, and Aleuts, 1969–1983: Implications for Etiology and Control," D. Snider, L. Salinas, and G. Kelley, "Tuberculosis: An Increasing Problem Among Minorities in the United States," and K. Toomey, A. Oberschelp, and J. R. Greenspan, "Sexually Transmitted Diseases and Native Americans," in *Public Health Reports*, 104 (November-December 1989): 527–35, 627–31, 621–26, 658–64, 646–53, and 566; R. J. DiClemente, C. B. Boyer, and E. S. Morales, "Minorities and AIDS: Knowledge, Attitudes and Misconceptions Among Black and Latino Adolescents," and R. Selik, K. Castro, and M. Pappaioanou, "Racial-Ethnic Differences in the Risk of AIDS in the United States," in *American Journal of Public Health* 78 (1988): 55–57, 1539–45; D. E. Hayes-Bautista, "Identifying 'Hispanic' Populations: The Influence of Research Methodology on Public Policy," *American Journal of Public Health* 70, no. 4 (April 1980): 353–56; M. Muecke, "Caring for Southeast Asian Refugee Patients in the USA," *American Journal of Public Health* 73 (1983): 431–38; and D. Strogatz, "Use of Medical Care for Chest Pain: Differences Between Blacks and Whites," *American Journal of Public Health* 80 (March 1990): 290–94.

Examples of literature directed to various types of health professionals include A. Antle, "Ethnic Perspectives of Cancer Nursing: The American Indian," *Oncology Nursing Forum* 14 (1987): 70–73; J. Boehnlein, "Clinical Relevance of Grief and Mourning Among Cambodian Refugees," *Social Science and Medicine* 25 (1987): 765–72; H. J. Chung, "Understanding the Oriental Maternity Patient," *Nursing Clinics of North America* 12 (1977): 67–75; S. D. Cochran, V. M. Mays, and V. Roberts, "Ethnic Minorities and AIDS," in *Nursing Care of the Patient with AIDS/ARC* ed. A. Lewis (Rockville, Md.: Aspen, 1988), pp. 17–24; C. De Monteflores, "Conflicting Allegiances: Therapy Issues with Hispanic Lesbians," *Catalyst* 12 (1981): 33–44; P. G. Higgins, "Pueblo Women of New Mexico: Their Background, Culture and Childbearing Practices," *Topics in Clinical Nursing* 4 (1983): 69–78; H. G. McComb, "The Application of an Individual/Collective Model to the Psychology of Black Women," *Women and Therapy* 5 (1986): 67–80; C. Milligan, "Nursing Care and Beliefs of Expectant Navajo Women," *American Indian Quarterly* 8, no. 2 (1984); C. Nelson and M. Hewitt, "An Indochinese Refugee Population in a Nurse-Midwife Service," *Journal of Nurse-Midwifery* 28 (9): 9–14. P. Pedersen, "Ten Frequent Assumptions of Cultural Bias in Counseling," *Journal of Multicultural Counseling and Development* (January 1987): 16–24; G. Romero, F. G. Castro, and R. C. Cervantes, "Latinas Without Work," *Psychology of Women Quarterly* 12 (Summer 1988): 429–43, 281–97; R. Saenz, W. J. Goudy, and F. O. Lorenz, "The Effects of Employment and Marital Relations on Depression Among Mexican American Women," *Journal of Marriage and the Family* 51 (February 1989): 239–51; K. Satz, "Integrating Navajo Tradition into Maternal-Child Nursing," *Image* 14 (1982): 89–91; E. Smith, "Mental Health and Service Delivery Systems for Black Women," *Journal of Black Studies* 12, no. 2 (1981): 126–41; E. Soto and P. Shaver, "Sex-Role Traditionalism, Assertiveness, and Symptoms of Puerto Rican Women Living in the United States," *Hispanic Journal of Behavioral Sciences*, 4, no. 1 (1982): 1–19; A. Torres and S. Singh, "Contraceptive Practice Among Hispanic Adolescents," *Family Planning Perspectives* 18 (1986): 193; L. Wadd, "Vietnamese Postpartum Practices: Implications for Nursing in the Hospital Setting," *Journal of Gynecological Nursing* 12 (1983): 252–58; and G. Wasserman, V. Rauh, S. Brunelli, M. Garcia-Castro, and B. Necos, "Pyschosocial Attributes and Life Experiences of Disadvantaged Minority Mothers: Age and Ethnic Variations," *Child Development* 61 (April 1990): 566–80.

Articles concerning women of color and the issues of domestic violence, drug use, alcoholism, and AIDS include: H. Amaro, "Considerations for Prevention of HIV Infection Among Hispanic Women," *Psychology of Women Quarterly* 12 (1988): 429–43; L. Arguelles and A. M. Rivero, "HIV Infection/AIDS and Latinas in Los Angeles County: Considerations for Prevention, Treatment and Research Practice," *California Sociologist* 11 (1988): 69–89; N. K. Bell, "AIDS and Women: Remaining Ethical Issues," *AIDS Education and Prevention* 1 (1989): 22–30; M. E. Guinan and A. Hardy, "Women and AIDS," *Journal of the American Medical Women's Association* 42 (1987): 157–58; V. Kanuha, "Sexual Assault in Southeast Asian Communities: Issues in Intervention," *Response* 10 (1987): 3–4; T. A. Lai, "Asian Women: Resisting the Violence," *Working Together to Prevent Sexual and Domestic Violence* 5, no. 5 (June 1985); J. E. Levy and S. J. Junitz, *Indian Drinking: Navajo Practices and Anglo-American Theories* (New York: John Wiley and Sons, 1974); D. Lewis and J. K. Watters, "Human Immunodeficiency Virus Seroprevalence in Female Intravenous Drug Abusers: The Puzzle of Black Women's Risk," *Social Science and Medicine* 29 (1989): 1071–76; V. Mays and S. D. Cochran, "Issues in the Perception of AIDS Risk and Risk Reduction Activities by Black and Hispanic-Latina Women," *American Psychologist* 43 (November 1988): 949–57; J. Mondanaro, "Strategies for AIDS Prevention: Motivating Health Behavior in Drug Dependent Women," *Journal of Pyschoactive Drugs* 19 (1987): 143–49; J. W. Moore and A. Mata, *Women and Heroin in Chicano Communities* (Washington, D. C.: National Institute on Drug Abuse, Chicano Pinto Research Project, 1982); B. Richie, "Battered Black Women: A Challenge for the Black Community," *The Black Scholar* 16 (1985): 2–40; M. Rosenbaum, *Women on Heroin* (New Brunswick, N. J.: Rutgers University Press, 1981); E. White, *Chain, Chain Change: For Black Women Dealing with Physical and Emotional Abuse* (Seattle: Seal Press, 1985); D. Worth, "Minority Women and AIDS: Culture, Race, and Gender," in *Culture and AIDS*, ed. D. Felman (New York: Praeger, 1990); S. B. Yim, "Korean Battered Wives: A Sociological and Psychological Analysis of Conjugal Violence in Korean Immigrant Families," in *Korean Women: In a Struggle for Humanization*, eds. H. H. Sunoo and D. S. Kim (Korean Christian Scholars Publication No. 3, Spring 1978); and M. Zambrano, *Mejor Sola Que Mal Acompanada: Para la Mujer Golpeada / For the Latina in an Abusive Relationship* (Seattle: Seal Press, 1985).

INDEX

Abuse: Black women and, 56. *See also* Domestic violence; Violence
Adolescents: cultural dilemmas among, 106; emotional problems of, 101–2; menstrual disorders among, 101; social problems among, 101; traditional explanations of problems among, 102
Adoption: African Americans and, 211
African-American beneficial societies, 187
African-American churches: aid to African-American women from, 187
African-American family: adoption and, 211; African-American organizations and, 218; misconceptions of, 211; poverty and, 211
African-American folk medicine: misconceptions of, 44; syncretic elements in, 45; women in, 43–44, 49
African-American midwifery: cultural context of, 210; resurgence of, 210. *See also* Granny midwives
African-American politicians: support of medical establishment by, 219
African-American psychologists: African-American artists and, 36
African Americans: access to hospital care among, 181; discrimination and health among, 61; Eurocentric psychology and, 29, 30, 31, 33; genocide of, 56; hypertension among, 59; mortality rates among, 56, 58, 180, 182; number of medical

personnel among, 182; oppression and mortality rate of, 215; psychoanalysis and, 50; psychosocial problems and health among, 61; public health officials and, 218; repressed anger and health problems among, 62; White medical personnel's treatment of, 188
African-American women: abuse as slaves and, 195; access to outpatient care by, 182; African-American beneficial societies and, 187; African-American churches and, 187; age and health correlation among, 63; AIDS and, 57, 312, 313, 314, 318, 319, 333, 335, 337, 340, 361; alcoholism and, 57; biological predisposition to breast cancer and, 244; breast cancer among, 244, 245, 253; breast self-examination among, 245, 250, 251, 252; cocaine and, 322; condoms and, 323; deference required of, 184, 189; depression and, 62, 63; detoxification programs and, 315, 317, 318, 319, 321, 322, 323, 325, 326n.8, 326n.9; discrimination against, 183, 185, 187; dispensaries used by, 182; drugs and AIDS among, 57; drugs used by, 57, 315, 330; employment and, 55, 186; family support systems and, 186, 187; granny midwives and, 192; group identity and health among, 64; home vs. hospital care of, 185, 186, 188; incidence of breast cancer among, 245; infant mortality rate among, 57;

383

as health concept among, 259; family
and illness among, 262, 263, 266,
267, 268–69; fatalism among, 259;
gossip and contraception among,
306; health care and, 257, 265; magic
and illness among, 260; religion
and health among, 259; sexual
proscriptions among, 303; social
definition of illness among, 262. *See
also* Latin Americans; Mexican men;
Mexican women
Hispanic teenagers (adolescents): birth
control among, 300; condoms and,
308; Dominican teenagers, 302;
early childbearing among, 300;
encouragement of birth control
among, 307; fears of birth control
among, 304–5; ignorance of birth
control among, 303, 307; language
barriers to birth control among, 306;
money and birth control among,
305–6; parents and birth control
among, 305–6; pregnancy and, 304,
307; Puerto Rican teenagers, 302;
sexual ignorance among, 303, 309;
shame and contraception among, 306,
307, 309; virginity and, 303–4
Hispanic women: age and attitudes
among, 265, 267; AIDS and, 340,
341, 342, 343, 344, 345, 346,
347, 350, 351; AIDS education
and, 343, 344, 346, 350; AIDS-
infected children and, 348, 349;
AIDS-infected spouses and, 349;
attitudes toward breast cancer among,
259–60, 263–64, 264, 265, 266, 267;
breast cancer symptoms and, 260;
breast self-examination among, 266;
childbearing and, 304, 348; Cuban
women and adolescents, 302; cultural
differentiations among, 341–42,
342; empowerment of, 350; family
networks and, 261–62, 263, 267,
268–69, 304, 346, 347, 348; folk
remedies for cancer among, 261;
general health and cancer among,

265; interpersonal relationships and
cancer among, 260, 269; lesbianism
and, 343, 344, 345, 350; male risk
behaviors and, 345, 346, 349, 350;
mammography and, 266; perceived
causes of breast cancer among, 260;
preventative medicine and, 261,
265, 267; risk perceptions of AIDS
among, 344; sexuality of, 342, 343,
349. *See also* Mexican women;
Women of color

HIV. *See* AIDS
Holy Spirit, 47
Home birthing: African-American babies
and, 208; decline in, 208; increased
rate of, 204; infant mortality and,
220–21; normal pregnancy and, 220;
public health officials' opposition to,
220; White vs. African-American
reasons for choosing, 217
Homelessness, 294
Hoo doo, 42, 48. *See also* Voodoo
Hospitals: African-American women's
access to, 188; nineteenth-century
attitudes towards, 180; segregation
and, 181; White personnel in, 189
"Hot/cold" health concepts: breastfeeding
and, 233, 234; Haitian culture and,
233–34; Khmer medicine and, 94,
98, 101, 102, 103; Latin American
cultures and, 232, 233; Mexican-
American medicine and, 113, 114;
pregnancy and, 233; Southeast Asian
cultures and, 234; traditional healing
systems and, 232, 233; yin yang
as, 234
Humoral medicine, 232; yin yang as, 234
Hypertension, 59

Illness: loss of religious faith and, 49;
"natural" vs. "unnatural," 42, 48, 50;
social definition of, 328
Immigrants to the U.S.: demography of,
226; health problems among, 227
Immune deficiencies and psychological
stress, 58

"Indian way," 125–26

Infant mortality, 222n.2; African Americans and, 57, 199, 213, 222n.3; Alabama and, 199; breastfeeding and, 227–28; home birthing and, 220–21; midwives blamed for, 198; nutrition and, 227; poor women and, 212–13; poverty and, 213; use of prenatal care services and, 199

Influenza, 175, 179n.1

Inner city health problems, 211

Insurance: African American access to, 214; Hispanic breast cancer and, 265, 267; midwifery and, 220

Intravenous drugs (IV): addiction to, 330; African-American women and, 313, 314, 315, 319, 324; AIDS and, 312, 313, 318, 322, 326n.4, 335, 345, 354; alcohol and, 324; crime and, 319, 321; demographics of, 313, 314, 357; detoxification programs for, 315, 317, 319, 321, 323, 326n.8, 326n.9; emotional release and, 336, 338n.5; health problems and, 323; minority communities and, 312; money spent on, 321; prostitution and, 316–17, 317, 321, 329, 331, 332, 333, 336, 338n.2; sexual partners of users of, 354, 355, 356, 357, 358; social context of, 324; social networks and, 315, 324, 325, 331, 336; socioeconomic status and, 336; women and, 313, 314, 315, 319, 324, 329. *See also* Cocaine; Crack cocaine; Drugs; Heroin; Marijuana

Khmer: adolescent health problems among, 101–2; attitude toward infant death among, 99; childbirth and pregnancy among, 103–4; coin rubbing among, 95, 99, 100, 105; disequilibrium and illness among, 95; elderly health problems among, 105; equilibrium as health concept among, 94; food and health among, 105; men's health problems among, 104–5; reconciliation of traditional and Western medicines among, 98–99; refugees to the U.S., 93; spirits and health among, 95; stress and male, 104; treatment of children's illness among, 100–1; use of U.S. medical system by, 96; war victims in Cambodia, 93–94; women and health-care decisions, 97–98; women's health problems among, 102; worldview and health among, 94

Kodiak Island, 148, 166n.1

Kodiak Island Resource Center, 149

Koniag, 164n.1. *See also* Alutiiq

Kru Khmer: changes in training of, 96; in Cambodia, 95

Lactation counseling, 230

Lakota, 170

Latin Americans: *espiritismo* among, 235; "hot/cold" health concepts among, 232, 233; *santeria* among, 235. *See also* Hispanics; Mexican men; Mexican women

Latinas. *See* Hispanic women; Mexican women

Lesbianism: AIDS and, 345; domestic violence and, 296; Hispanic women and, 343–44, 345, 350

Magic, 260

Malcolm X, 28, 32, 36

Mammography: African-American women and, 266, 267, 269; cost of, 246; early breast cancer detection and, 245, 246; Hispanic women and, 266, 267, 269

Marijuana, 316, 319, 320, 332

Mastectomy: as mutilation, 277; husband's reaction to, 274; social shame of, 275, 279; woman's reaction to 274, 277

Maternal death rate: African-American vs. White, 220; hospital vs. home birth and, 220; in early 20th-century U.S., 197

sexism and, 292, 293; undocumented immigrant status and, 295–96. *See also* African-American women; Hispanic women; Mexican women

Women's health: emerging group identity and, 54; experience as insight to, 123; inadequate study of, 54; poverty and, 54, 56